Radiotherapy
and
Cancer Immunology

Volume I

Editor

Naresh Prasad, Ph.D.

Associate Professor
Department of Radiology
Baylor College of Medicine
Houston, Texas
Director, Radiobiology Research Laboratory
Veterans Administration Medical Center
Houston, Texas

Editor-in-Chief
CRC Series in High Level
Radiation and Immunology
Naresh Prasad, Ph.D.

RC 268.3
R3
v.1
1981

CRC Press, Inc.
Boca Raton, Florida

Library of Congress Cataloging-in Publication Data
Main Entry under title:

Radiotherapy and cancer immunology

(CRC series in high level radiation and immunology)
    Bibliography: p.

    Includes index.
    1. Cancer—Immunological aspects. 2. Cancer—Radiotherapy—Complications and sequelae.
3. Immunosuppression. 4. Radiation immunology. I. Prasad, Naresh. II. Series. [DNLM:
1. Neoplasms—Immunology. 2. Neoplasms—Radiotherapy.
3. Radiotherapy—Adverse effects.
QZ 269 R131] RC268.3.R3   616.99'40642   81-864
ISBN 0-8493-5901-5   AACR2

Direct all inquiries to CRC Press, Inc., 2000 N.W. 24th Street, Boca Raton, Florida 33431.

© 1981 by CRC Press, Inc.

International Standard Book Number 0-8493-5901-5

Library of Congress Card Number 81-864
Printed in the United States

PREFACE

It is quite apparent now that the host immune system plays an important role in combatting malignant diseases. While radiotherapy is effective in controlling the non-disseminated malignant tumor, it also exerts a negative influence on the host immune system. A large volume of precise and valuable information has accumulated in a short time, but unfortunately the information is scattered. In this book attempts have been made to pull together in compact form the state of our knowledge about the impact of radiotherapy on the immunology of patients with cancer of the head and neck, lung, breast, uterus, prostate and urinary bladder, lymphomas, Hodgkin's disease, and leukemia. This book should be a valuable source of information for clinical and experimental oncologists, radiation therapists, and immunologists.

I would like to thank our editors at CRC Press for their consistent and professional assistance. I also would like to particularly thank Dr. James E. Harrell, Professor and Chairman, Department of Radiology at Baylor College of Medicine, for his constant encouragement and to my colleagues, Dr. John I. Thornby, Dr. Stewart C. Bushong for many suggestions.

Naresh Prasad

THE EDITOR

Naresh Prasad, Ph.D. is an Associate Professor in the Department of Radiology at Baylor College of Medicine in Houston, Texas and Director of Radiobiology Research Laboratory at Veterans Administration Medical Center in Houston, Texas.

Dr. Prasad received his B.S. degree with honors and M.S. degree both from Patna University (India) in 1959 and 1961, respectively, and his Ph.D. degree from North Dakota State University in 1967.

Dr. Prasad is a member of various scientific societies, including the Radiation Research Society and American Association for Cancer Research.

His present research concerns the experimental radiation oncology and biology.

CONTRIBUTORS

Donald E. Carlson, Ph.D.
Associate Professor of Radiology
University of Texas Health Science
  Center at Dallas
Dallas, Texas

Vernon K. Jenkins, Ph.D.
Associate Professor
Department of Radiology
University of Texas Medical Branch
Galveston, Texas

Eva Lotzová, Ph.D.
Associate Professor and Associate
  Immunologist
Department of Developmental
  Therapeutics
The University of Texas System Cancer
  Center
M.D. Anderson Hospital and Tumor
  Institute
Houston, Texas

Kenneth J. McCormick, Ph.D.
Associate Laboratory Director
The Stehlin Foundation for Cancer
  Research
Houston, Texas, and
Adjunct Associate Professor of
  Experimental Biology
Department of Surgery
Baylor College of Medicine
Houston, Texas

Nancy McCormick, M.S.
Department of Obstetrics & Gynecology
Baylor College of Medicine
Houston, Texas

Luka Milas, M.D., Ph.D.
Radiotherapist and Professor of
  Radiotherapy
Chief, Section of Experimental
  Radiotherapy
The University of Texas System Cancer
  Center
M.D. Anderson Hospital and Tumor
  Institute
Houston, Texas

David M. Mumford, M.D.
Professor
Department of Obstetrics & Gynecology
Baylor College of Medicine
Houston, Texas

Naresh Prasad, Ph.D.
Associate Profesor
Department of Radiology
Baylor College of Medicine
Houston, Texas, and Director,
  Radiobiology Research Laboratory
Veterans Administration Medical
  Center
Houston, Texas

Sameer Rafla, M.D., Ph.D.
Director of Radiation Therapy
Methodist Hospital
Brooklyn, New York,
and State University of New York
  College of Medicine,
Brooklyn, New York,
Clinical Associate Professor of
  Radiology
State Universtiy of New York
College of Medicine
Brooklyn, New York

Donthamsetti S. Rao, M.D.
Associate Director
Department of Radiation Oncology
Mount Sinai Hospital
Chicago, Illinois

Julianne Souchek, Ph.D.
Biostatistian
Veterans Administration Medical
  Center
Hines, Illinois

Stefano S. Stefani, M.D.
Professor of Therapeutic Radiology
Rush Medical College
Chicago, Illinois, Director of Radiation
  Oncology
Mount Sinai Hospital
Chicago, Illinois, and Chief,
  Therapeutic Radiology Service
Veterans Administration Hospital
Hines, Illinois.

Paul H. Sugarbaker, M.D.
Senior Investigator
Surgery Branch, N.I.H.
Bethesda, Maryland

Shung-Jun Yang, Ph.D.
Clinical Assistant and Professor
Department of Radiology
Downstate Medical Center
State University of New York
College of Medicine
Brooklyn, New York
Chief, Radiation Biology
Department of Radiation Therapy
Methodist Hospital
Brooklyn, New York

TABLE OF CONTENTS

Chapter 1

EXPERIMENTAL RADIATION AND IMMUNE DEFENSE INTERACTIONS

Eva Lotzová

TABLE OF CONTENTS

I. INTRODUCTION

In spite of the lengthy and rich history and background of experimental radiation research, this area of investigation is still very actual and of great importance, especially in the view of its cancer-related therapeutic potential. It has been generally accepted that radiotherapy can very effectively control tumor growth without disturbing the integrity of normal tissues.[1-3] The ionizing radiation, however, despite its beneficial therapeutic effect in diminishing tumor burden, can exert a negative influence on the immune system, certainly a very important component of anticancer defense. Consequently, the injured immune system may be inefficient in detecting and/or destroying residual tumor cells (that have not been eliminated by irradiation), and thus, contributing to the dissemination of the tumor. Moreover, the immune system-impaired individual may be more prone to the unrelated type of malignancy, because of the radiation-caused damage to the immunosurveillance mechanism. Another negative effect of irradiation could be activation of a latent virus genome that may lead to the induction of leukemia. This possibility is indicated by experimental animal studies and can be pertinent also for humans, since an excess frequency of leukemia has been found in many humans exposed to radiation either occupationally, medically, or in the war or accidents.

Altogether, it is clear that radiation can interact with the tumors as well as with tumor immunity on various (negative and positive) levels, and that such interaction does not occur in simple but in a rather complex manner. It is important to study and understand these multifacet effects radiation exerts, so the radiation therapy can be approached in a most efficient and least harmful way. Especially important is evaluation of the effect of irradiation not only on the immune system in general, but also on its individual members. In the light of relatively recent advances in immunology, it has been realized that not only T lymphocytes are involved in tumor immunity, but also other populations of cells, e.g., macrophages, various types of killer cells (natural killer cells and antibody dependent killer cells) are most likely very important counterparts of tumor surveillance and defense. In addition, it has become obvious that distinct populations and subpopulations of lymphocytes with divergent functions and different relevance for cancer immunity exist and that these may express different radiation sensitivity. Ad hoc, it is pertinent to reevaluate carefully and systematically the effect of ionizing radiation in the light of our new knowledge of the immune system, and its functions in various immune phenomena.

II. COMPLEXITY OF THE IMMUNE SYSTEM

For the purpose of a better understanding of the radiation-immune system interactions, the complexity of immune responses and the heterogeneity of lymphocyte subpopulations will be briefly discussed. It is generally believed that the lymphocytic stem cells are present in the yolk sac and fetal liver during the embryonic life and in bone marrow in adult life. These stem cells then follow at least two different pathways; one pathway is migration through the thymus, in which organ these cells are exposed to various influences (including, e.g., thymic hormones) and undergo a series of maturational events. In the thymus they also acquire specific cell surface antigens. At this stage, these cells are most likely irreversibly to play a role of T cells. The substantial fraction of thymocytes then migrates from the thymus into peripheral lymphoid tissues, such as lymph nodes, spleen, and gut-associated lymphoid tissues and some of them also circulate in peripheral blood. T cells are prevailing in paracortical areas of lymph nodes, also designated thymic-dependent areas. To a lesser extent, T cells are found in the cortex and in the medullary cords. In the spleen, most of the T cells are localized in the dense white pulp, but some are also present in the loose white pulp and the red pulp.[4,5] The other pathway of lymphocytic stem cells in mammals is unknown, but it is believed that these cells are educated by the organ similar to that of avian bursa of Fabricius, to become B cells. Much attention has been paid to gut-associated lymphoid tissues as the mammalian equivalent of bursa of Fabricius. Similarly to cells of T cell lineage, members of B cell lineage then migrate to peripheral lymphoid organs, and settle in so called B cells-dependent areas. In the peripheral lymphoid tissues, B cells are intermixed with T cells. T cells can be distinguished from B cells by various parameters, between others by cell surface and functional characteristics. In the mouse, the Thy-1 antigen is T cell-specific antigen, found on both cells within the thymus and on all peripheral T cells. Such T cell-specific antigen is not restricted to murine specie, but has also been found in rats; moreover, in man, specific antihuman T cell sera were produced by several laboratories. In mice, another antigen is expressed on thymocytes of certain (not all) strains of mice, but not on peripheral T cells. This antigen (actually series of antigens) is designated thymus leukemia (TL) antigenic system. Furthermore, irrespective of whether TL antigen is expressed on normal thymocytes of a given strain, all strains of mice are expressing TL antigens on leukemic cells. Expression of TL antigen on normal thymocytes is a reflection of maturational events in the T cell lineage (i.e., stem cells lack this antigen, lymphocytes maturing within the thymus express it, and this antigen is not expressed by mature T cells in peripheral lymphoid organs). There is another series of antigens expressed on T cell membranes or their precursors. These are Ly-1, Ly-2, Ly-3, and Ly-5.

The typical marker of B cell lymphocytes is a membrane-bound immunoglobulin. B cells express, however, also various other antigens, such as Ly-4, Ly-6, Ly-7, Lyb-8, mouse-specific B lymphocyte antigen (MLBA), etc. Functionally, the T cells can be recognized from B cells by their primary involvement in cell-mediated immunity, the latter cells being the main factors of humoral immunity. Also, these two cell populations exhibit different reactivity to mitogenic stimulus, B cells responding primarily to LPS and dextran sulfate (the latter response is apparently mediated by less mature B cells) and T cells responding primarily to phytohemagglutinin (PHA) and concanavalin A (ConA). However, the above mentioned functional division of T cells and B cells is only arbitrary, since as will be seen later different subpopulations of B cells and T cells exist and these are not compatible with regard to their functions. Moreover, it has been recognized by now that for some of the functions, e.g., antibody production, B cells cooperation with T cells is necessary. The phenomenon of cell cooperation became increasingly evident after the initial observations of Claman and Chaperson,[6] and shortly thereafter by Miller and Mitchell[7] and Davis[8] indicating requirement of T and B cell cooperation for optimal antibody response. At the same time Roseman[9] reported that for the induction of antibody response another cell population, i.e., macrophage (also called "accessory" cell), was necessary. It has been recognized that all of these cell populations differ with regard to their functions in antibody production; specifically, T cells assist and/or help B cells by reacting to carrier proteins in particular antigens (thus, they received designation helper T cells) while B cells react to the hapten of the same antigenic molecule and become antibody-forming cells. Macrophage plays a role in processing the antigen and through cooperation with T cells presenting it to B cells. A few years later similar interaction between T cell subpopulations was observed in various immune phenomena.[10,11] It was realized that except for helper T cells augmenting antibody formation, the subpopulation of T cells existed that could very effectively suppress immune response; the latter subpopulation of T cells, suppressing the immune response, was designated suppressor T cells. Suppressor T cells were found to operate not only in humoral immunity but also in cell-mediated immunity.[12]

Similarly, various types and subtypes of B cells involved in various functions can be distinguished; precursors B lymphocytes, which are not sensitive to antigen, precursors of antibody-forming cells which are sensitive to antigen, antibody forming cells (plasma cell), and finally suppressor B cells.[13] It has also been indicated that the B cells responding to thymus dependent antigens differ from B cells responding to thymus independent antigens.

Macrophages appear also to represent rather heterogeneous cell population involved in both facilitation of immune response as well as in its suppression. Beside T cells, B cells, and macrophages, another population of cells appear to represent an important component in immunity, especially in tumor immunity. These cells were designated natural killer (NK) cells because of their natural occurrence (no immunization for their function is required) and tumor killing activities. NK cells may represent also a very important counterpart of immunosurveillance mechanism; in fact, their prompt and strong reactivity to various types of malignancies, presence in T cell-deficient animals (which do not experience higher incidence of malignancies, in spite of the lack of mature T cell functions) poses NK cells in superior position to T cells as immunosurveillance candidates. Despite their lymphoid-like morphology, murine NK cells cannot be classified as typical mature B cells, T cells, or macrophages because of the lack of cell surface markers, specific for T and B cells and macrophage properties.[14] Some investigators believe that NK cells could represent less mature members of a T cell lineage because of the small amount of Thy-1 antigen (specific T cell antigen) detected by some (but not all) of the anti-Thy-1 sera preparations. Although most of the NK cell antitumor activity was detected in vitro, these cells appear to operate also in resistance to tumors in vivo, especially in resistance to leukemias. This is indicated, for example, by the fact that mice with high spontaneous tumor incidence are low NK cells responders in vitro and vice versa.[14] There is another feature of NK cells that makes them interesting for immunologists, i.e., their resemblance of cells involved in rejection of histoincompatible bone marrow transplants. Thus, NK cells may have dual functions, one in tumor defence and the other in controlling the take of bone marrow grafts. Another population of cells which is also involved in immunity, are killer (K) cells. In contrast to NK cells, which operate without contribution of antibody, cytotoxic function of K cells is antibody dependent.

Because of the variety of the cell populations composing the immune complex, (allowing and/or regulating the immunocompetence of the individual), it is important to evaluate the radiation effect on each of these immune components separately in order to obtain a realistic picture on the radiation-immune system relationship. For example, if one studies the radiation influences on antibody response to various antigens, it must be realized that such response is mediated through cooperation of at least three cell types, T cells, B cells, and macrophages. If any two of these three cell populations will be radioresistant and one radiosensitive, the antibody response will not occur or will be suboptimal. However, this type of experiment does not provide any information on which of the three cell types was damaged by irradiation. Similarly, the radiation damage to various T cell subpopulations need not have the same results; if, for instance, suppressor cells were radiation sensitive, the decline of immune responses may not occur (actually, it could be augmented). On the contrary, if helper T cells were radiosensitive, immunity will certainly decline. These facts must be kept in mind when radiation studies are performed.

III. IMMUNE SYSTEM AND RADIATION

A. Lymphoid Tissues and Radiation

Already at the beginning of the 19th century the damaging effect of radiation on the thymus was reported by Heineke[15] and Rudberg,[16] although at that time the thymus was not recognized as an important counterpart of the immunological system. The radiosensitive nature of thymic lymphocytes, in contrast to reticulum cell components, and their destruction after irradiation (especially those in the thymic cortex and to a lesser extent those in the medulla) was observed consequently by several groups of investigators.[17-19] The early studies exploring radiation effect on lymphoid organs other than thymus revealed that all lymphoid tissues were severely impaired after irradiation, as shown by their histological appearance as well as by their defective function.[19]

Recently Sharp and Thomas[20] made a comprehensive study of the effect of whole body X-irradiation on various components of the murine lymphomyeloid system, i.e., thymus, lymph nodes, spleen, and bone marrow. This study showed that all tissues of the lymphomyeloid compartment were negatively affected by irradiation, but the degree of radiation damage was dependent on the radiation dose used and the type of the tissue studied. All organs retained regeneration potential up to the dose of 200 rads of X-irradiation; above this dose, however, obvious differences in radiosensitivity among individual tissues were observed. The lymph nodes represented apparently the most radiation-sensitive tissue, since they failed to exhibit any regeneration capacity after irradiation with 400 rads. The spleen, bone marrow, and thymus exhibited regeneration potential up to doses of 500 rads and the doses of 650 rads, although not affecting regeneration of the thymus (which retained its regeneration capacity up to doses approaching 800 rads), did prevent regeneration of bone marrow and spleen. No correlation was found between radiation sensitivity and the age and/or sex of the animals in these studies. In the other series of experiments, the same authors studied systematically time-related changes in various lymphomyeloid tissues caused by total body irradiation in the dose of 750 rads. These experiments showed a marked reduction in the weights, cellularity, and histological appearance of spleens, lymph nodes, thymus, and femoral bone marrow during the first 4 days after irradiation.[20] In contrast to the other lymphomyeloid organs, in which these changes were irreversible, thymus weight and cellularity increased in subsequent 6 days and reached maximum regeneration in 10 days postirradiation. There was also an active DNA synthesis in the thymus beginning day six, as judged by extensive thymidine incorporation. No DNA synthesis reflecting cell proliferation was observed in any other tissue tested. On the 10th day the histological appearance of the irradiated thymus was essentially comparable to that of normal thymus. Thus, thymic regeneration occurred in the absence of regeneration of other compartments of lymphomyeloid complex. The regeneration of the thymus after this rather high dose of irradiation suggests that adult thymus, unlike other lymphoid tissues, possesses a relatively radioresistant precursor cell population. The existence of radioresistant thymic precursor cell population is compatible with the observation of Kubai and Auerbach.[21] The latter investigators during their experimentation on in vitro T cells differentiation observed that in vitro irradiation of thymus rudiments obtained from 12 to 13-day-old mouse embryos with doses of 1000 rads did not prevent subsequent differentiation of lymphoid cells.

Surprisingly, in spite of the presence of radioresistant thymic precursors allowing thymic recovery from irradiation, such recovery was not a permanent phenomenon; the initial phase of thymus regeneration was followed later by a secondary thymic atrophy, as judged by both histological appearance of the thymus and its weight. Takada et al.[18] studied more systematically and for a longer time period the pattern of thymic regeneration after administration of intermediate doses of irradiation (in the range of 300 to 500 rads). These investigators reported that thymic regeneration followed a biphasic pattern. They observed in accordance with Sharp and Thomas[20] initial fall in thymic weight a few days after irradiation, then consecutive increase in mitotic index and almost complete thymic restoration within 10 to 15 days. Thymic restoration was, however, followed by a secondary temporary fall in thymic appearance, weight, and cellularity and then by a secondary recovery phase at about 30 days after irradiation. This biphasic pattern of thymic regeneration after whole body irradiation was confirmed by several other investigators.[22,23] It was consequently reported that the second (but not the first) radiation-caused thymic atrophy was greatly diminished by transplantation of syngeneic bone marrow cells and/or by shielding of the hind limbs of the animal during the irradiation.[18,24-26] On the basis of these observations it was concluded that the second thymic atrophy could be caused by the lack of thymic precursors due to the inadequate traffic of stem cells from radiation-injured bone marrow to the thymus. Since further experiments showed that thymic atrophy was not observed after small doses of radiation (in the range of 50 to 200 rads), the doses which were insufficient in causing significant bone marrow injury, this explanation appeared logical.

Additional studies evaluating the effect of radiation on thymic tissue have shown that thymus was composed of two populations of lymphocytes with different sensitivity to radiation. Thymic medulla was described to be comprised of radioresistant population of thymocytes (apparently the population involved in the first phase of thymic regeneration) and the cortex of the radiosensitive thymocyte population.[17,27] Similarly, taking advantage of different cell surface and cell density characteristics of thymic lymphocytes, Konda et al.[28] subdivided thymic lymphocytes into two populations, one of which was radiosensitive and the other radioresistant. The radiosensitive population presented the majority of thymic lymphocytes and was composed of cells of relatively high density, expressing high concentration of Thy-1 antigen, TL antigen (thymus leukemia), G_{Ix} (Gross virus) antigen, and Ly-A, Ly-B, and Ly-C antigens (series of T cell antigens), and practically no H-2 antigens. Moreover, this population did not exert any responsiveness to PHA and did not possess any alloantigen recognition capabilities. The second radioresistant population of thymocytes represented minor thymic population and was of low cell density, large concentration of H-2 antigens, and low concentration of thymus antigens; in addition this population was PHA responsive and expressed alloantigen recognition properties.[28] Furthermore, these authors observed that the radiation-sensitive thymic population was also sensitive to cortisone, while the radioresistant population was not. Compatible observation, indicating correlation between radiation sensitivity and cortisone sensitivity of thymocytes was made by another group of investigators.[27] The heterogeneity of thymocytes with regard to their radiation sensitivity was also shown by Warner and Anderson[29] in experiments involving transfer immunoglobulin system.

As indicated earlier, lymph nodes and spleen are also sensitive to irradiation as shown by rapid appearance of advanced morphological damage and hypocellularity observed in these tissues following shortly after irradiation. As will be shown later, however, different degrees of radiation sensitivity are expressed by individual cell populations within each of these tissues. One of the most radiation-susceptible structures of the murine spleen and lymph nodes are germinal centers.[30,31] Shortly after irradiation necrosis of germinal centers is observed and is, in general, more pronounced in nonthymic-dependent areas of outer lymph node and spleen cortex. In parallel with these findings is the observation of Anderson et al.[32] who studied histological changes and functional characteristics of murine lymph nodes, spleen, and Peyer's patches after whole body irradiation. In splenic tissue he observed greater susceptibility of bone marrow-dependent lymphocyte population than thymus-dependent lymphocyte population, to irradiation. The histological observation indicating higher susceptibility of splenic B cells than T cells to irradiation were confirmed by experiments employing immunofluorescence technique. The latter studies showed that depletion of B cells was not only more pronounced but also occurred earlier. For example, significant decrease in B cells was evident as soon as 24 hr after irradiation with 5.50 and 500 r, while comparable decrease of T cells was seen only after 500 r of total body irradiation.[32]

Also in lymph node tissue, B cell-dependent areas were the primary radiation target when compared with T cell-dependent areas. When comparison in radiation sensitivity between short-lived and long-lived lymph node lymphocytes was made, the former appeared to be less radioresistant.[33] The pathological changes of lymph node lymphocytes initiated by total body of irradiation were found to be closely accompanied by the failure of the major lymph nodes functions. No development of antibody-forming cells in response to antigenic stimulus was detected.[27] In general, the radiation-caused changes in lymph nodes were of a greater degree than those in the spleen and occurred earlier. In contrast to lymph node and splenic lymphocytes which were destroyed after whole body irradiation, the stromal cell components, reticuloendothelial cells, and plasma cells proved to be relatively radioresistant.[35] Histological examination of Peyer's patches at various times after irradiation also showed great damage to this tissue which was radiation dose-dependent and reversible up to 500 rads of irradiation.

Analogously to mice, rabbit lymphoid tissues including spleen, lymph nodes, and appendix were showed also to be susceptible to irradiation in the dose range of 500 rads. Moreover, in this specie the radiation damage was more pronounced in B cell compartment than in T cell compartment.[31,36,37]

B. Antibody Response and Radiation

The sensitivity of the lymphocyte functions to irradiation is a phenomenon recognized for many years. As early as at the beginning of the 19th century the suppressive effect of irradiation on antibody formation was described by various investigators.[38] The initial studies also showed that an early phase of antibody formation was more radiosensitive than the consequent phase, i.e., antibody production. Benjamin and Sluka[38] reported that irradiation of rabbits a few days before injection of antigen inhibited antibody formation, whereas antibody formation was not affected when irradiation was administered after injection of antigen. These findings have been later confirmed and extended by several other investigators in various animal species.[8,39-43] The extreme sensitivity of the early phase of antibody formation to irradiation was lucidly shown by Dixon et al.[40] who studied the effect of various doses of irradiation administered prior to antigen injection on antibody formation. These investigators observed depression of antibody formation with doses of irradiation as low as 75R and 125R and almost complete inhibition with the escalated doses (in the range of 200 to 300 R). Observations of Jacobson et al.,[44,45] showing that the shielding of the appendix or spleens of rabbits during irradiation resulted in a nearly normal titer of antibodies, showed clearly that the depression of antibody formation was due to the damage to lymphocytes. Similar results indicating abolition of suppressive effect of irradiation by shielding of the spleen were obtained by Wissler et al.[46] and Nagareda[47] in rats.

In contrast to total body irradiation, studies employing local irradiation do not indicate any decline in antibody response. In fact, local body irradiation was found sometimes to increase antibody response.[48] For instance, Graham et al.[49] reported an enhancement of both circulating and local antibody titers in rabbits after irradiation of the site that has been injected intradermally with antigen. In other investigations, Taliaferro and Taliaferro[50] studied the effect of local splenic irradiation of the rabbits on the response to sheep red blood cells (SRBC). Spleens were irradiated locally with the dose ranging from 50 to 10,000 R and 2 days later the animals received a single i.v. injection of SRBC. Significant increase in antibody titers was observed despite local irradiation up to the dose of 2000 R in these studies. Another group of investigators[51] tested the capacity of irradiated sheep's popliteal lymph nodes to respond to killed typhoid bacilli and found that the antibody titer from irradiated lymph node lymphoctes was of the same magnitude as that of unirradiated lymph nodes cells. Benninghoff et al.[52] made comparison between the effects of local versus total body irradiation on rat lymph nodes. They observed that after local irradiation with 300R the cervical lymph nodes were not significantly depleted of lymphocytes, although there was a temporary dip in lymphocyte population shortly after irradiation. Within 48 hr after irradiation, however, the lymphocytes equaled that of controls. In contrast, lymph nodes of animals receiving the same dose of total body irradiation were severely depleted.

Even though total body irradiation appears to have, in general, a damaging effect on lymphoid organs and consequently on antibody production, it was also shown to augment antibody formation under certain conditions. Such radiation-mediated enhancement of antibody response was observed either when low doses of irradiation (25 to 200 r) were administered before antigen injection and/or when relatively high doses of irradiation (over 400 R) were administered after antigen injection.[53] The example of the former situation is represented by experiments of Taliaferro et al.[53] who observed extended production of high titers of antibodies when rabbits were irradiated with 25 to 100 R given a week before antigen administration. In mice, 150 to 175 R of irradiation administered for 4 weeks prior to antigen injection was reported to increase primary antibodies directed against hemocyanin.[54] Higher doses of irradiation (150 to 300 R) were, however, suppressive under the same experimental conditions. Radiation-caused augmentation of the secondary immune response was observed by some but not by the other investigators.[54-56] The latter phenomenon appeared to vary significantly with regard to the type of antigen and schedule of irradiation.[57]

Secondary antibody response is considered in general to be more radioresistant than primary antibody response.[40,58,59] Nevertheless, some investigators reported that secondary response can be decreased by irradiation to the same extent as primary antibody response. Tao and Leary,[60] for instance, observed that the primary and secondary response to bacteriophage antigen declined in a similar level after irradiation in vitro. Similar observation was made by Makinodan et al.[41] in cell transfer experimental system in vitro. Tada et al.[61] reported that the enhancement of antibody formation by irradiation was not a general phenomenon involving all classes of antibodies and showed certain restriction with regard to the antibody involved. For instance, whole body irradiation with 400 R administered a few days after antigen injection augmented production of hemocytotropic antibody, but apparently suppressed IgG response in the same animal.[61]

Whereas the inhibitory effect of irradiation on antibody is to be expected, because of the detrimental effect of ionizing radiation on lymphoid cell populations involved in antibody production, the mechanism underlying the augmentation of antibody response is unknown. Anderson and Warner[19] summarized various possibilities which could underly the mechanisms of radiation-induced immune enhancement: (1) unequal repopulation of radiation-depleted lymphoid tissues by rapidly dividing antigen-stimulated cells, (2) increase in antibody production in response to endotoxin released from the gut tissue after irradiation, (3) increase in proliferation and differentiation of immunocompetent cells stimulated by factors released from radiation damaged cells, (4) disturbed feedback regulation of antibody response[62,63] (IgG antibody is considered to control feedback regulation of antibody response and thus changes in IgG levels — caused by irradiation — could inhibit IgG feedback control), and (5) inhibition of suppressor cells regulating immune functions which could result in increased immune responsiveness. The experiments of Dixon and McConahey,[56,64] designed to study the kinetics of the effect of X-irradiation on antibody production, eliminated the possibility that the adjuvant properties of endotoxin are responsible for radiation-caused enhancement of immune response. There are the other possibilities that could be involved in immune enhancement, e.g., the increased function of macrophages after irradiation could lead to augmentation of antibody formation. The radiation effect on macrophages can be direct and/or indirect (i.e., mediated by various factors released from cells after radiation caused damage). It is reasonable to postulate that various factors and/or their combination may be involved in augmentation of antibody response. One of the above-mentioned possibilities involved in radiation-mediated augmentation of antibody response, i.e., elimination of suppressor cells, was already experimentally supported, as will be shown later.

IV. RADIATION AND VARIOUS SUBPOPULATIONS OF LYMPHOCYTES

From previous sections, it is obvious that in general immune responsiveness of the individual is negatively influenced by irradiation and that lymphocytes are the primary targets of radiation effect (Table 1). However, most of the experiments studying the effect of irradiation on immune competence were done before new concepts of immunology were developed and the heterogeneity of lymphocyte populations and subpopulations realized. Hence, the observation that radiation is damaging for, e.g., antibody response or for other immune phenomena (most of which are mediated through cell cooperations), does not provide any information on the radiosensitivity (radioresistance) of specific populations or subpopulations of lymphocytes. In this section we will review the radiation effect on individual subsets of lymphocytes. We will also report on macrophages in this section since these cells, even though they do not belong to lymphocyte lineage, represent an important component in various immune phenomena.

A. Macrophages

Macrophages are considered to represent a rather radioresistant population of cells. Histological studies indicate that radiation does not cause any apparent morphological damage to these cells[65] and functional studies indicate that macrophages retain their phagocytic and migratory capacity despite relatively high doses of irradiation.[66-69] Macrophages have been found to be morphologically and functionally intact after doses of irradiation in vivo and in vitro in the range of 600 to 800 R. For instance, it has been reported that the ability of the reticuloendothelial system to clear bacteria from the blood of mice, rats, and rabbits was not affected by X-irradiation in the range of 600 to 800 R.[70] Similarly, clearance of colloidal carbon from the circulation of mice was not affected by these doses of irradiation[71] and in vitro capacity of mouse peritoneal macrophages to engulf SRBC was resistant to kiloroentgen doses of X-irradiation.[68] In vitro irradiation in the dose of 10,000 R, however, resulted in macrophage damage.[69] Macrophage function in immune response in vitro was reported also to be radioresistant. The function of macrophages in the primary antibody response in vitro to SRBC was resistant to doses of irradiation which abolished the response of lymphocytes.[9,72] In fact, increased immunogenicity and binding of the antigen by macrophages irradiated in vitro has been observed.[69] Also in vitro blastogenic response to purified protein derivative (PPD) was markedly facilitated by irradiated macrophages.[73] On the contrary, some reports indicated that macrophages from X-irradiated animals lost their capacity to participate in antibody production to Shigella,[74,75] bovine serum albumin (BSA),[76] and bovine gamma globulin (BCG).[77] Macrophages represent the heterogeneous population of cells not only with regard to their location (they are present in peritoneal cavity, lungs, spleens, liver, etc...) but also with regard to their functions. These cells were reported not only to facilitate various immune phenomena but also to suppress immune response. Weiss and Fitch[78] demonstrated that macrophages present in normal rat spleens suppressed both the generation of plaque-forming cells to SRBC in vitro and the generation of cytotoxic lymphocytes in mixed lymphocytes cul-

TABLE 1
RADIATION EFFECT ON LYMPHOCYTE
SUBPOPULATIONS

Cell type	Radiation sensitivity

T Cells

Helper cells	Radioresistant (possibly radiosensitive subpopulation)
Suppressor Cells	Radiosensitive
DTH effector	Radioresistant
GvH effectors	Radioresistant
HvG effectors	Radiosensitve
CTL lymphocytes (in vitro)	Radioresistant

B Cells

Unprimed B cells	Radiosensitive
Primed B cells	Radiosensitive (possibly radioresistant subpopulation)
Suppressor B cells	Radiosensitive
Plasma cells	Radioresistant

Other Cell Types

Macrophages	Radioresistant
NK cells	Radioresistant
K cells	Radioresistant
BM-E cells	Radioresistant

tures in vitro. The suppressive function of macrophages was in these studies radioresistant indicating that also suppressor macrophages pertain their functions despite irradiation. Similar observation was made by Oehler et al.[79]

B. Helper T Lymphocytes

The T lymphocytes, designated helper T cells, function in facilitating (both qualitatively and quantitavely) the antibody response to various antigens. These cells are also involved in augmenting or amplifying various cellular immunity-mediated phenomena, such as allograft rejection and generation of cytotoxic lymphocytes.[12] Because of these properties, helper T cells are important for optimal humoral and cell-mediated immune responsiveness, and the effect of radiation on these cells is of utmost interest. In the initial studies, Claman and his colleagues reported that the murine helper T cells activity was radiosensitive.[80] It was shown later, however, by Kettman and Dutton[81-83] that the murine helper T cells were rather radioresistant. These authors studied the effect of irradiation on helper T cells which participate in the in vitro primary antibody response to SRBC and to 2,4, 6-trinitrobenzenesulfonic acid hapten (TNP)-SRBC (hapten-carrier) complexes and showed that these cells were radioresistant. Specifically, in vitro primary anti-TNP response of splenocytes from normal (not primed) mice to TNP-SRBC complexes was greatly augmented by addition of splenocytes from carrier (SRBC) primed mice. In vitro X-irradiation (4000 R) of these splenocytes prevented the development of antibody response, but did not eliminate their function as helper cells in the anti-TNP response of normal spleen cells. This observation, indicating radioresistance of murine helper T cells, was confirmed by other investigators.[84,85] Similar studies were performed in guinea pigs by Katz et al.[86] These investigators determined that guinea pig lymphocytes which were primed with carrier (bovine gamma globulin) and then exposed to irradiation in vitro (1000 to 5000 R) were effective as "helpers" in augmenting the secondary anti-2,4, dinitrophenyl (DNP) hapten antibody response when transferred to DNP-primed syngeneic guinea pigs. It is important, however, to mention here that the helper T cells are radioresistant only after they are primed with antigen and are allowed some time to proliferate and differentiate into functionally mature helper cells. The requirement of maturity for the expression of radioresistance explains the discrepancy between the observations of Kettman and Dutton,[81] indicating radioresistance of helper T cells and that of Claman et al.,[80] suggesting radiosensitivity of helper T cells. In the latter situation the helper T cells were not yet fully primed and thus required proliferation, the function that is sensitive to irradiation. It has been shown by two groups of investigators[7,87] that approximately 3 days of interaction between T cells and antigen (in this situation SRBC) was required before T cells could cooperate with B cells. When the X-irradiation was administered at the time of T cell-antigen interaction, helper function of T cells was abolished. The observations indicating radioresistance of helper T cells can seemingly be in contrast to those of Anderson et al.[88] whose experiments indicated relative radiosensitivity of primed helper T cells involved in antibody response in mice. Irradiation with 1000 R in vitro practically abrogated the capacity of fowl γ-globulin (FγG)-primed thoracic duct T cells or splenocytes to cooperate with DNP-primed B lymphocytes in antibody response to DNP-FγG. Similar observation was made by Hamaoka et al.[89] who, however, noticed that it was not a helper function of primed mouse T cells which was affected by irradiation but the radiation-caused change in migration pattern of T cells. This conclusion was made on the basis of the following observations: (1) carrier-specific helper function remained unchanged in carrier primed mice after X-irradiation, and (2) adoptively transferred carrier primed lymphocytes were effective helper cells after in vitro irradiation. It was reported later by Anderson et al.[90] that radiation indeed influenced the migratory properties of lymphocytes. These authors showed that when [51]chromium-labeled T lymphocytes were irradiated in vitro prior to i.v. adoptive transfer, they expressed reduction in migration pattern to spleen and lymph nodes within 4 to 24 hr. In addition, lymph node homing pattern of irradiated lymphocytes was totally abolished by maintaining these cells in vitro for 7 hr before adoptive transfer in vivo. Hence, there are no discrepancies between above-mentioned reports with regard to the radioresistance of helper T cells.

An interesting observation with regard to the effect of radiation on helper T cells was made recently by Lawrence et al.[91] They reported that SRBC-sensitized T cells, primed by two different methods, had differential sensitivities to radiation. The first type of primed T cells was prepared by injection of thymocytes together with SRBC into lethally-irradiated syngeneic mice and was designated antigen-activated T cells (ATC). The second type of primed T cells was isolated from SRBC-immunized mice and was designated primed T cells (pT); pT cells were found radiosensitive, losing 50% of their activity after 500 R of irradiation and more than 80% of activity after administration of 1000 R. The ATC were, on the contrary, relatively radioresistant; in fact, their activity was slightly enhanced after 500 r and more than 50% of activity was still expressed after irradiation with 1000 R. Similar radiation sensitivity patterns of ATC and pT were also observed by these investigators when hapten carrier (TNP-SRBC) system was used. These data indicate that various subpopulations of helper T cells, expressing differential radiosensitivity, may exist. Nonetheless, concluding from all experimental data described above, most of the helper T cells appear to be radioresistant.

C. Suppressor T Cells

With increased experimentation on T cell functions, it has been realized that T cells not only augment immune responses but could also exert suppressive influences on immune system.[92,93] Contrasted with the relative radioresistance of helper T cells functions is relative radiosensitivity of suppressor T cells functions. The first observation of the deleterious effect of irradiation on suppressor cells was demonstrated by Tada et al.[61] They noted that administration of 400 R of X-irradiation to rats shortly before primary immunization with DNP-ASC plus Bordetella pertussis resulted in an increase in anti-DNP antibody response of IgE class, but not of the IgM of IgG antibody classes. Other groups of investigators[94] observed also that in the murine system, X-irradiation efficiently augmented IgE antibody response against rabbit antilymphocyte serum. Similar augmentation of both primary and secondary murine IgE antibody response was reported in DNP-carrier conjugate system.[95,96] Moreover, experiments of Okumura and Tada[97] showed that the enhanced IgE antibody response of rats after X-irradiation could be abolished by adoptive transfer of syngeneic carrier primed rats' spleen cells or thymocytes. However, this effect was expressed only by carrier-primed rats (the T cell function) and not by hapten-primed animals (the B cell function). On the basis of these experiments it was postulated that augmentation of IgE response by X-irradiation was due to the elimination of suppressor T cell controlling antibody response activities in this system. Similar enhancement of antibody response to various antigens was reported by several other investigators.

Rotter and Trainin[98] reported that suppressor T cells involved in T cell-independent antibody response of mice to polyvinylpyrolidone (PVP) were radiosensitive, since X-irradiation resulted in increased antibody response to PVP. Suppressor cells regulating helper T cell responses in SRBC antibody formation system were also described to be radiosensitive[99] and so were the antigen-specific suppressor cells involved in regulation of antibody response to synthetic random terpolymer of glutamic acid, alanine, and tyrosine (GAT).[100] Eardley and Gershon[99] reported that the suppressor cells activities were totally abolished by exposure to 400R of X-irradiation in vitro.

Nevertheless, in contrast to radiosensitive suppressor cells population, there is an indication that the functions of suppressor cells stimulated by ConA mitogen are relatively radioresistant in regulating in vivo antibody responses.[101,102] Similarly ConA-activated suppressor T cells, operating in murine mixed lymphocyte reaction, were described to be radioresistant.[103] Radioresistant suppressor T cells were also reported to be involved in graft-vs-host reaction[104] and in generation of cytotoxic T lymphocytes.[104]

To summarize, the suppressor T cells appear to be relatively radiosensitive, even though some of them, especially those activated by mitogens, express certain degrees of radioresistance. The radiation-related changes in suppressor cells activities may reflect stages of maturation of these cells; in general, suppressor cells may be more sensitive to irradiation prior to antigen activation and during subsequent proliferation and differentiation state, whereas already activated suppressor T cells (e.g., with ConA) could be more radioresistant.

D. Effector T Cells

T cells are not involved only in regulation of antibody production (i.e., perform either helper or suppressor functions) but are also involved in cell-mediated immune reactions, such as cytotoxicity of normal and tumor tissues, graft-vs-host reaction (GVHR), and delayed type hypersensitivity reactions (DTHR).

T cells involved in DTHR in various species appear to express a low sensitivity to irradiation. It has been shown, for example, that exposure of guinea pigs to single dose of 250 R did not suppress allergic contact dermatitis to dinitrochlorbenzene.[105] Similar observation was made by Uhr and Scharf in rabbits.[106] In the latter experiments 400 r given to rabbits did not significantly suppress DTHR. In cell transfer systems, guinea pigs' DTHR could be transferred with cells which were irradiated in vitro with 1000 R.[107] In rats, radiation dose as high as 6000 R of X-irradiation was reported not to prevent lymphocytes' capacity to transfer DTHR.[108] In the mouse, cells transferring DTHR to SRBC were fully functional even after irradiation with 1500 rads in vitro under the condition that the cells were injected directly into the site of antigen challenge;[109] i.v. cell transfer was not successful. Similar observation was made by Hamaoka et al.[89] The failure to transfer the DTHR intravenously, but not locally, could be contributed to the changes in homing in vivo properties of in vitro-irradiated lymphocytes.

Cytotoxic T lymphocytes (CTL) were also reported to be relatively radioresistant. Using the [51]chromium-release cytotoxicity assay, it has been shown that previously sensitized CTL expressed their activities in spite of their previous irradiation.[110] In contrast to mature CTL, however, CTL precursors appear to be radiosensitive, since X-irradiation was reported to prevent their differentiation and maturation into fully effective effector cells.[111,112]

Similar observations were made in the GVHR system. It has been shown that GVHR of parental cells against F_1 hybrid tissues were abolished by their prior irradiation.[113] Radiation-caused inhibition of GVHR was also reported by Biggar et al.[114] in murine system and by Blackett[115] in rats. Sprent and his colleagues[113] made comparisons between unprimed and alloantigen-sensitized T cells with regard to their radiation sensitivity and GVHR functions. They found that irradiated, unprimed alloantigen-reactive T lymphocytes were radiosensitive; such irradiated cells were incapable either to induce GVHR or undergo DNA synthesis. On the other side, alloantigen activated T cells were fully active in GVHR and DNA synthesis, despite their irradiation with 5000 R of X-irradiation.

Ad hoc, it appears that radiation sensitivity of cytotoxic T lymphocytes is also a reflection of their maturity.

E. Natural Killer (NK) Cells

Murine NK cells represent a population(s) of cells expressing a relatively high degree of resistance to radiation. NK cells cytotoxic potential to tumors as well as to normal tissues is preserved despite the lethal doses of total body irradiation. We have observed that the in vivo irradiation in the range of 900 to 1200 R or in vitro irradiation up to 1500 R, did not inhibit NK cells activities, provided that these were tested within 24 hr after irradiation.[14,116] However, within 2 to 3 days after irradiation, NK cells lost their cytotoxic potential.[133]

The systematic study on murine NK cells radioresistance have shown that for the first 12 days after 700 r of total body irradiation NK cell cytotoxicity of B6C3F_1 mice against YAC-1 lymphoma was comparable to, or was above control levels. Then the cytotoxicity declined sharply and remained low until day 25. Beginning day 28, the activity was slowly increased, reaching near normal levels within 5 to 8 weeks.[117] This data indicates the relative radioresistance of mature NK cells to moderate doses of irradiation. However, the fall in NK cells activities around 14 days indicates that the NK cell precursors are rather sensitive to and temporarily arrested by irradiation. We have observed in our laboratory similar decline in NK cells cytotoxicity of B6DF_1 mice to YAC-1 after total body irradiation with 700 r; no change in cytotoxic potential was observed after 500 r of total body irradiation.[134] Nevertheless, even though the in vitro cytotoxic potential of mature NK cells is relatively radioresistant there is nothing known about radiation sensitivity of in vivo NK cells' antitumor activities.

The antibody dependent killer cells, although not studied so sytematically were reported also to be relatively radioresistant.[118]

F. B Cells

Effect of radiation of B cells, especially on various B cell subpopulations, has not been studied so extensively as that of T cells. As indicated earlier, however, B lymphocytes are relatively radioresistant and certainly more sensitive to ionizing effects of X-irradiation than are T lymphocytes. Fox et al.[95] observed that there is a difference in radiosensitivity between various B lymphocyte subpopulations. These authors studied the effect of radiation on B lymphocytes by measuring the production of hapten-specific IgG and IgE antibody-irradiated B lymphocytes. Their results showed that both primed and unprimed B lymphocytes of IgG class were more radiosensitive than primed and unprimed IgE-B lymphocytes. Moreover, primed IgG-B lymphocytes were found by these authors more radioresistant than unprimed IgG-B lymphocytes. In contrast, unprimed IgE-B lymphocytes showed comparable radioresistance with primed IgE-B lymphocytes. For example, in the cell transfer system, it has been shown that irradiation of 300 R inhibited production of IgG anti-DNP antibody, but not IgE anti-DNP antibody. Recently, it has been shown that the B cells can express suppressive activities. B cells residing in bone marrow were reported to suppress in vitro antibody response to SRBC.[13] The latter functions were found to be diminished after irradiation with 2000 R.

The antibody-producing cells, plasma cells, express a great radioresistance; no change in numbers of long-lived plasma cell population following 800 r was found by Miller and Cole.[119] It has been shown also by other groups of investigators that neither the rate of antibody synthesis, nor the integrity of cytoplasmic structures of plasma cells was affected by 10,000 R of irradiation.[120,121] The IgM and IgG production by plasma cells was found also to be relatively radioresistant.[121]

V. TRANSPLANTATION AND RADIATION

A. Solid Tissue Transplantation

The protective effect of irradiation on rabbit skin allografts rejection was shown by Dempster as early as 1950.[122] In these experiments radiation dose as low as 250 R, administered to rabbits prior to allogeneic skin graft transplantation, significantly prolonged graft survival. In the murine system, prolonged rejection of male skin isografts transplanted into females was induced by 300 r of irradiation.[123] Extended survival of murine allogeneic skin grafts was also reported.[124] In the latter experiments, the time of survival was in direct relationship with the dose of irradiation, i.e., the greater the dose, the longer the survival of the graft. It has also been shown that the dose of irradiation was related to the genetic difference between the donor and the recipient; the greater the genetic difference, the larger were the radiation doses required for suppression.[125] In contrast to rather high radiosensitivity of cells mediating rejection of primary grafts (i.e., the grafts transplanted into naive, nonsensitized animals) second-set responses (i.e., the responses of animals presensitized by previous grafts) were found to be more radioresistant. The doses of 670 to 850 r were practically ineffective in the latter situation.[125]

For its protective effect in allogeneic graft rejection, irradiation has been used as a conditioning regimen for various types of transplantation.

B. Bone Marrow Transplantation

The cells responsible for rejection of parental, allogeneic, or xenogeneic bone marrow transplants (hemopoietic transplants) differ by various parameters from cells mediating rejection of solid tissue grafts, and from those involved in other types of cellular and humoral immunity.[126-128] Except for other differences, bone marrow effectors (BM-E) in contrast to solid tissue graft effector cells are relatively radioresistant; resistance to hemopoietic transplants is expressed even after lethal doses of total body irradiation in the range of 1000 to 1500 R. However, the radioresistance of BM-E cells is not an absolute phenomenon since it has been shown that resistance to parental marrow can be abrogated by doses of irradiation ranging from 2000 to 5000 R[126,133] and xenogeneic resistance by doses in the range of 6600 to 8000 R.[129] Resistance to hemopoietic grafts can be also abrogated by increasing the time interval between irradiation (in the range of 900 to 1100 R) and marrow transplantation. Specifically, when transplantation is performed 6 to 24 hr after irradiation, hybrid and xenogeneic resistance are fully expressed. If, however, transplantation follows 5 days after irradiation, hybrid resistance and allogeneic resistance are abrogated.[130] The precursors of BM-E cells express less radioresistance, however, than mature BM-E cells since preirradiation with 500 to 700 R, 10 to 14 days before lethal dose of irradiation and bone marrow transplantation prevented rejection of bone marrow grafts.[131] As to the nature of BM-E cells, these have not yet been characterized with certainty; in fact, bone marrow graft rejection appears to be mediated through cell cooperation. One of the cell types involved in antibone marrow reactivity resembles subpopulations of macrophages[130] and the other type could be the NK cell, since the latter cell shares the following characteristics with BM-E cells: natural occurrence, relative radioresistance, late maturation, prompt reactivity, lack of reactivity in bone marrow tolerant mice, and sensitivity to the same agents.[14,132]

VI. CONCLUDING REMARKS

In the present chapter an attempt has been made to highlight the complexity of the immune system and the diverse effects radiation exerts on heterogeneous population of immunocompetent cells. It should be rather obvious that radiation-immune interaction is not a simple one, and in order to develop the most efficient protocols for radiation therapy, more research in this area is needed. It is not unreasonable to hope that our understanding of the mechanism of such interactions may allow us not only to effectively eliminate tumor cells by irradiation, but also to manipulate the immune system (effector vs suppressor cell populations) in the most effective antitumor direction.

It should be stressed that it was not attempted here to give a comprehensive review of the area of irradiation, since it would be an impossible task with regard to the space limitation. It is hoped that the readers interested in radiation research will find sufficient information through the references cited in this article.

REFERENCES

1. Suit, H. D. and Kastelan, A., Immunological status of host and response of a methylcholanthrene-induced sarcoma to local X-irradiation, *Cancer*, 26, 232, 1970.
2. Suit, H. D., Considerations in the interactions of radiation and immunotherapy, in *Interaction of Radiation and Host Defense Mechanisms in Malignancy*, Brookhaven Natl. Lab. Assoc. Univ. Inc., United States Atomic Energy Commission, Upton, N.Y., 1974, 130.
3. Withers, R. H., Radiobiological basis of radiotherapy, in *Interaction of Radiation and Host Defense Mechanisms in Malignancy*, Brookhaven Natl. Lab. Assoc. Univ. Inc., United States Atomic Energy Commission, Upton, N.Y., 1974, 119.
4. Chanana, A. D., Schaedeli, J., Hess, M. W., and Cottier, H., Variations in expression of θ C3H alloantigen on thymic and peripheral blood lymphocytes of newborn and young adult mice, *Cell. Immunol.*, 2, 216, 1974.

5. Joel, D. D., Hess, M. W., and Cottier, H., Magnitude and pattern of thymic lymphocyte migration in neonatal mice, *J. Exp. Med.*, 135, 907, 1972.

6. Claman, H. N. and Chaperson, E. A., Immunologic complementation between thymus and marrow cells. A model for the two-cell theory of immunocompetence, *Transpl. Rev.*, 1, 92, 1969.

7. Miller, J. F. A. P. and Mitchell, G. F., Interaction between two distinct cell lineages in an immune response, in *Lymphatic Tissue and Germinal Centers in Immune Response*, Vol. 5, Fiore-Donati, L. and Hanna, M. G., Eds., Plenum Press, New York, 1969, 455.

8. Davis, A. J. S., The thymus and the cellular basis of immunity, *Transplant. Rev.*, 1, 43, 1969.

9. Roseman, J., X-ray resistant cell required for the induction of *in vitro* antibody formation, *Science*, 165, 1125, 1969.

10. Cantor, H. and Asofsky, R., Synergy among lymphoid cells mediating the graft-versus-host response, *J. Exp. Med.*, 131, 235, 1970.

11. Cantor, H. and Asofsky, R., Synergy among lymphoid cells mediating the graft-versus-host response III. Evidence for interaction between two types of thymus-derived cells, *J. Exp. Med.*, 135, 764, 1972.

12. Katz, D. H., Functional properties of T lymphocytes, in *Lymphocyte Differentiation, Recognition and Regulation*, Academic Press, New York, 1977, 247.

13. Fuchs, B. B., Khaitov, R. M., Petrov, R. V., Atanllakhanov, R. I., Sidorovich, I. G., Vanho, L. V., and Malaitsev, V. V., Bone marrow suppressor B cells *in vitro*, *Immunology*, 35, 997, 1978.

14. Lotzová, E. and McCredie, K. B., Natural killer cells in mice and man and their possible biological significance, *Cancer Immunol. Immunother.*, 4, 215, 1978.

15. Heineke, H., Uber die eiwerkung der rontgenstrahlen aus tire, *Muench. Med. Wochenschr.*, 1, 2090, 1903.

16. Rudberg, H., Studien uber die thymus involution. I. Die involution nach rontgenbestrahlung, *Arch. Anat. Physiol. (Leipzig)*, Suppl. 123, 1907.

17. Trowell, O. A., Radiosensitivity of cortical and medullary lymphocytes in the thymus, *Int. J. Radiat. Biol.*, 4, 163, 1961.

18. Takada, A., Takada, Y., Huang, C. C., and Ambrus, J. L., Biphasic pattern of thymus regeneration after whole body irradiation, *J. Exp. Med.*, 129, 445, 1969.

19. Anderson, R. and Warner, N. L., Ionizing radiation and the immune response, *Adv. Immunol.*, 24, 215, 1976.

20. Sharp, J. G. and Thomas, D. B., Thymic regeneration in lethally X-irradiated mice, *Radiat. Res.*, 64, 293, 1975.

21. Kubai, L. and Auerbach, R., Radiation-resistant thymic stem cells, *Proc. Soc. Exp. Biol. Med.*, 142, 554, 1973.

22. Haran-Ghera, N., The effects of ionizing radiation on growth and regeneration of intrarenal thymus grafts in mice, *Radiat. Res.*, 26, 442, 1965.

23. Brecher, G., Endicott, K. M., Gump, H., and Brawner, H. P., Effects of X-rays on lymphoid and hemopoietic tissues of albino mice, *Blood*, 2, 1259, 1948.

24. Takada, A., Takada, Y., Kim, U., and Ambrus, J., Bone marrow, spleen and thymus regeneration pattern in mice after whole body irradiation, *Radiat. Res.*, 45, 522, 1971.

25. Blomgren, H., The role of bone marrow of X-irradiated mice in thymic recovery, *Cell Tissue Kinet.*, 4, 443, 1971.

26. Decleve, A., Gerber, G. V., Leonard, A., Lambiet-Collier, M., Sassen, A., and Maisin, J. R., Regeneration of thymus, spleen and bone marrow in X-irradiated AKR mice, *Radiat. Res.*, 51, 318, 1972.

27. Blomgren, H. and Anderson, B., Characteristics of the immunocompetent cells in the mouse thymus cell population changes during cortisone-induced atrophy and subsequent regeneration, *Cell Immunol.*, 1, 545, 1971.

28. Konda, S., Nakao, Y., and Smith, R. T., Immunological properties of mouse thymus cells. Identification of T cell functions withing a minor low-density subpopulation, *J. Exp. Med.*, 136, 1461, 1972.

29. Warner, N. L. and Anderson, R. S., Helper effect of normal and irradiated thymus cells on transferred immunoglobulin production, *Nature (London)*, 254, 604, 1975.

30. Jordan, S. W., Ultrastructural studies on spleen after whole body irradiation of mice, *Exp. Mol. Pathol.*, 6, 156, 1967.

31. Durkin, H. G. and Thorbecke, G. J., Preferential destruction of germinal centers by prednisolone and X-irradiation, *Lab. Invest.*, 26, 53, 1972.

32. Anderson, R. E., Olson, G. B., Autry, R. J., Howarth, J. L., Troup, G. M., and Bartels, P. H., Radiosensitivity of T and B lymphocytes. IV. Effect of whole body irradiation upon various lymphoid tissues and numbers of recirculating lymphocytes, *J. Immunol.*, 118, 1191, 1977.

33. Miller, J. J., III and Cole, L. J., The radiation resistance of long-lived lymphocytes and plasma cells in mouse and rat, *J. Immunol.*, 98, 982, 1967.

34. Weissman, I. L., Nord, S., and Ellis, R., Radiolabeled antibodies: their potential as quantitative tools for *in vitro* and *in vivo* tumor diagnosis, in *Interaction of Radiation and Host Immune Defense Mechanisms in Malignancy,* Brookhaven Natl. Lab. Assoc. Univ., Inc., U.S. Atomic Energy Commission, Upton, N.Y., 1974, 379.

35. Congdon, C. C., The destruction effect of radiation of lymphoatic tissue, *Cancer Res.,* 26, 1211, 1966.

36. Blythman, H. E. and Waksman, B. H., Effect of locally administered endotoxin on regenerating appendix structure and responses of appendix cells to mitogens, *J. Immunol.,* 11, 108, 1973.

37. Keuning, F. J., Van der Meer, J., Niehwenhuis, P., and Oudenijk, P., The histopathology of the antibody response. II. Antibody responses and splenic plasma cell reactions in sublethally X-irradiated rabbits, *Lab. Invest.,* 12, 156, 1963.

38. Benjamin, S. and Sluka, E., Antikorperbildung nach experimenteteller schadigung des hematopoietischen systems durch rontgenstrahlen, *Wien. Klin. Wochenschr.,* 21, 311, 1908.

39. Taliaferro, W. H. and Taliaferro, L. G., Effect of X-irradiation on immunity: a review, *J. Immunol.,* 66, 181, 1951.

40. Dixon, F. J., Talmage, D. W., and Maurer, P. H., Radiosensitive and radioresistant phases in the antibody response, *J. Immunol.,* 68, 693, 1952.

41. Makinodan, T., Kastenbaun, M. A., and Peterson, W. J., Radiosensitivity of spleen cells from normal and pre-immunized mice and its significance to intact animals, *J. Immunol.,* 88, 31, 1962.

42. Kohn, H. I., The effect of X-rays upon the hemolysin production in the rat, *J. Immunol.,* 66, 525, 1951.

43. Stoner, R. D. and Hale, W. M., Radiation effects on primary and secondary antibody responses, in *Effects of Ionizing Radiation on Immune Processes,* Leone, C. A., Ed., Gordon & Breach, New York, 1962, 183.

44. Jacobson, L. O., Robson, M. J., and Marks, E. K., The effects of X-irradiation on antibody function, *Proc. Soc. Exp. Biol. Med.,* 75, 145, 1950.

45. Jacobson, L. O. and Robson, M. J., Factors effecting X-ray inhibition of antibody function, *J. Lab. Clin. Med.,* 39, 167, 1952.

46. Wissler, R. W., Robson, M. J., Nelson, W., Fitch, F., and Jacobson, L. O., The effects of spleen-shielding and subsequent splenectomy upon antibody formation in rats receiving total body X-irradiation, *J. Immunol.,* 70, 379, 1953.

47. Nagareda, C. S., Antibody formation and the effect of irradiation on circulating antibody levels in the hypophysectomized rat, *J. Immunol.,* 73, 88, 1954.

48. Sussdorf, D. H., Partial body irradiation and antibody response, in *Effects of Ionizing Radiations on Immune Processes,* Leone, C. A., Ed., Gordon & Breach, New York, 1962, 335.

49. Graham, J. B., Graham, R. M., Neri, L., and Wright, K. A., Enhanced production of antibodies by local irradiation. I. Measurement of circulating antibodies, *J. Immunol.,* 76, 103, 1956.

50. Taliaferro, W. H. and Taliaferro, L. G., X-ray effects on hemolysin formation in rabbits with the spleen shielded or irradiated, *J. Infect. Dis.,* 99, 109, 1956.

51. Hall, J. G. and Morris, B., Effect of X-irradiation of the popliteal lymph node on its output of lymphocytes and immunological responsiveness, *Lancet,* 1, 1077, 1964.

52. Benninghoff, D. L., Tyler, R. W., and Everett, N. B., Repopulation of irradiated lymph nodes by recirculating lymphocytes, *Radiat. Res.,* 37, 381, 1969.

53. Taliaferro, W. H., Taliaferro, L. G., and Jaroslaw, B. N., The hemolysin response in rabbits irradiated with 500R, in *Radiation and Immune Mechanism,* Academic Press, New York, 1964, 17.

54. Hoffstein, P. E. and Dixon, F. J., Effect of irradiation and cyclophosphamide on anti-KLH antibody formation in mice, *J. Immunol.,* 112, 564, 1974.

55. Taliaferro, W. H. and Taliaferro, L. G., Effects of irradiation on initial and anamnestic hemolysin responses in rabbits: antigen injection before X-rays, *J. Immunol.,* 104, 1364, 1970.

56. Dixon, F. J. and McConahey, P. J., Enhancement of antibody formation by whole body X-irradiation, *J. Exp. Med.,* 117, 833, 1963.

57. Schmidtke, J. R. and Dixon, F. J., Effects of sublethal irradiation on the plaque-forming cell response in mice, *J. Immunol.,* 11, 691, 1973.

58. Taliaferro, W. H., Taliaferro, L. G., and Janssen, E. F., The localization of X-ray injury to the initial phases of antibody response, *J. Infect. Dis.,* 91, 105, 1952.

59. Silverman, M. S. and Chin, P. H., Quantitative serological determination of antibody formation in X-irradiated rabbits, *J. Immunol.,* 73, 120, 1954.

60. Tao, T. W. and Leary, P. L., Radiation-induced depression of primary and secondary antibody responses to bacteriophage ϕX 174 *in vitro, Nature (London),* 223, 306, 1969.

61. Tada, T., Taniguchi, M., and Okumura, K., Regulation of homocytotropic antibody formation in the rat, *J. Immunol.,* 106, 1012, 1971.

62. Uhr, J. W. and Moller, G., Regulatory effect of antibody on the immune response, *Adv. Immunol.,* 8, 81, 1968.

63. Diener, E. and Feldmann, M., Relationship between antigen and antibody-induced suppression of immunity, *Transplant. Rev.,* 8, 76, 1972.

64. Dixon, F. J. and McConahey, P. J., X-ray enhancement of antibody formation, *Immunopathol. Int. Symp.,* 158, 1963.

65. Bloom, M. A., Bone marrow, in *Histopathology of Irradiation from Internal and External Sources,* McGraw-Hill, New York, 1948, 162.

66. Smith, E. B., White, D. C., Hartsock, R. J., and Dixon, A. C., Acute ultrastructural effects of 500 roentgens on the lymph node of the mouse, *Am. J. Pathol.,* 50, 159, 1967.

67. Gadeberg, O. V., Rhodes, J. M., and Larson, S. O., The effect of various immunosuppressive agents on mouse peritoneal macrophages and on the *in vitro* phagocytosis of Escherichia Coli O4:K3:H5 and degradation of ^{125}I-labeled HSA-antibody complexes by these cells, *Immunology,* 28, 59, 1975.

68. Perkins, E. H., Nettesheim, P., and Morita, T., Radioresistance of the engulfing and degradative capacities of peritoneal phagocytes to kiloroentgen X-ray doses, *J. Reticuloend. Soc.,* 3, 71, 1966.

69. Schmidtke, J. R. and Dixon, F. J., The functional capacity of X-irradiation macrophages, *J. Immunol.,* 108, 1624, 1972.

70. Benacerraf, B., Influence of irradiation on resistance to infection, *Bacteriol. Rev.,* 24, 35, 1960.

71. Benecerraf, B., Kivy-Rosenberg, E., Schestyen, M. M., and Zweibach, B. W., The effect of high doses of X-irradiation on the phagocytic, proliferative and metabolic properties of the reticuloendothelial system, *J. Exp. Med.,* 110, 49, 1959.

72. Cosenza, H., Leserman, L. D., and Rowley, D. A., The third cell type required for the immune response of spleen cells *in vitro, J. Immunol.,* 107, 414, 1971.

73. Schechter, G. P. and McFarland, W. J., Interaction of lymphocytes and a radioresistant cell in PPD-stimulated human leukocyte cultures, *J. Immunol.,* 105, 661, 1970.

74. Gallily R. and Feldman, M., The role of macrophages in the induction of antibody in X-irradiated animals, *Immunology,* 12, 197, 1967.

75. Geiger, B. and Gallily, R., Effect of X-irradiation on various functions of murine macrophages, *Clin. Exp. Immunol.,* 16, 643, 1974.

76. Mitchison, N. A., The immunogenic capacity of antigen taken up by peritoneal exudate cells, *Immunology,* 16, 1, 1969.

77. Prinbow, J. F. and Silverman, M. S., Studies on the radiosensitive phase of the primary antibody response in rabbits, *J. Immunol.,* 98, 225, 1967.

78. Weiss, A. and Fitch, F., Suppression of the plaque-forming cell response by macrophages present in the normal rat spleen, *J. Immunol.,* 120, 357, 1978.

79. Oehler, J. R., Herberman, R. B., Campbell, D. A., Jr., and Djeu, J. Y., Inhibition of rat mixed lymphocyte cultures by suppressor macrophages, *Cell. Immunol.,* 29, 238, 1977.

80. Claman, H. N., Chaperson, E. A., and Triplett, R. F., Immunocompetence of transferred thymus-marrow cell combinations, *J. Immunol.,* 97, 828, 1969.

81. Kettman, J. and Dutton, R. W., Radioresistance of the enhancing effect of cells from carrier-immunized mice in an *in vitro* primary immune response, *Proc. Natl. Acad. Sci.,* 68, 699, 1971.

82. Hirst, J. A. and Dutton, R. W., Cell components in the immune response. III. Neonatal thymectomy restoration in culture, *Cell. Immunol.,* 1, 190, 1970.

83. Dutton, R. W., Campbell, P., Chan, E., Hirst, J., Hoffman, H., Kettman, J., Lesley, L., McCarthy, M., Mishell, R. I., Raidt, D. J., and Vann, D., Cell cooperation during immunological responses of isolated lymphoid cells, in *Cellular Interactions in the Immune Response,* Cohen, S., Cudkowicz, G., and McCluskey, R. T., Eds, Karger, Basel, 1970, 83.

84. Haskill, J. S., Byrt, P., and Marbrook, J., *In vitro* and *in vivo* studies of the immune response to sheep erythrocytes using partially purified cell preparations, *J. Exp. Med.,* 131, 57, 1970.

85. Osoba, D., Some physical and radiobiological properties of immunobiologically reactive mouse spleen cells, *J. Exp. Med.,* 132, 368, 1970.

86. Katz, D. H., Paul, W. E., Goidl, E. A., and Benacerraf, B., Radioresistance of cooperative function of carrier-specific lymphocytes in anti-hapten antibody responses, *Science,* 170, 462, 1970.

87. Shearer, G. M. and Cudkowicz, G., Distinct events in the immune responses elicited by transferred marrow and thymus cells. I. Antigen requirements and proliferation of thymic-reactive cells, *J. Exp. Med.,* 130, 1243, 1969.

88. Anderson, R. E., Sprent, J., and Miller, J. F. A. P., Cell to cell interaction in the immune response. VIII. Radiosensitivity of thymus-derived lymphocytes, *J. Exp. Med.,* 135, 711, 1972.

89. Hamaoka, T., Katz, D. H., and Benacerraf, B., Radioresistance of carrier-specific helper thymus-derived lymphocytes in mice, *Proc. Natl. Acad. Sci.,* 69, 3453, 1972.

90. Anderson, R. E., Sprent, J., and Miller, J. F. A. P., Radiosensitivity of T and B lymphocytes. I. Effect of irradiation on cell migration, *Eur. J. Immunol.,* 4, 199, 1974.

91. Lawrence, D. A., Eastman, A., and Weigle, W. O., Murine T-cell preparations radiosensitivity of helper activity, *Cell. Immunol.,* 36, 97, 1978.

92. Gershon, R. K. and Kondo, K., Cell interactions in the induction of tolerance: the role of thymic lymphocytes, *Immunology*, 18, 723, 1970.
93. Gershon, R. K. and Kondo, K., Infectious immunological tolerance, *Immunology*, 21, 903, 1971.
94. Kind, L. S. and Macedo-Sobrinho, B., Reaginic antibody formation in mice injected with rabbit anti-mouse thymocyte serum, *Int. Arch. Allergy Appl. Immunol.*, 45, 780, 1973.
95. Fox, D., Chiorazzi, N., and Katz, D. H., Hapten specific IgE antibody responses in mice. V. Differential resistance of IgE and IgG B lymphocytes to X-irradiation, *J. Immunol.*, 117, 1622, 1976.
96. Chiorazzi, N., Fox, O., and Katz, D. H., Hapten-specific IgE antibody responses in mice. VI. Selective enhancement of IgE antibody production by low doses of X-irradiation and by cyclophosphamide, *J. Immunol.*, 117, 1629, 1976.
97. Okumura, K. and Tada, T., Regulation of homocytotropic antibody formation in the rat. VI. Inhibitory effect of thymocytes on the homocytotropic antibody response, *J. Immunol.*, 107, 1682, 1971.
98. Rotter, V. and Trainin, N., Thymic cell population exerting a regulatory function in the immune response of mice to polyvinylpyrrolidone, *Cell. Immunol.*, 13, 76, 1974.
99. Eardley, D. D. and Gershon, R. R., Induction of specific suppressor T cells *in vitro*, *J. Immunol.*, 117, 313, 1976.
100. Benacerraf, B., Kapp, J. A., Debré, P., Pierce, C. W., and De la Croix, F., The stimulation of specific suppressor T cells in genetic non-responder mice by linear random copolymers of L-amino acids, *Transplant. Rev.*, 26, 21, 1975.
101. Dutton, R. W., Inhibitory and stimulatory effects of concanavalin-A on the response of mouse spleen cell suspensions to antigen, *J. Exp. Med.*, 136, 1445, 1972.
102. Dutton, R. W., Suppressor T cells, *Transplant. Rev.*, 26, 39, 1975.
103. Rich, R. R. and Rich, S. S., Biological expressions of lymphocyte activation. IV. Concanavalin-A-activated suppressor cells in mouse mixed lymphocyte reactions, *J. Immunol.*, 114, 1112, 1975.
104. Gershon, R. K., Liebhaber, S., and Ryu, S., T-cell regulation of T-cell responses to antigen, *Immunology*, 26, 909, 1974.
105. Schipior, P. and Marguire, H. C., Resistance of the allergic contact dermatitis sensitization reaction to whole body X-ray in the guinea pig, *Int. Arch. Allergy Appl. Immunol.*, 29, 447, 1966.
106. Uhr, J. W. and Scharff, M., Delayed hypersensitivity. V. The effect of X-irradiation on the development of delayed hypersensitivity and antibody formation, *J. Exp. Med.*, 112, 65, 1960.
107. Asherson, G. L. and Loewi, G., The effect of irradiation on the passive transfer of delayed hypersensitivity, *Immunology*, 13, 509, 1967.
108. Feldmann, J. D., The role of proliferation in delayed hypersensitivity, *J. Immunol.*, 101, 563, 1968.
109. Kettman, J. and Mathews, M. C., Radioresistance of cells for delayed hypersensitivity reactions in the mouse, *J. Immunol.*, 115, 606, 1975.
110. DeLuca, D., Miller, A., and Sercarz, E., Antigen binding to lymphoid cells from unimmunized mice. IV. Shedding and reappearance of multiple antigen binding Ig receptors of T- and B-lymphocytes, *Cell. Immunol.*, 18, 286, 1975.
111. Cantor, H. and Jandinski, K. F., The relationship of cell division to the generation of cytotoxic activity in mixed lymphocyte culture, *J. Exp. Med.*, 140, 1712, 1974.
112. Peavy, D. L. and Pierce, C. W., Cell-mediated immune responses *in vitro*. III. Elimination of specific cytotoxic lymphocyte responses by ³H-thymidine suicide, *J. Immunol.*, 115, 1521, 1975.
113. Sprent, J., Anderson, R. E., and Miller, J. F. A. P., Radiosensitivity of T and B lymphocytes. II. Effect of radiation on response of T cells to alloantigen, *Eur. J. Immunol.*, 4, 204, 1974.
114. Biggar, W. D., Menurssen, H. J., and Good, R. A., Effect on *in vitro* irradiation of cells in graft-versus-host reactions, *Proc. Soc. Exp. Biol. Med.*, 137, 1274, 1971.
115. Blackett, N. M., Effect of radiation on the parent to F₇ hybrid graft-versus-host reaction, *Int. J. Radiat. Biol.*, 3, 323, 1965.
116. Lotzová, E. and Savary, C. A., Possible involvement of natural killer cells in bone marrow graft rejection, *Biomedicine*, 27, 341, 1977.
117. Hochman, P. S., Cudkowicz, G., and Dausset, J., Decline of natural killer cells activity in sublethally irradiated mice, *J. Natl. Cancer Inst.*, 61, 265, 1978.
118. Herberman, R. B., Djeu, J. Y., Kay, H. D., Ortaldo, J. R., Riccardi, C., Bonnard, G. D., Holden, H. T., Fagnani, R., Santoni, A., and Puccetti, P., Natural killer cells: characteristics and regulation of activity, *Immunol. Rev.*, 44, 43, 1979.
119. Miller, J. J., III and Cole, L. J., The radiation resistance of long-lived lymphocytes and plasma cells in mouse and rat lymph nodes, *J. Immunol.*, 98, 982, 1969.
120. Vaun, D. C. and Makinodan, T., *In vitro* antibody synthesis by diffusion chamber cultures of spleen cells. I. Methods and effect of 10,000R on antibody synthesis, *J. Immunol.*, 102, 442, 1969.
121. Sado, T., Functional and ultrastructural studies on antibody-producing cells exposed to 10,000R in millipore diffusion chambers, *Int. J. Radiat. Biol.*, 15, 1, 1969.
122. Dempster, W. J., Lennox, B., and Boag, J. W., Prolongation of survival of skin homotransplants in rabbit by irradiation of host, *Br. J. Exp. Pathol.*, 31, 670, 1950.

123. Kelly, W. D., McKneally, M. F., Oliveras, F., Martinez, O., and Good, R. A., Cell-free antigenic material employed to produce tolerance to skin grafts tissue sources, preservation, dose requirements and the effects of combined use with azathioprine and sublethal irradiation, *Ann. N.Y. Acad. Sci.,* 129, 210, 1966.

124. Micklem, H. S. and Brown, J. A. H., Rejection of skin grafts and production of specific iso-hae-magglutinins by normal and X-irradiated mice, *Immunology,* 4, 318, 1961.

125. Tyan, M. L. and Cole, L., Differential radiosensitivity of first and second-set responses to allogeneic and xenogeneic skin grafts in sublethally irradiated mice, *Transplantation,* 1, 546, 1963.

126. Lotzová, E., Involvement of MHC-linked hemopoietic histocompatibility genes in allogeneic bone marrow transplantation in mice, *Tissue Antigens,* 9, 148, 1977.

127. Lotzová, E., Resistance to parental, allogeneic and xenogeneic hemopoietic grafts in irradiated mice, *Exp. Hematol.,* 5, 215, 1977.

128. Lotzová, E., Dicke, K. A., Trentin, J. J., and Gallagher, M. T., Genetic control of bone marrow transplantation classification of mouse strains according to their responsiveness to bone marrow allografts and xenografts, *Transplant. Proc.,* 9, 289, 1977.

129. Rauchwerger, J. M., Gallagher, M. T., Monie, H. J., Lotzova, E., and Trentin, J. J., Abrogation of genetic resistance to murine bone marrow transplantation by high radiation exposures, *Exp. Hematol.,* 2 (Abstr.), 294, 1977.

130. Lotzová, E., Gallagher, M. T., and Trentin, J. J., Macrophages involvement in genetic resistance to bone marrow transplantation, *Transplant. Proc.,* 8, 477, 1976.

131. Lotzová, E. and Cudkowicz, G., Hybrid resistance to parental bone marrow grafts. Association with genetic markers of linkage group IX, *Transplantation,* 13, 256, 1972.

132. Lotzová, E. and Savary, C. A., Possible involvement of natural killer cells in bone marrow graft rejection, *Biomedicine,* 27, 341, 1977.

133. Lotzová, E., unpublished observations, 1979.

134. Savary, C. A. and Lotzova, E., unpublished data, 1979.

Chapter 2

HOST-TUMOR INTERACTIONS AND METHODS OF EVALUATING IMMUNOCOMPETENCE IN HUMANS

Kenneth J. McCormick*

TABLE OF CONTENTS

*   Present address: Department of Otolaryngology and
                      Maxillofacial Surgery
                      The University of Iowa Hospitals and Clinics
                      Iowa City, Iowa

I. INTRODUCTION

Immunological studies of tumor-bearing hosts have been intensively carried out in recent years. The considerable body of work in human systems evolved directly from basic investigations of experimental animal models. The implications of such studies have great potential in therapeutic manipulation, and, therefore, the immediate application of this information to treatment in man is also increasing. However, the complex interactions between cancer cells and the *human* host must be clearly understood before the utilization of immunological concepts is securely established in multidisciplinary approaches to cancer therapy.

The following will be attempted in this chapter: (1) to concisely review the relationships and interactions between the immune system and cancer, and (2) to present the various methods now available to estimate immunocompetence in man. The future should present ample opportunities to combine standard therapeutic approaches with the immunological principles now being formulated in the area of *human* tumor immunology.

II. EVIDENCE FOR IMMUNOLOGICAL INTERACTIONS BETWEEN HOST AND TUMOR

The following discussion is designed to present the links which have been observed between the immune system and the oncogenic process in man. However, one must realize that these links are presumptive evidence for an immune involvement in the process and cannot be separated from physiologic or other co-varying host factors. The wealth of information available was stimulated by the hypothesis of immunological surveillance which was initiated by Ehrlich[1] and developed through the ideas of Thomas[2] and Burnet.[3]

I will proceed from a summary of the individual clinical observations to a statement of the immune surveillance theory. This approach may tend to "select" results which support such a theory without appropriate discussion of negative evidence. However, the justification for this approach lies in a concise presentation of the material and, hopefully, in the clarity thus obtained.

A. Correlates of the Host Immune System and Cancer
1. Age
The age distribution in incidence of malignant neoplasms in man demonstrates a small increase in the very young, followed by a decrease, until the incidence curve again rises in older age groups. This generalized distribution, which has many exceptions when viewed as incidence of specific types of tumors, suggests a cumulative effect which is dependent on duration of exposure, e.g., to environmental carcinogens.[4] It was recognized that this distribution might also be explained by perinatal immunological insufficiencies followed, in older age groups, by waning immunological competence.[3] Variations[5] in immune reactivity with age are, or can be, reflected in thymic atrophy; in decreases in delayed hypersensitivity to microbial antigens or to de novo sensitization with new antigens; in decreases in lymphocyte responses to plant mitogens; and in decreases in the circulating levels of naturally occurring isoantibodies. However, these changes do not occur in all individuals and the degree of correlation between functional loss in immunoreactivity and causality of malignant disease may be extremely small in the general population.

2. Genetic Immunodeficiency
Inherited immune deficiency diseases have been associated with increased incidence of cancer in many case reports. This group of genetic diseases may severely limit the life span of affected individuals and, consequently, decrease the likelihood of obtaining a true picture of cancer incidence in this population. However, diseases such as the Bruton-type (sex-linked) agammaglobulinemia or Wiskott-Aldrich syndrome (sex-linked thrombocytopenia, eczema, and recurrent infection) have been associated with increased frequencies of neoplasms. Lymphoid cancers predominate in patients with genetic immunodeficiency and, therefore, the genetically diseased tissue is the site of the malignant transformation. If cancer, in general, were related to a depressed immune system, one would expect malignancies to develop in all tissues depending on cell turnover, exposure to carcinogen, etc. The "pros and cons" of the relationship between primary immunodeficiency disease and cancer have been reviewed extensively.[6]

3. Immune Suppression
Immunosuppressive drugs are currently used in treating cancer patients, patients

with autoimmune or related diseases, and in patients who have received organ allografts. In the latter group, enhanced incidence (approximately 5%) of cancer was reported.[7] In contrast to patients with genetic immunodeficiency (see above), the predominant histologic type of tumor was epithelial in origin. Lymphomas, however, represented the majority of mesenchymal tumors found. After thorough review, Stutman[6] stated "...patients who are immunodepressed for organ transplantation have an increased risk for development of certain malignancies, especially atypical lymphomas, which does not seem to be the case for patients with other diseases who are submitted to chronic immunodepressive treatments." It is obvious that these patients receive, in addition to immunosuppression, chronic antigenic stimulation derived from the allografted organ.

4. Spontaneous Regression

Although rare, spontaneous regression of malignant neoplasms does occur.[8] Adenocarcinoma of the kidney, neuroblastoma, malignant melanoma, and choriocarcinoma are known to regress, in that order of frequency. The mechanisms of such regressions are unclear, but immunological, endocrine, and psychological factors, as well as fever, have been suggested to play a role.[9]

A peripheral infiltrate of reactive mononuclear cells may be observed around many types of tumors. Patients with these infiltrates at the tumor site appear to have a better prognosis than those without such a reaction, although this is limited to a few types of tumors, e.g., carcinomas of the breast and stomach, Hodgkin's disease, and neuroblastoma.[10] During regression, the tumor itself becomes infiltrated wtih macrophages and lymphocytes. Again, these phenomena suggest a correlation with an immune function.

5. Trophoblastic Carcinoma

Choriocarcinoma is the equivalent of a semiallogeneic tissue graft which is derived from trophoblastic tissue and carries genes of both parents. The tumors are curable by chemotherapy, even, in some instances, when using a less than intense course of treatment.[11] In addition, it was suggested that survival following chemotherapy was enhanced for women who had greater genetic incompatibility with their husbands.[12] This has led to the assumption that the mother's ability to recognize paternal antigens on the cancer cells aids in the overall efficiency of chemotherapy. Although this hypothesis is unproven, Mathé et al.[13] demonstrated the presence of antibodies in these women which reacted against paternal tissue antigens.

6. Response to Treatment

a. Nonimmunological Therapy

Objective regressions of malignant neoplasms subsequent to treatment which was noncurative have been reported following surgery[9] and less than intense chemotherapy for Burkitt's lymphoma[14] and choriocarcinoma.[11] In addition, hyperthermic perfusion of an extremity for malignant melanoma, a completely local treatment, can result in regression of distant skin metastases.[15] Such reports suggest that a host factor(s) in addition to the primary therapy may be operating in these patients. Although it has not been proven that the factor(s) is immunological, each of these tumors has been shown to elicit either antibodies or cell-mediated immune responses in the host.

b. Immunotherapy

The various approaches used in this new modality of treatment have been clearly stated by Hersh et al.[16] These may include attempts: (1) to nonspecifically stimulate the host's general immune mechanism (e.g., *Bacille Calmette-Guerin (BCG)* or *Coryne bacterium parvum),* (2) to stimulate *specific* immunity to a particular type of tumor (e.g., nonviable tumor cells or tumor extracts), (3) to restore depressed immunocompetence (e.g., levamisole, thymosin), (4) to utilize adoptive or passive transfer of lymphoid cells or serum which are specifically reactive to the tumor, or (5) to induce local or regional nonspecific reactivity against the cancer cell by local injection of antigenic materials (e.g., *BCG, C. parvum,* purified protein derivative of *Mycobacterium tuberculosis).*

Certain of these approaches have borne fruit and are exemplified in the pioneering work of Edmund Klein on local immunotherapy of skin cancers[17] and of Georges Mathé on systemic immunotherapy of acute lymphocytic leukemia.[18] The ability of certain forms of immunotherapy to effect regressions illustrates an intimate relationship between the host's immune system and cancer. The current effectiveness of this type of therapy can be assessed in several recent publications.[19,20]

B. Immunological Surveillance

Thomas[2] proposed that the phenomenon of homograft rejection, a cell-mediated immune function, evolved as a primary natural defense against neoplasia. His proposal resembled an earlier suggestion of Ehrlich[1] that a natural immune mechanism to control cancer existed and was cellular in origin. Burnet expanded these concepts into a theory of immune surveillance[3,21,22] which dealt with a host's ability *to prevent* the outgrowth of malignant cells, not with its ability to induce regression of an established tumor. Surveillance presupposes, of course, that a majority of tumors are antigenic and that tumor antigens can invoke a host immune response. Burnet[3] proposed that this response is a thymus-dependent cell-mediated reaction and that tumor regression resembled homograft rejection. His concepts were based on the facts that oncogenic agents can depress immune responses, that immunodeficient hosts may have an increased incidence of tumors, and that the highest incidence of tumors in man occurs at times when the immune system is depressed (early in life and in old age).

Although clinical observations may support this hypothesis (see above Section A, 1-3), critical examination of all the data suggested that immunosurveillance, as proposed, should be revised.[6,23] In fact, Prehn demonstrated that a weak, but specific, immunological response could lead to stimulation of tumor growth in a murine system.[24] Since many spontaneously occurring murine tumors have little or no antigenicity,[25] a surveillance mechanism which depends on the sensitization of the thymus-dependent lymphocyte system may be ineffective in preventing proliferation of a clone of tumor cells. Immunosurveillance does occur, however, in certain animal systems and, probably, in Burkitt's lymphoma in man.[26] These models involve viral-induced tumors with "strong" tumor antigenicity. The mass of information concerning destruction of tumor cells by specifically or nonspecifically cytotoxic macrophages,[27] by antibody-dependent cell-mediated cytotoxic mechanisms,[28] and by the recently described class of natural killer lymphocytes,[29,30] increases the mechanisms which must be considered in any revised surveillance theory. In the future, an improved theory of immunosurveillance will certainly evolve.

C. Immune Response of the Host
1. Humoral Antibodies
a. Specific (Tumor-Associated)

Antibodies to a variety of tumors have been found in sera of patients bearing the corresponding neoplasm.[31] The antibodies are synthesized by the more differentiated form of B lymphocytes, the plasma cells. Antibody-mediated reactions are detected by various serologic techniques; however, the essential question is whether the antigen to which the antibody reacts is actually tumor-associated. Specificity is usually determined by showing that sera from normal individuals react less frequently and, perhaps, at lower titer than sera obtained from patients. Absorption of sera with antigen or testing of the sera with other types of tumor and normal cells aid in demonstrating the specificity of the reactions observed.

The necrotic area found in the central portion of growing tumors may serve as a reservoir of intracellular antigenic components which, on dissemination, can stimulate the host's immune response. In animal systems, the amount of antibody formed against intracellular tumor antigen may parallel the size of the tumor.[32] Similarly, we have found that the titer of antibodies to intracellular antigen(s) of malignant melanoma cells (Figure 1) increased with the stage of disease which probably reflects the total tumor burden experienced by the patient (Table 1). Approximately 50% of normal individuals had low titers (1:6) of these antibodies and patients with localized melanoma (Stage I) were similar to normal individuals in titer and percent of positive reactions. As the disease progressed, both the titer and the percent of positive sera increased and the geometric mean titer at Stage IV was 8 times higher than that at Stage I disease. Although occasional antinuclear antibodies were found, none of the sera tested, from either normal individuals or patients, reacted with melanocytes cultured from fetal uveal tissue. These results suggest that the cytoplasmic antigen(s) is not a fetal antigen and that dissemination of tumor enhances the formation of these antibodies.

When one considers the localization of tumor antigen within the cell, it becomes obvious that only antigens which are presented to the host on the external cell membrane could be important in the defense against tumor. Antibodies to intracellular antigens, though reflecting tumor burden, cannot attack tumor cells because they cannot penetrate an intact cell membrane. The presence of antigen on the cell surface would permit both stimulation of the host and ready access of antigen to antibody for defense purposes. Immunoglobulins are bound within tumors[33] and serum antibodies to membrane antigens tend to disappear as a tumor enlarges.[34] The absorption of antibody by the tumor mass could explain both of these phenomena.

In one of the most thoroughly studied systems, it was found that the *cytoplasmic* antigen of human melanoma is cross-reactive from tumor to tumor.[35,36] Of 10 cell lines derived from melanomas, we found each to react by indirect immunofluorescence with antibody-containing patients' sera.[37] However, exhaustive serological studies of *membrane* antigens in melanoma indicated that: (1) some tumor cells bear membrane antigens which cross-react serologically with other melanomas, (2) some tumor cells bear membrane antigens which react only with autologous sera, and (3) some tumor cells bear membrane antigens which cross-react serologically with antigens found on normal allogeneic or xenogeneic cells.[38]

In vitro, specific antibodies can damage viable tumor cells in the presence of complement or can act in conjunction with a class of lymphocytes which destroy tumor cells if the latter are coated with antibodies. Nevertheless, the role of humoral antibodies in tumor rejection in vivo is unclear.

b. Nonspecific

Nontumor-associated antibodies may also increase in some cancer patients. Antinuclear antibodies are found in a high percentage of patients with carcinoma of the postnasal space[39] and autoantibodies also become evident in other types of cancer.[40] We have reported an increase in antibodies to Epstein-Barr virus (EBV) in sera from cancer patients who produced antinuclear antibodies (Table 2).[41] Since the cancer sera were from diseases unrelated to EBV infection, the increase in antibody probably resulted from a nonspecific immunological disorder characterized both by formation of antinuclear antibodies and stimulation of anti-EBV titers. The specificities of antibodies found in patients' sera may thus reflect processes other than antitumor reactions.

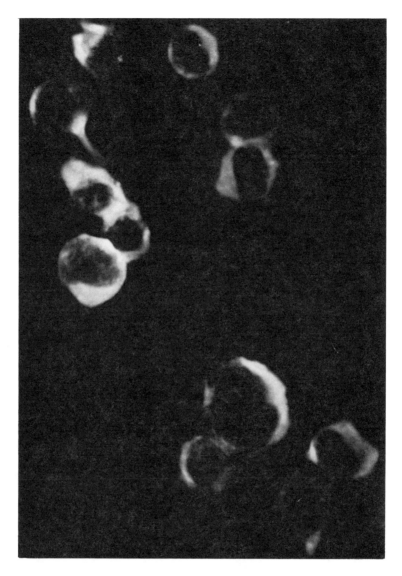

FIGURE 1. Indirect immunofluorescence micrograph demonstrating a reaction between antibodies in a melanoma patient's serum and an antigen(s) in the cytoplasm of a melanoma cell line, SW 691.

2. Cell-Mediated Reactions

a. T Lymphocytes

The T lymphocyte matures under the influence of the thymus and is responsibile for cell-mediated immune reactions, e.g., skin test hypersensitivity of the delayed type, and homograft rejection. As in other immune phenomena, T cells must be presensitized to an antigen in order to react against it. Ample evidence exists which demonstrates the reactivity of patients' lymphocytes against autologous or allogeneic tumors utilizing skin test procedures or in vitro cytotoxicity tests.[42] The tumor-specific nature of such reactions is, however, problematic. An example of tumor-directed preferential cytotoxicity to autologous melanoma cells in vitro is shown in Table 3. In this case, lymphocytes from the patient were capable of killing his own tumor cells, but not his normal fibroblastic cells. In another example (Table 4), the autologous cytotoxicity

TABLE 1
GEOMETRIC MEAN TITERS (GMT) OF ANTIBODIES IN HUMAN SERA TO CYTOPLASMIC ANTIGEN IN THE MELANOMA CELL LINE, SW 691,[a] BY INDIRECT IMMUNOFLUORESCENCE[166]

Sera	Stage[b]	SW 691			Fetal Melanocytes		
		No. tested	% Positive[c]	GMT	No. tested	% Positive[d]	GMT
Mela-	I	66	44	1:4[e]	55	0	—
noma	III A	9	78	1:12	6	0	—
	III B	27	81	1:22	27	0	—
	III AB	12	83	1:27	8	0	—
	III, total	48	81	1:21	41	0	—
	IV	22	86	1:32	20	0	—
Normal	—	54	50	1:6[f]	38	0	—

[a]   Obtained from A. Leibovitz, Scott-White Clinic, Temple, Texas.
[b]   Staging,[15] I local; III A, intransit metastases; III B, metastasis to regional nodes; III AB, both intransit and nodal (regional) metastases; IV, extraregional metastasis.
[c]   Titer positive sera, ≥ 1:8.
[d]   Negative at a dilution of 1:2.
[e]   Significantly lower than GMT of Stages III B, III AB, III total, and IV, $P < 0.001$.
[f]   Significantly lower than GMT of Stages III B, III AB, III total, and IV, $P < 0.01$.

TABLE 2
ANTIBODIES TO EPSTEIN-BARR VIRUS (EBV) IN NORMAL HUMAN SERA AND IN SERA FROM CANCER PATIENTS AS DETECTED BY INDIRECT IMMUNOFLUORESCENCE[41]

Group	No. tested	Antinuclear antibodies present	% Positive[a]	Anti-EBV titer[b]
Normal	70	—	51	1:52
Cancer	21	—	100	1:48
	28	+	89	1:143[c]

[a]   Positive sera had titers ≥ 1:10.
[b]   Geometric mean titer of positive sera.
[c]   Significantly elevated ($P < 0.01$) when compared to other groups.

demonstrated is nonspecific, i.e., the effector lymphocytes killed both tumor and normal cells in a similar fashion. In our experience,[43] 85% of melanoma patients (9/11) with advanced disease (Stages III and IV) produced lymphocytes which were cytotoxic to their own tumor; however, parallel assessment on *both* autologous tumor and autologous normal skin cells showed that only about one half of the reactions were preferentially cytotoxic to tumor cells. Since lymphocytes from normal individuals may also be cytotoxic in in vitro assays, the significance of in vitro tests must still be assessed. However, the rejection of inadvertently transplanted tumor cells by organ allograft recipients who no longer received immunosuppressive therapy demonstrated that the homograft reaction in man is capable of inducing regression of a growing cancer.[44]

b. *Lymphocytes Bearing Fc Receptors*

K cells — The antibody-dependent cell-mediated cytotoxic (ADCC) reaction is me-

TABLE 3
PREFERENTIAL CYTOTOXICITY OF MONONUCLEAR CELLS FROM PATIENT GI TO AUTOLOGOUS MELANOMA AND SKIN CELLS[a]

Mononuclear cell/target cell	Melanoma cells[b]		Skin fibroblasts[c]	
	$-x \pm s_{-x}$	% Reduction[e]	$-x \pm s_{-x}$	% Reduction[e]
50:1	20.3 ± 1.9^{f}	57	98.5 ± 12.8	2
25:1	29.0 ± 3.6^{f}	39	95.5 ± 12.4	5
12:1	39.3 ± 3.3^{g}	17	94.5 ± 4.3	6
—	47.5 ± 1.7	—	100.9 ± 6.7	—

[a] The microcytotoxicity test was used.[160]
[b] Passage 12.
[c] Passage 7.
[d] Mean number of cells remaining after incubation with effector cells (± standard error).
[e] % reduction = (number of cells in control-number of cells in test) 100/(number of cells in control).
[f] $P < 0.001$.
[g] $P < 0.05$.

TABLE 4
NONSPECIFIC CYTOTOXICITY OF MONONUCLEAR CELLS FROM PATIENT BU TO AUTOLOGOUS MELANOMA AND SKIN CELLS[a]

Mononuclear cells/target cell	Melanoma cells[b]		Skin fibroblasts[c]	
	$-x \pm s_{-x}$	% Reduction	$-x \pm s_{-x}$	% Reduction
400:1	56.1 ± 7.2^{d}	55	62.8 ± 8.7^{d}	49
200:1	88.8 ± 4.9^{d}	28	86.6 ± 7.9^{d}	29
100:1	99.1 ± 8.3^{e}	20	101.9 ± 10.5^{f}	17
—	123.9 ± 4.0	—	122.8 ± 3.7	—

[a] See footnotes, Table 3.
[b] Passage 23.
[c] Passage 2.
[d] $P < 0.001$.
[e] $P < 0.01$.
[f] $P < 0.05$.

diated by a subpopulation of lymphocytes which can kill target tumor cells coated with antibodies.[28] The lymphocytes, designated K cells, are not specifically sensitized to tumor antigen; the specificity of the cytotoxic reaction depends on humoral antibodies which can recognize and coat the antigen-bearing tumor cell target. K lymphocytes then become associated with the antibody-target cell complex by virtue of lymphocyte membrane receptors for the Fc portion of the immunoglobulin molecule. This type of activity has now been demonstrated in bladder cancer,[45] melanoma,[46] and leukemia.[47] Recently, the ADCC reaction was shown to correlate with prognosis in nasopharyngeal carcinoma, i.e., patients with a high antibody titer in the ADCC test had a longer survival than did those with low antibody titer.[48]

Natural killer (NK) cells — These lymphocytes are responsible for non-T cell-mediated spontaneous cytotoxicity found in normal individuals or patients with cancer.[29,30] In mice, NK cells are neither mature T nor B cells when assayed for surface markers,[49] but, in the peripheral blood of man, they bear Fc receptors.[50] The degree of cytoxicity exhibited by this population of lymphocytes varies from individual to individual and from target cell to target cell.[51] At present, it is unclear if the K cell and the NK cell represent the same or different lymphocyte populations. It has been suggested that this type of cell may be involved in the immune surveillance system.[29]

c. Macrophages

The macrophage plays an important role in the processing of antigen during the immune response. In animal systems, these cells were shown to be differentially cyto-toxic or cytostatic to tumor, but not to normal, cells.[52] In addition, macrophages may become ''armed'' and specifically cytotoxic to a particular antigenic tumor.[53] The arming factor, which is responsible for the specificity of the reaction, is produced by antigen-sensitized lymphocytes. Macrophages, as represented by peripheral blood monocytes, may also take part in ADCC-type reactions.[54] The relationships between macrophages and cancer were recently reviewed;[55] however, the importance of these cells in human neoplasia is unclear. Nevertheless, large numbers of these cells are attracted to sites of tumor destruction following injection of BCG into localized melanomas of the skin.[56]

d. Granulocytes

Neutrophilic polymorphonuclear leukocytes (PMN) also demonstrate cytotoxic effects in appropriate in vitro situations. Burton et al.[57] have shown that the PMN of mice were cytotoxic to various types of murine lymphoid tumors. The importance of this cell type in antitumor reactions in man is not known.

3. Summary

Although the host responds to its cancer by production of antibodies and sensitized lymphocytes, the relative effectiveness of these defense systems against a *proliferating* tumor is not immediately apparent. For example, at the time that a tumor is detected clinically, an effective immune defense is already breached. In addition, the ability to demonstrate a myriad of cytotoxic reactions in vitro does not mean that the mechanism is operative and/or effective in vivo. Immunological manipulation by use of tumor cell vaccines and nonspecific immune stimulants may enhance the course of disease at the expense of the host.[58] However, the relatively large inoculum needed to obtain growth on reimplantation of autologous cancer cells in humans indicates that man can resist growth of his own tumor.[59]

The host defense mechanism may be thought of as a series of immunological barriers operating at different levels of complexity. Those mechanisms which require no apparent previous exposure to antigen, e.g., cytotoxic reactions produced by macrophages, NK cells, or granulocytes, represent a first barrier to the outgrowth of a transformed cell. More specific barriers are erected by those reactions which require sensitization to tumor antigen, and are mediated by antibodies, sensitized T lymphocytes, or specifically armed macrophages. The basic availability of most of these systems has now been demonstrated in man; their importance in human neoplasia, however, must still be determined.

D. If There is an Immune Defense, How Do Tumors Break Through?

Klein has discussed the escape of tumors from surveillance.[60] He has listed five phenomena which could account for the appearance of clinically detectable tumors. These are (1) inadequate recognition, (2) immunoresistance, (3) immune deficiency of the host, (4) sneaking through, and (5) malfunctioning of antitumor effector mechanisms. Although each phenomenon has been demonstrated in animal models, their operation in man is, for the most part, undocumented.

The possibility that the immune system may not recognize a clone of newly transformed cells is not unlikely. The variations in antigenicity of chemically induced murine tumors, as well as the lack of antigenicity of spontaneous[61] and some carcinogen-induced[25,62] murine tumors, suggest that weak or nonexistent antigenicity might explain the de novo development of tumor. Although most human tumors tested are susceptible to lymphocytotoxicity in vitro, the inability to correlate the in vitro reaction with rejection mechanisms in vivo suggests that the antigens detected in these tests are tumor-associated, but not responsible for rejection.

The ability of tumors to develop immunoresistance has been described in several species. It is not difficult to assume that this could happen in man. If evolving cancers are constantly being subjected, by an immunocompetent host, to selection of progressively less antigenic tumor cell populations, the clinically detectable tumor might become less susceptible to an immune attack.

Immunodeficiency has been discussed above. Cessation of immunosuppression in organ transplant patients can result in the regression of metastasizing tumor allografts that were unwittingly transplanted with the normal organ.[44] This clinical example illustrates the point that correction of an immune deficiency, in this case iatrogenic, may produce rejection of tumor grafts.

Sneaking through[63] is a term used to describe the situation in murine tumors wherein small numbers of antigenic tumor cells grow in a host; moderate numbers of these cells do not; large numbers of cells again can form a tumor. It would appear that when small numbers of cells are inoculated, the rate of growth of the tumor outruns the ability of the host's immune system to recognize the small cell inoculum and destroy it. However, if moderate cell numbers are used, the host mounts a more rapid immune response and no tumor develops. With large doses of tumor cells, the immune system is overcome. In more recent studies, Prehn has demonstrated that a weak immune response may specifically stimulate tumor growth, although a strong response inhibits the tumor.[24] The exact mechanism of sneaking through is unknown, yet, certainly, an analogous situation might be present in man.

Malfunctioning of the antitumor effector mechanism could result from abnormalities of the effector cells or antibodies or from faulty interactions between the various components of the effector mechanism. Sera from patients with various types of tumors have been shown to block the cytotoxic activity of patients' lymphocytes.[64,65] Blocking factors can be either circulating antigen or antigen-antibody complexes.[66] These tumor-associated antigens are probably shed from the tumor cell surface into the general circulation and produce a *specific* inhibition of the host's immune defense. Antigen-antibody complexes are found in the sera of many tumor patients,[67] but their function is often not definable.

E. Effect of Tumor Growth on the Host

1. Depressed Immunological Reactivity

A decline in immune function has been observed in patients with lymphoid or solid tumors.[68] Depressions were noted in both B and T cell functions including: humoral responses to sheep erythrocytes or tetanus toxoid; cell-mediated recall responses to common skin test antigens; de novo sensitization to skin-sensitizing chemicals; in vitro responses to polyclonal mitogens such as phytohemagglutinin; and in the speed with which skin allografts were rejected. These changes in reactivity reflected a generalized inability to deal with antigenic stimuli in a normal manner. In addition, monocytes from cancer patients may have a depressed chemotactic response and a defect in maturational activity.[69] Thorough immunological evaluations have shown that good immunocompetence is related to a better prognosis for the patient.[70]

Although decreased immune responses could be expected to fluctuate with the number of the host's functional T and B lymphocytes, circulating T and B cells are only rarely affected by nonlymphoid neoplastic disease. However, "active" T cells, a subset of T lymphocytes, are apparently related to immunocompetence and are decreased in cancer patients.[71]

a. Suppressor Cells

Immunological responses can be regulated by positive (helper activity) or negative (suppressor activity) interactions of subsets of T lymphocytes with other types of functional lymphocytes.[72] In addition to suppression by T cells, suppressive activity also may be mediated by glass-adherent cells which resemble peripheral blood monocytes or macrophages.[73,74] Lymphocytes from patients with Hodgkin's disease[75] or other cancers[74] have been shown to inhibit T cell responses in vitro. Cell-mediated suppression of immunoglobulin synthesis in myeloma patients[76] has also been reported. Although these regulatory effects are nontumor directed, specific suppression of antitumor responses can certainly be expected. Yu et al.[77] have described the simultaneous presence of tumor-specific cytotoxic and inhibitory (regulatory) lymphocytes in patients with osteogenic sarcoma.

b. Humoral Immunosuppressive Factors

Naturally occurring immunosuppressive factors have been found in serum, amniotic fluid, and extracts of lymphoid tissues.[78] The factors may exert their suppressive effects selectively on T cells, on B cells, or on macrophages. Although demonstrating selectivity for the inhibited target cell, the suppressive action of the substances is not antigen-specific. The factors isolated from serum are predominantly α-globulins and their isolation and assay were recently catalogued.[78] Antigenic stimulation may induce production of α_2-globulins and these immunoregulatory proteins can be increased in patients with various types of cancer.[79] An immunosuppressive polypeptide has also been found in sera from cancer patients.[80]

The acute phase C-reactive protein (CRP) appears in high concentration in sera of individuals during acute febrile reactions or chronic illnesses characterized by tissue damage and inflammation. The protein is synthesized in the liver[81] and was recently shown to be a normal serum component[82] which increases in quantity under the stimulation of certain disease processes. CRP can modulate a number of immunologic T cell functions[82,83] and is known to be elevated in sera from patients with lymphoid[84] or nonlymphoid cancer.[85] Proteins such as CRP may, perhaps, act as immune modulators during the course of neoplastic disease.

The foregoing "normal" humoral immunosuppressive factors act as nonspecific inhibitors of various immune responses. Substances such as tissue polypeptide antigen, α-fetoprotein, and perhaps, carcinoembryonic antigen may also suppress T cell function.[68] However, in these cases, the inhibiting molecules are synthesized by the neoplastic tissues. Both α-fetoprotein and carcinoembryonic antigen are normal fetal antigens which can also be synthesized by tumor cells in an adult host (see below).

Specific inhibition of antitumor immune reactivity may occur through the action of circulating unbound specific tumor antigen or through the action of complexes of specific tumor antigen and its corresponding antibodies (see above). Immune complexes appear to decrease after tumor resection in patients who have a good prognosis.[86] Measurement of immune complexes during therapy may become important as an quantitative indicator of tumor burden.

F. Effect of Therapeutic Intervention on Tumor Immunity

1. Surgery

Fisher has discussed the developing concept of an oncological surgery based on biological, as well as anatomical, foundations.[87] Ultimately, this approach aims at decreasing the bulk of tumor in order to present the host with a quantity of tumor cells which can be destroyed by host factors, adjuvant chemotherapy, or both.

Surgical procedures have been shown to produce several alterations in the host immune mechanism. As noted above, spontaneous regression of metastatic tumors may follow surgery. Although blocking factors are often found in the serum of patients with a growing tumor, this activity may be difficult to detect in patients with a minimal tumor burden.[65] In this instance, "debulking" of tumor would quantitatively decrease the mass of tumor from which specific blocking activity could be released.

Transient postsurgical suppression of T cell response to mitogen has also been noted in cancer patients.[88] Depression in T cell-mediated antitumor reactivity recovers within 3 weeks after surgery.[89] The role of anesthesia or postsurgical steroid levels in transient immunosuppression is still unresolved.

2. Radiotherapy

This subject has been recently reviewed.[90,91] Following radiotherapy, there is a prolonged decrease in the number of circulating lymphocytes and a decrease in the absolute number of T lymphocytes.[91] Since the lymphocyte is the basic functional unit of the immune system, its depletion would be expected to adversely affect the host's defense mechanism. However, various factors influence the effect of radiotherapy on immune function. These factors[92] include: (1) dose, (2) previous immune status, (3) size and location of the treated area, (4) the repopulation of treated sites by progenitor stem cells, and (5) compensatory proliferation of the hematopoietic system.

Functional changes in T cell activity suggest that there is a depressed response to phytohemagglutinin which, however, has not been observed in all studies.[91] Skin tests to recall antigens, a T cell-mediated function, may be enhanced by therapy. Lymphocyte-mediated reactivities to tumor-associated antigens are also depressed following radiotherapy,[93,94] but may increase within 1 week after treatment.[93]

The number of circulating B lymphocytes was reported to be increased[95] or be depressed[96,97] by therapy. The response of lymphocytes to pokeweed mitogen (PWM), a stimulator of both B and T lymphocytes, was enhanced in the studies of Blomgren et al.[98] The quantities of serum immunoglobulins are relatively unaffected by local radiotherapy, but decrease following whole-body radiation.[99]

There appears to be no directly lethal effect on peripheral blood monocytes or neutrophilic polymorphonuclear leukocytes, although the latter may decrease as a result of damage to stem cell precursors in bone marrow. An eosinophilic response has been noted following radiotherapy[100] and may be related to an immune response. It was suggested that eosinophilia may be an indicator of favorable prognosis for the patient.[101]

3. Chemotherapy

In addition to the antineoplastic effectiveness of chemotherapeutic agents, one of the primary concerns of the cancer chemotherapist is the immunosuppressive characteristics of the drug.[102] Besides the acute problem of increased susceptibility to infectious agents,[103] the long-term effects of immunosuppression combined with the potential carcinogenic activity of some of these drugs may be hazardous.[104]

Depressions in leukocyte and lymphocyte numbers result from treatment with most of these agents. Depressed lymphocyte function in vitro, however, is less prolonged than that following irradiation.[105] Both B and T lymphocytes, as well as monocytes, can be affected.[106]

Immune parameters which must be evaluated in vivo to determine the suppressive activity of the drugs have been discussed recently.[107] These include effects on antibody responses to primary and secondary antigenic stimulation, as well as effects on de novo induction of delayed hypersensitivity, on established delayed hypersensitivity, and on nonimmunological (nonspecific) inflammatory responses. The suppressive action of these agents depends on the stage at which they interfere with the immune response. Interference[108] may occur at the level of: (1) antigen uptake or processing, (2) antigen recognition, (3) blastogenesis, (4) proliferation, (5) antibody production, or (6) effector reactions. Intensive, yet intermittent, administration of chemotherapeutic drugs does not inhibit de novo induction of delayed hypersensitivity and produces only transient suppression of established cell-mediated immunity.[108] Continuous therapy is more suppressive of de novo induction of cell-mediated hypersensitivity. Therefore, the schedule for administration of drug becomes as important to minimize depressions in immune function as is the type of drug employed. Although B cell function is affected by certain forms of chemotherapy e.g., cyclophosphamide, the importance of the B cell system to tumor immunity is unclear. Immunotherapy interspersed with chemotherapy may perhaps prolong remission and survival of patients treated with both types of agents.[108]

4. Immunotherapy

This treatment, either specific or nonspecific, is directed toward stimulating the host's immune defense. Since the immune system is the target for drug action, immune modulations would be expected to occur and vary with the drug chosen. Hersh et al.[110] have provided examples of the immunological monitoring which should accompany therapeutic trials and have presented some of the immunological modulations observed during treatment. To date, it has been difficult to obtain consistent results in such monitoring because of the many variations used in the therapy itself. However, the development of antibodies to organisms, e.g., *C. parvum,* used to stimulate the host's defenses,[111] and, more recently, the activation of monocytes in patients treated with intravenous bacteria or their products[112,113] have been found to be markers for those forms of immunotherapy.

Data from recent clinical immunotherapeutic trials have been published.[19,20] The proposals of Israel et al.[114] may well reflect the most important future course for immunotherapy. These authors suggest that assay of immune defects for each patient will lead to individualization of treatment for the particular immune deficit(s). This becomes an attractive approach and challenge for the future.

III. ASSESSMENT OF IMMUNOLOGICAL COMPETENCE

A. Introduction

When immunological competence is assessed in the cancer patient, one must differentiate between general immune functions and those immune functions which are directed toward tumor. The former are nonspecific with regard to cancer, yet they have an important place in determining the overall immunological status of the patient. The latter functions, the tumor-related, are often more difficult to test in the laboratory. They can, in some instances, however, be regarded as "tumor-specific" and are probably the most informative tests in a patient's evaluation.

Although adequate immunological competence can be a factor in prognosis,[70] this is not always the case. Nevertheless, monitoring of immunological parameters, both specific and nonspecific, are useful in assessing the effect of various therapies on the immune system. Evaluation of procedures for testing tumor-directed immune reactions in cancer patients was recently reviewed.[115,116] It should be stressed that these assays are useful for research purposes, but they have not yet become valuable clinical tools which aid the practicing physician. In this section, the basic tests available are described; detailed methodologies may be found in laboratory manuals of clinical immunology.[117]

B. Nonspecific Parameters
1. Humoral Assays in Vitro
a. Immunoglobulins

The immunoglobulins (Ig) are classified into five groups according to the antigenic structure of the heavy chain of the Ig molecule.[118] The classifications are IgG, IgA, IgM, IgD, and IgE. Ig of the first three classes, G, A, and M, are the predominant immunoproteins found in human serum and are present at levels of approximately 1000, 200, and 120 mg/dl, respectively. Elevations in both IgG and IgA have been observed in certain types of nonlymphoid-cancers,[119] but others have reported a decline in concentrations of Ig.[120]

Ig are quantitated by single radial immunodiffusion.[121] In this test, human serum is placed in a well cut into an agar medium which contains antibodies to the specific Ig being assayed. A ring of precipitate of antigen and antibody forms around the well as a result of diffusion. The diameter of the ring is related to the concentration of Ig and the time of diffusion. The amount of Ig present can be determined by comparison with standard preparations assayed at the same time.

The rather wide variations in Ig concentration in normal individuals makes it difficult to assess the meaning of a single patient's serum unless the sample is extremely atypical. Studies of Ig are, therefore, except in myeloma patients (see below), more useful in population studies. It should be kept in mind that increases in Ig in cancer patients do not necessarily reflect enhanced synthesis of antibodies specific for tumor.

b. Complement

Functional activity of complement may be expected to decrease in cancer patients who present with circulating immune complexes of antibodies and tumor-associated antigens. Depletion of activity occurs by binding of complement to antigen-antibody complexes *via* the classical complement pathway. The ability of complement (a series of 11 complement proteins) to lyse sheep erythrocytes sensitized with antibodies is a simple method which detects a deficiency in total complement activity.[122] The relative quantitation in these functional tests is derived from the amount of hemoglobin released by a dilution of the test serum.

Specific complement proteins may also be assessed in radial immunodiffusion plates which are commercially available. In this case, the quantities of individual complement proteins are measured, but their functional capacity is not assayed. Cancer patients have been observed to have abnormalities in the quantities of various proteins of this system.[119] However, since complement levels vary in many diseased states,[122] the interpretation of changes in these proteins may be difficult.

c. Acute Phase Proteins

These proteins, which include α_1-acid glycoprotein, α_1-antitrypsin, transferrin, and C-reactive protein, appear in serum from patients with acute infections or diseases with extensive tissue damage. Certain of these substances may act as immunoregulatory proteins and Israel et al.[114] have suggested that plasmapheresis of immunodepressed patients with large amounts of these humoral factors may reverse suppression. The proteins may be assayed by radial immunodiffusion, but their relation to immune deficits in cancer is unproven.

d. Humoral Suppressors of Lymphocyte Blastogenesis

The lymphocyte blastogenic (transformation) assay in response to mitogenic or antigenic stimulation is described below. Incorporation of patient's serum or plasma into the reaction mixture will demonstrate any inhibitory effect of autologous serum when compared to normal homologous serum incubated with the same lymphocytes. Such humoral inhibitory factors have been described in sera from various types of cancer.[68]

2. Cell-Mediated Assays in Vitro

a. Membrane Receptors on Mononuclear Cells

Mononuclear cell preparations are separated from peripheral blood by centrifugation on buoyant density-gradients of Ficoll-sodium metrizoate.[123] Enumeration of the various lymphocyte populations can then be performed on the resultant lymphocyte-monocyte preparation.[124]

Differentiation of lymphocyte populations is based on identification of receptors found on the cell membranes (Table 5) and have proved useful in classifying leukemias.[125] The T lymphocyte, which is thymus-dependent and responsible for delayed hypersensitivity and homograft rejection reactions, is assayed by using membrane receptors for sheep erythrocytes (SRBC). T lymphocytes bind SRBC, forming spontaneous rosettes (E rosettes) of red blood cells attached to a central mononuclear cell. "Active" T cells[126] are a subgroup of T lymphocytes which bind SRBC under conditions of short-term incubation in which the total T cell population does not rosette. The number of circulating "active" T cells was reported to be depressed in cancer patients.[71]

B lymphocytes develop under the influence of the bone marrow, and, under appropriate stimulation, may differentiate into antibody-secreting plasma cells. B lymphocytes produce Ig molecules that are localized on the cell membrane. This Ig may be detected by fluorescent antibody techniques. Mixtures of fluorochrome-labeled antisera to human IgM and IgD are used to produce membrane immunofluorescence on viable membrane Ig-bearing lymphocytes. Ig-bearing lymphocytes may also be detected with polyacrylamide beads coated with antiserum to human Ig.[127] Human B cells have also been reported to form rosettes with mouse erythrocytes.[128]

Mononuclear cells which bear receptors for the Fc fragment of the IgG molecule may be detected by a membrane immunofluorescent method or by a modification of the rosette assay. In the former, fluorochrome-labeled antibodies are either heat-aggregated or complexed with the corresponding antigen, e.g., fluorescein-labeled goat anti-rabbit IgG complexed with rabbit IgG, and the complexes are incubated with the lymphocyte preparation. The rosette assay (EA rosette) utilizes erythrocytes, e.g., ox, coated (complexed) with subagglutinating amounts of IgG antibodies against the red blood cells. Both assays depend on the binding of the Fc portion of the aggregated or complexed reagents to Fc receptors on the mononuclear cell membrane. Monocytes must be carefully differentiated (see below) from lymphocytes since both possess Fc receptors.

Complement receptors are found on B lymphocytes. A rosette assay (the EAC rosette) is used to identify these cells. SRBC are coated with a subagglutinating amount of IgM antibody to SRBC. The sensitized cells are then treated with complement which is nonlytic because of depletion of various components. The coated cells are used to assay the presence of receptors. Two types of complement receptors have been recognized and each requires a separate EAC reagent for its detection. Monocytes also possess complement receptors and must be differentiated from lymphocytes for this test.

Lymphocytes which possess none of the above markers are termed "null" cells and are differentiated by lack of membrane receptors.

The monocyte is the only mononuclear cell which exhibits phagocytic activity. How-

TABLE 5
CHARACTERIZATION OF PERIPHERAL BLOOD MONONUCLEAR
CELLS

| Cell type | Membrane receptors | | | Rosette-formation Erythrocytes | | Phagocytosis |
	Immunoglobulin	Fc	Complement	Sheep	Mouse	
T	−	−	−	+	−	−
B	+	+	+	−	+	−
K	−	+	+	−	−	−
NK	−	+	±	−	−	−
Null	−	−	−	−	−	−
Monocyte	−	+	+	−	−	+

ever, together with certain types of lymphocytes, monocytes possess both Fc and complement receptors. Latex particles are used to label and identify phagocytic cells in the foregoing assays. In addition, a histochemical stain for nonspecific esterase detects monocytes in a preparation of mononuclear cells.[129]

Values[124] for distribution of receptor-bearing cells in the peripheral blood of normal individuals are: E rosette, 85%; membrane Ig, 1 to 15%; Fc receptors, 5 to 20%; and complement receptors, 5 to 20%. These values are not absolute and various minor subpopulations, e.g., E-rosetting cells with Fc receptors, may also be detected in peripheral blood. The distribution[130] of T lymphocytes in tissues is: peripheral blood, 55 to 75%; bone marrow, < 25%; lymph nodes, 75%; spleen, 50%; and thymus, > 75%. B cells are distributed as follows: peripheral blood, 1 to 15%; bone marrow, > 75%; lymph node, 25%; spleen, 50%; and thymus, < 25%.

b. Lymphocyte Blastogenesis

This assay is easy to perform and detects the functional activity of lymphoid populations in response to stimulation by nonspecific mitogenic substances or specific antigens.[123] Nonspecific mitogens, such as phytohemagglutinin and concanavalin A, stimulate T lymphocytes. Pokeweed mitogen, another nonspecific agent, produces a blastogenic response in both B and T cells. Antigens, which include purified protein derivative, streptolysin-O, streptokinase-streptodornase, or *Candida albicans,* can be used to specifically activate T lymphocytes of presensitized individuals. Lipopolysaccharide, however, stimulates previously sensitized B cells only in the presence of T lymphocytes.

During incubation, responding lymphocytes undergo a blastogenic transformation. Affected lymphocytes enlarge, vacuolate, and the cytoplasm becomes more basophilic. Protein and DNA synthesis are increased and the cells divide. Results of these tests may be estimated morphologically or by radioactive techniques.

The assays are performed using dilutions of whole blood,[131] or mononuclear cells isolated from the blood.[123] Since the test depends both on the number of lymphocytes present and the density of the cell population per unit volume, the use of isolated mononuclear cells is advantageous. In addition, excessive numbers of polymorphonuclear leukocytes interfere with the response.

The cultures of blood or mononuclear cells are incubated at 37°C in the presence of antigen or mitogen for an optimal period of time. Prior to harvest, dividing cells are labeled with tritiated thymidine and the amount of radioactive label incorporated into DNA is determined.

The mixed lymphocyte reaction is also a sensitive indicator of T cell function.[132] In this case, the stimulant is a population of lymphocytes which has been treated with radiation or mitomycin C to inhibit their ability to synthesize DNA. When mixed with test lymphocytes, the nonreplicating stimulator cells act as antigen to which the responder test cells react by blastogenesis and proliferation. DNA synthesis may be used to estimate the response of the test population.

c. K Cells

The K cell is responsible for ADCC reactions and can be quantitated by radioactive chromium release assays for cell-mediated cytotoxicity.[133] In this instance, the target cells, e.g., the Chang liver cell line, are labeled with ^{51}Cr. Target cells are coated with antibodies and mixed with the effector lymphocyte population. Control preparations contain ^{51}Cr-labeled target cells and medium. Cytotoxic activity is shown by the release of ^{51}Cr to the supernatant fluid. The difference in cytotoxicity between effector cell-treated targets and control cultures indicates the degree of K cell-mediated toxicity.

d. NK Cells

The human NK cell is usually assayed by the chromium release method, using the sensitive human chronic myeloid leukemia cell line, K562.[30] This type of spontaneous cytotoxic activity occurs without the mediation of humoral antibodies or previous exposure to antigen. Spontaneous cytotoxicity to other types of target cells derived from solid tumors may also be produced by this type of lymphocyte. However, the characteristics of NK populations responsible for "natural" cytotoxicity to solid tumor cell targets have not yet been compared to those of cells responsible for toxicity to lymphoid cell targets. It is possible that the effector cell populations differ from each other in some parameters.

e. Lymphokines

Other tests of nontumor-directed lymphocyte function evaluate the elaboration of lymphokines from sensitized T lymphocyte populations. These molecules, which are released on exposure to antigens, act as mediators of in vitro activities such as macrophage migration inhibition. The importance of these substances to clinical evaluation of nonspecific immunocompetence in cancer patients has not yet been determined. The topic of soluble mediators of immune phenomena has been reviewed.[134]

f. Monocytes and Macrophages

The functional activity of peripheral blood monocytes may be assessed by phagocytic, chemotactic, or microbial killing responses, as well as by ADCC reactions. For the first three tests, monocytes are obtained by adherence to glass of mononuclear cell suspensions from peripheral blood.[135] The monocytes are freed from the glass substrate by trypsinization or by scraping. The cells are then mixed with the appropriate microorganisms for tests of phagocytic function or killing capacity. Chemotaxis is studied in special chambers in which quantitative chemotactic migration across a filter can be assessed by direct counts of migrating cells.

Human monocytes have been shown to function in ADCC reactions when antibody-coated human erythrocytes are used as target.[54] It is not necessary to purify monocytes from a mononuclear cell suspension in order to perform the ADCC test. Cancer patients have increased monocyte-mediated ADCC activity and increased expression of surface Fc receptors on peripheral blood monocytes.[69]

Lysozyme is synthesized by macrophages and was shown by Currie and Eccles to increase in serum during the growth of animal tumors or following treatment of animals with *BCG* or *C. parvum*.[136] Application of these results to man indicated that intravenous injection of microbial products in cancer patients, as well as cutaneous treatment with *BCG,* enhanced the levels of serum lysozyme.[112,113,137] The elevation of serum lysozyme in monocytic leukemias is well-known.

g. Granulocytes

Functional activity of neutrophilic leukocytes can be assessed by various tests including phagocytic assays (qualitative or quantitative), evaluation of the degranulation process, and assays of neutrophile oxygen metabolism *via* nitroblue tetrazolium reduction.[138] Although consistent defects in these leukocytes have been observed only in certain genetic diseases, a complete immunological workup should probably include functional tests of the granulocytic cell series. As noted above, cytotoxicity has been demonstrated for this cell type in animals[57] and, recently, in man.[139]

3. Assays In Vivo
a. Humoral Antibody Synthesis

The ability of patients to synthesize specific antibodies is a function of the differentiated B lymphocyte, the plasma cell. Interference with humoral immune responses can be affected by various therapies and the degree of interference may be assessed by immunization with antigens to which the patient has never been exposed (de novo sensitization). Such antigens may include microbial vaccines and products, or keyhole limpet hemocyanin.[107]

b. Cell-Mediated Immunity — de novo Sensitization

The ability of an individual to recognize a new antigen and to react against it by a cell-mediated immune response is a function of the T cell system. It has been recognized as a factor of prognostic value in cancer-related surgery.[140] Thus patients who responded to de novo sensitization with dinitrochlorobenzene (DNCB) were, as a group, better able to handle their disease postsurgery than were those whose immune system could not respond to de novo stimulation. In addition to DNCB, keyhole limpet hemocyanin or picryl chloride can be used as antigen in this test.[107]

c. Cell-Mediated Immunity — Recall Antigens

The use of microbial antigens in testing for delayed type hypersensitivity is well established.[141] These antigens, e.g., tuberculin, candida, and mumps, detect the ability of the patient's immune system to recall and to respond to antigens that were previously encountered through natural exposure or immunization. A positive skin test is one in which both erythema and induration can be observed. Cancer patients can often present with erythematous responses in which the test area is flat and induration cannot be felt. Normal responses are usually maximal at 48 hr, but responses in patients may be more evanescent. The response of cancer patients to recall antigens may be of some prognostic value in surgical oncology.[140]

C. Tumor-Associated Parameters
1. Humoral Assays in Vitro
a. Antibodies to Tumor-Associated Antigens

The complement-fixation test has been used to some extent to assay antitumor antibodies.[116] Extracts of tumor cells serve as antigen(s) and, in the presence of specific antibodies, fix complement. The fixation is detected by addition, to the reaction mixture, of a hemolytic indicator system composed of SRBC sensitized with antibodies to SRBC. Presence or absence of hemolysis indicates a negative or positive reaction, respectively.[142] Tests must be carefully controlled to eliminate false positive reactions.[143] Since crude extracts are used, the localization of the antigen(s) within the tumor cell and the number of such antigens in the extract are unknown.

The immunofluorescence reaction[144] not only detects antibodies, but also visualizes the location of antigen within a cell. The most common fluorochrome used for these tests is fluorescein isothiocyanate. The fluorescent compound is conjugated to the antibody-containing globulin fraction of serum. In the direct test, fluorochrome is conjugated to the test serum; in the indirect test, the fluorochrome is conjugated to anti-human globulin (or to anti-Ig of the individual classes). The indirect test employs only one reagent, the fluorochrome-labeled antiglobulin, to test many sera. The direct test requires that each unknown serum be individually labeled with fluorochrome. After staining of viable cells (to study membrane antigens) or fixed cells (to study internal antigens), the preparations are viewed by dark-field microscopy with a source of ultraviolet or blue light. When an appropriate system of exciter and barrier filters is used, the fluorochrome bound to antigen *via* antibody is excited and fluoresces intensely. Adequate controls must be performed to assure the specificity of the reactions.

Immune adherence is a sensitive serologic method which depends on the binding of primate erythrocytes to antigen-antibody-complement complexes *via* complement receptors ($C'3$) on the erythrocyte membrane.[116] The assay is used to detect antigens that are located on the surface of target cells. The test is 100 times more sensitive than complement-fixation and 1000 times more sensitive than bacterial agglutination.

Cytotoxicity can be mediated either by serum antibodies or cellular reactions. In the case of humoral cytotoxic activity, killing is complement dependent and can be assessed by morphological criteria (uptake of trypan blue dye by nonviable cells[145]), release of radioactivity from damaged cells (e.g., release of ^{51}Cr, solubilization of damaged cells by enzymatic activity[146]), uptake of tritiated actinomycin-D into the DNA of damaged cells[147], or detachment of viable tumor cells from a culture vessel.[148] Although each of these tests is not suitable for a given target cell, an adequate technique can be devised for most types of experiments.

The immunodiffusion-in-agar technique is used to detect the number of antigens reacting in an immunological system.[149] The antigen and antibody solutions are allowed to diffuse in agar, forming lines of precipitation which identify common antigenic components in various antigen preparations. The sensitivity of this method, however, is less than that of other tests and it is not used extensively in tumor immunology.

b. Antigen-Antibody Complexes

Antigen-antibody complexes in sera from cancer patients have been assayed by a number of techniques, including the Raji cell assay, C1q binding, and complement consumption methods.[150] The Raji lymphoblastoid cell line derived from Burkitt's lymphoma is composed of cells which lack membrane-bound Ig, but synthesize Fc receptors and a large number of complement receptors.[151] Antigen-antibody complexes in human sera are treated with complement and can then be adsorbed to Raji cells by way of the complement receptors. Adsorption is detected by immunofluorescence or radioimmunoassay using either fluorescein- or radio-labeled antihuman IgG, respectively.

The ^{125}I-C1q binding test is a radioimmunoassay which measures the amount of C1q (a subunit of the C1 protein of complement) bound to macromolecular substances in human sera.[152] Although DNA or endotoxin may also bind C1q, the system, when properly used, detects binding to antigen-antibody complexes. Radioactive C1q is added to serum and, following incubation, polyethylene glycol is added to precipitate high molecular weight materials which have bound labeled C1q.

The complement consumption (fixation) test[122] measures the spontaneous binding of complement by human sera and this inherent binding is known as anticomplementary activity. The activity is higher in cancer patients than in normal individuals and correlates with tumor burden, but not with clinical staging of the disease.[150]

Circulating immune complexes can be associated with a variety of autoimmune and infectious diseases. Therefore, detection of complexes in the sera of cancer patients may be totally unrelated to the neoplastic disease.

c. Tumor Products

Measurement of tumor products in serum is an aid in diagnosis, and, in certain instances, in following the course of disease. The monoclonal gammopathies, determined by serum electrophoresis on cellulose acetate membranes, are characterized by a homogeneous spike of protein located in the γ, γ-β, or, rarely, in the β-α_2 regions of the electrophoretic pattern.[153] A monoclonal peak results from overproduction of a single class and antigenic type of Ig by an abnormal plasma cell clone. These gammopathies are associated with multiple myeloma, macroglobulinemia, and, occasionally, malignant lymphoma. The specific antigenic class of Ig involved is ascertained by immunoelectrophoresis. Serum (antigen) is added to several wells cut into an agar medium and the samples are treated with an electrical current to separate serum proteins. After electrophoresis, troughs are cut into the agar and each is filled with antiserum to the various classes of Ig. The monoclonal protein is identified by enhanced formation of precipitin bands.

Alpha-fetoprotein (AFP) is a glycoprotein which is synthesized by cells in the liver and yolk sac of the human fetus.[154] Although synthesis is decreased by the fortieth week of fetal development, it continues to decline until the levels found in normal human serum (1 to 30 ng/mℓ) by 2 years of age are attained. AFP is elevated in adult serum from 70 to 90% of individuals with hepatocellular carcinoma and in 50 to 70% of individuals with germ cell tumors. Assays of AFP may aid in diagnosis of suspected hepatocellular carcinoma, but its chief use is in following the course of an AFP-producing malignancy after surgical resection. Successful resection is followed by a decrease in circulating AFP; increases precede clinical recurrence of tumor. Elevations in AFP may also be present in nonmalignant liver diseases as well as in other types of cancer. Although AFP can be detected by a relatively insensitive immunodiffusion assay, either radioactive or enzymic immunoassays are preferred for adequate quantitation.

Carcinoembryonic antigen (CEA) is a nonspecific marker which may be present in sera of patients bearing several types of adenocarcinomas.[155] It is found in 60 to 70% of sera from individuals with colon carcinoma. However, metastatic disease increases the positivity to 96%. Diagnostically, the presence of the antigen is a better indicator of metastatic disease than of early cancer. CEA has been reported in more than 50% of patients with carcinoma of the breast or bronchus and in 30 to 40% of those with bladder or prostatic cancer. The antigen is a carbohydrate-containing protein with a molecular weight of approximately 200,000. CEA is a fetal antigen found in the gut, liver, and pancreas of fetuses between the second and sixth month of development. Low levels of CEA ($\leqslant$ 10 ng/mℓ) are present in normal sera, but elevations are found in heavy cigarette smokers and in patients with non-neoplastic liver disease. The antigen is detected by radioimmunoassay and, as described for AFP, serial determinations, especially in patients with colon carcinoma, reflect the progress of disease after surgical resection.

2. Cell-Mediated Assays In Vitro

a. Lymphocyte Blastogenesis

The basic lymphocyte stimulation technique was described above. However, the antigens in tumor-directed assays are either crude extracts of tumors,[156] irradiated tumor cells,[157] mitomycin-C-treated tumor cells,[158] or 3M KCl-extracts of tumor cells.[157] Tests utilizing allogeneic combinations of tumor cells and either normal lymphocytes (for control) or patients' lymphocytes may be difficult to interpret because of histocompatibility differences in addition to tumor-associated antigenic differences. However, the tests can also be performed in autologous situations which may identify tumor-specific reactivity.[158]

b. Cytotoxicity

The techniques used to assess cell-mediated cytotoxicity have been reviewed recently.[159] The problems of appropriate control and patient populations were also discussed. Experimentally, cytotoxicity tests are divided into isotope release, isotope incorporation, or visual assays.

Target cells can be labeled with isotopes prior to assessing the cytotoxic activity of mononuclear cell preparations. Various isotopes have been used, including: ^{51}Cr which labels the cytoplasm of cells by binding to macromolecules; ^{3}H-thymidine which is incorporated into DNA; ^{3}H-proline which is incorporated into protein; or ^{125}I-iodo-deoxyuridine (IUDR) which is incorporated into DNA. Mixing of prelabeled target cells with attacker lymphocytes results, after incubation, in the release of radioactivity to the supernatant fluid. Specific cytotoxicity can then be calculated by comparison of release in test cultures to that in cultures receiving control lymphocytes.

Postlabeling experiments reserve isotope incorporation until after incubation of attacker and target cells. Cytotoxicity is assessed by determining the number of viable target cells remaining which can incorporate a radioactive label. For these experiments, ^{3}H-proline, ^{3}H-thymidine, and $^{125}IUDR$ have been used.

The microcytotoxicity test of Takasugi and Klein[160] is used as a nonisotopic technique to determine cytotoxicity to target cells which grow adherent to a plastic substrate. The target cells are incubated in microwells to which effector lymphocytes are added. Following incubation, the microcultures are washed to remove dead target cells and lymphocytes and the remaining cells are stained and counted microscopically. Both this assay and postlabeling assays measure target cell death, as well as effects on target cell growth and adherence to the plastic substrate.

c. Lymphokines

These tests assess the ability of sensitized lymphocytes to specifically release soluble factors (lymphokines) which can be assayed by their nonspecific functional effects on leukocyte activities in vitro. Lymphokines which can inhibit the migration of leukocytes or the adherence of leukocytes to glass have been used to assay the reactions of patients to tumor antigens.

In the direct migration assay,[161] peripheral blood leukocytes are collected and aliquots of the cells are incubated with tumor and control extracts. The cells are then drawn into capillary tubes and centrifuged. The tube is cut at the interface of fluid and leukocytes. The portion of the capillary containing the cells is placed in a chamber with media to allow migration of leukocytes from the end of the capillary. The area of migration is then determined following incubation. If sensitized lymphocytes have reacted to the tumor extract, the area of migration is reduced significantly.

Inhibition of leukocyte adherence to glass hemocytometers depends on elaboration, following incubation with specific antigen, of a lymphokine from sensitized T lymphocytes.[162] This technique is being used extensively in tumor immunology.[163]

3. Assays In Vivo

a. Skin Tests

Skin testing to microbial antigens is used to assess general immunocompetence in cancer patients. However, if tumor-associated antigens are used, the assay may become a test for specific reactivity. Antigens can either be a tumor extract[164] or a cryostat section of autologous tumor.[165]

If an alcohol-ether fixed cryostat section is used, it is mounted on a coverslip and placed on an area of abraded skin, as in the Rebuck skin window technique. After remaining in place for 30 hr, the coverslip is removed and the degree of infiltration by host cells is assessed.

The use of crude tumor extracts as antigen presents several problems. Ethical considerations do not permit intradermal injection of such material into non-cancer patients or normal individuals for control purposes. In addition, much of the positive reactivity obtained may be related to nontumor-antigen-specific reactions, e.g., extracts of normal tissues may react.[164] Since the technique has potential utility in prognostic and diagnostic studies, the purification of tumor-associated antigens for this purpose is extremely important.

IV. COMMENT

In this article, I have attempted to present an overview of both the basic concepts in human tumor immunology and the methods which are available to assess immunocompetence in humans. The wealth of evidence which demonstrates the host's immune defenses against tumor illumine the complexities of the host-tumor relationship. Although the ultimate importance of the immune system in the prevention, diagnosis, and treatment of cancer must still be assessed, current information suggests that there is a bright future in the application of immunological concepts to neoplastic disease.

ACKNOWLEDGMENT

The work from this laboratory, the St. Joseph Hospital Laboratory for Cancer Research, Houston, Texas, was supported by the Stehlin Foundation for Cancer Research.

REFERENCES

1. Ehrlich, P., Ueber den jetzigen stand der Karzinomforschung, *Ned. Tijdschr. Geneeskd.*, 5, 1, 1909.
2. Thomas, L., Discussion, in *Cellular and Humoral Aspects of the Hypersensitive State*, Lawrence, H. S., Ed., Hoeber-Harper, New York, 1959, 529.
3. Burnet, F. M., The concept of immunological surveillance, *Progr. Exp. Tumor Res.*, 13, 1, 1970.
4. Doll, R. and Kinlen, L., Immunosurveillance and cancer: epidemiological evidence, *Br. Med. J.*, 4, 420, 1970.
5. Kay, M. M. B., Aging & the decline of immune responsiveness, in *Basic & Clinical Immunology*, Fudenberg, H. H., Stites, D. P., Caldwell, J. L., and Wells, J. V., Eds., Lange Medical Publ., Los Altos, Calif., 1976, chap. 23.
6. Stutman, O., Immunodepression and malignancy, *Adv. Cancer Res.*, 22, 261, 1975.
7. Penn, I., Occurrence of cancer in immune deficiencies, *Cancer (Philadelphia)*, 34, 858, 1974.
8. Everson, T. C. and Cole, W. H., *Spontaneous Regression of Cancer*, W. B. Saunders, Philadelphia, 1966.
9. Sindelar, W. F. and Ketcham, A.S., Regression of cancer following surgery, *Natl. Cancer Inst. Monogr.*, 44, 81, 1976.
10. Cochran, A. J., *Man, Cancer and Immunity*, Academic Press, New York, 1978, 18.
11. DeVita, V. T., Jr., Young, R. C., and Canellos, G. P., Combination versus single agent chemotherapy: a review of the basis for selection of drug treatment of cancer, *Cancer (Philadelphia)*, 35, 98, 1975.
12. Lawler, S. D., Klouda, P. T., and Bagshawe, K. D., The HL-A system in trophoblastic neoplasia, *Lancet*, 2, 834, 1971.
13. Mathé, G., Dausset, J., Hervet, E., Amiel, J. L., Colombani, J., and Brule, G., Immunological studies in patients with placental choriocarcinoma, *J. Natl. Cancer Inst.*, 33, 193, 1964.

14. Nkrumah, F. K. and Perkins, I. V., Burkitt's lymphoma. A clinical study of 110 patients, *Cancer (Philadelphia),* 37, 671, 1976.
15. Stehlin, J. S., Jr., Giovanella, B. C., De Ipolyi, P. D., and Anderson, R. F., Results of eleven years' experience with heated perfusion for melanoma of the extremities, *Cancer Res.,* 39, 2255, 1979.
16. Hersh, E. M., Mavligit, G. M., Gutterman, J. U., and Richman, S. P., Immunotherapy of human cancer, in *Cancer. A Comprehensive Treatise,* Vol. 6, Becker, F., Ed., Plenum Press, New York, 425, 1977.
17. Klein, E., Papermaster, B. W., Case, R. W., and Apisarnthanarax, P., Immunological aspects of neoplasia, in *Immunological Aspects of Neoplasia, A Collection of Papers Presented at the Twenty-Sixth Annual Symposium on Fundamental Cancer Research,* Williams & Wilkins Co., Baltimore, 549, 1975.
18. Mathé, G., Amiel, J. L., Schwarzenberg, L., Schneider, M., Cattan, A., Schlumberger, J. R., Hayat, M., and De Vassal, F., Follow-up of the first (1962) pilot study on active immunotherapy of acute lymphoid leukemia. A critical discussion, *Biomedicine,* 26, 29, 1977.
19. Terry, W. D. and Windhorst, D., Eds., Immunotherapy of cancer: present status of trials in man, in *Progress in Cancer Research Therapy,* Vol. 6, Raven Press, New York, 1978.
20. The University of Texas System Cancer Center M.D. Anderson Hospital and Tumor Institute 22nd Annual Clinical Conference on Cancer, *Immunotherapy of Human Cancer,* Raven Press, New York, 1978.
21. Burnet, F. M., Immunological factors in the process of carcinogenesis, *Br. Med. Bull.,* 20, 154, 1964.
22. Burnet, F. M., Immunological aspects of malignant disease, *Lancet,* 1, 1171, 1967.
23. Prehn, R. T., Immunological surveillance: pro and con, in *Clinical Immunobiology,* Vol. 2, Bach, F. H. and Good, R. A., Eds., Academic Press, New York, 1974, 191.
24. Prehn, R. T., The immune reaction as a stimulator of tumor growth, *Science,* 176, 170, 1972.
25. Prehn, R. T. and Main, J. M., Immunity to methylcholanthrene-induced sarcomas, *J. Natl. Cancer Inst.,* 18, 769, 1957.
26. Klein, G. and Klein, E., Immune surveillance against virus-induced tumors and nonrejectability of spontaneous tumors: contrasting consequences of host *versus* tumor evolution, *Proc. Natl. Acad. Sci. U.S.A.,* 74, 2121, 1977.
27. Alexander, P., The role of macrophages in the host defense against cancer, in *Host Defense against Cancer and its Potentiation,* Mizuno, D., Chihara, G., Fukuoka, F., Yamamoto, T., and Yamamura, Y., Eds., University Park Press, Baltimore, 1975, 113.
28. Pearson, G. R., *In vitro* and *in vivo* investigations on antibody-dependent cellular cytotoxicity, *Curr. Top. Microbiol. Immunol.,* 80, 65, 1978.
29. Lotzová, E. and McCredie, K. B., Natural killer cells in mice and man and their possible biological significance, *Cancer Immunol. Immunother.,* 4, 215, 1978.
30. Pross, H. F. and Baines, M. G., Spontaneous human lymphocyte-mediated cytotoxicity against tumor target cells. VI. A brief review, *Cancer Immunol. Immunother.,* 3, 75, 1977.
31. Cochran, A. J., *Man, Cancer, and Immunity,* Academic Press, New York, 1978, 34.
32. Van Hoosier, G. L., Jr., Trentin, J. J., Chenault, S. S., Bryan, M. E., and McCormick, K. J., Infrequent C-F antibody response in mice with adenovirus type 12 tumors, *Proc. Soc. Exp. Biol. Med.,* 124, 1053, 1967.
34. Witz, I. P., Tumor-bound immunoglobulins: *in situ* expression of humoral immunity, *Adv. Cancer Res.,* 25, 95, 1977.
34. Canevari, S., Fossati, G., Della Porta, G., and Balzarini, G. P., Humoral cytotoxicity in melanoma patients and its correlation with the extent and course of the disease, *Int. J. Cancer,* 16, 722, 1975.
35. Morton, D. L., Malmgren, R. A., Holmes, E. C., and Ketcham, A. S., Demonstration of antibodies against human malignant melanoma by immunofluorescence, *Surgery,* 64, 233, 1968.
36. Muna, N. M., Marcus, S., and Smart, C., Detection by immunofluorescence of antibodies specific for human malignant melanoma cells, *Cancer (Philadelphia),* 23, 88, 1969.
37. McCormick, K. J., Stehlin, J. S., Jr., Giovanella, B. C., and de Ipolyi, P. D., unpublished data, 1977.
38. Shiku, H., Takahashi, T., Resnick, L. A., Oettgen, H. F., and Old, L. J., Cell surface antigens of human malignant melanoma. III. Recognition of autoantibodies with unusual characteristics, *J. Exp. Med.,* 145, 784, 1977.
39. Yoshida, T. O., High incidence of antinuclear antibodies in the sera of nasopharyngeal cancer patients, in *Recent Advances in Human Tumor Virology and Immunology,* Nakahara, W., Nishioka, K., Hirayama, T., and Ito, Y., Eds., University Park Press, Baltimore, 1971, 433.
40. Yoshida, T. O., Autoantibodies in the sera of various cancer patients, *Gann, Mongr. Cancer Res.,* 16, 63, 1974.
41. McCormick, N. K., McCormick, K. J., and Trentin, J. J., Antinuclear antibodies and elevated anti-Epstein-Barr virus titers in cancer patients, *Infect. Immunol.,* 13, 1382, 1976.

42. Cochran, A. J., *Man, Cancer, and Immunity,* Academic Press, New York, 1978, 40.

43. McCormick, K. J., Giovanella, B. C., Stehlin, J. S., de Ipolyi, P. D., and Parsons, W. R., Cellular cytotoxicity against autochthonous human melanoma cells, in *Fed. Proc. Fed. Am. Soc. Exp. Biol.,* 38, 1105, 1979.

44. Penn, I. and Starzl, T. E., Immunosuppression and cancer, *Transplant. Proc.,* 5, 943, 1973.

45. O'Toole, C., Perlmann, P., Wigzell, H., Unsgaard, B., and Zetterlund, C. G., Lymphocyte cytotoxicity in bladder cancer, no requirement for thymus-derived effector cells? *Lancet,* 1, 1085, 1973.

46. Kodera, Y. and Bean, M. A., Antibody-dependent cell-mediated cytotoxicity for human monolayer target cells bearing blood group and transplantation antigens and for melanoma cells, *Int. J. Cancer,* 16, 579, 1975.

47. Hersey, P., MacLennan, I. C. M., Campbell, A. C., Harris, R., and Freeman, C. B., Cytoxicity against human leukaemic cells. I. Demonstration of antibody-dependent lymphocyte killing of human allogeneic myeloblasts, *Clin. Exp. Immunol.,* 14, 159, 1973.

48. Pearson, G. R., Johansson, B., and Klein, G., Antibody-dependent cellular cytotoxicity against Epstein-Barr virus-associated antigens in African patients with nasopharyngeal carcinoma, *Int. J. Cancer,* 22, 120, 1978.

49. Kiessling, R., Klein, E., Pross, H., and Wigzell, H., "Natural" killer cells in the mouse. II. Cytotoxic cells with specificity for mouse Moloney leukemia cells. Characteristics of the killer cell, *Eur. J. Immunol.,* 5, 117, 1975.

50. Eremin, O., Coombs, R. R. A., Plumb, D., and Ashby, J., Characterization of the human natural killer (NK) cell in blood and lymphoid organs, *Int. J. Cancer,* 21, 42, 1978.

51. Takasugi, M., Akira, D., Takasugi, J., and Mickey, M. R., Specificities in human cell-mediated cytotoxicity, *J. Natl. Cancer Inst.,* 59, 69, 1977.

52. Hibbs, J. B., Jr., Lambert, L. H., Jr., and Remington, J. S., *In vitro* non-immunological destruction of cells with abnormal growth characteristics by adjuvant activated macrophages, *Proc. Soc. Exp. Biol. Med.,* 139, 1049, 1972.

53. Evans, R. and Alexander, P., Rendering macrophages specifically cytotoxic by a factor released from immune lymphoid cells, *Transplantation,* 12, 227, 1971.

54. Holm, G. and Hammarstrom, S., Haemolytic activity of human blood monocytes, lysis of human erythrocytes treated with anti-A serum, *Clin. Exp. Immun.,* 13, 29, 1973.

55. Eccles, S. A., Macrophages and cancer, in *Immunological Aspects of Cancer,* Castro, J. E., Ed., University Park Press, Baltimore, 1978, 123.

56. Morton, D. L., Eilber, F. R., Holmes, E. C., Hunt, J. S., Ketcham, A. S., Silverstein, M. J., and Sparks, F. C., BCG immunotherapy of malignant melanoma: summary of a seven-year experience, *Ann. Surg.,* 180, 635, 1974.

57. Burton, R. C., Grail, D., and Warner, N. L., Natural cytotoxicity of haemopoietic cell populations against murine lymphoid tumours, *Br. J. Cancer,* 37, 806, 1978.

58. Hedley, D. W., McElwain, T. J., and Currie, G. A., Specific active immunotherapy does not prolong survival in surgically treated patients with stage IIB malignant melanoma and may promote early recurrence, *Br. J. Cancer,* 37, 491, 1978.

59. Braunschwig, A., Southam, C. M., and Levin, A. G., Host resistance to cancer, clinical experiments by homotransplants, autotransplants and admixture of autologous leucocytes, *Ann. Surg.,* 162, 416, 1965.

60. Klein, G., Immunological surveillance against tumors, in *Immunological Aspects of Neoplasia, A Collection of Papers Presented at the Twenty-Sixth Annual Symposium on Fundamental Cancer Research,* Williams & Wilkins, Baltimore, 1975, 21.

61. Hewitt, H. B., Blake, E. R., and Walder, A. S., A critique of the evidence for active host defence against cancer, based on personal studies of 27 murine tumours of spontaneous origin, *Br. J. Cancer,* 33, 241, 1976.

62. Baldwin, R. W. and Embleton, M. J., Immunology of 2-acetylaminofluorene-induced rat mammary adenocarcinomas, *Int. J. Cancer,* 4, 47, 1969.

63. Old, L. J., Boyse, E. A., Clarke, D. A., and Carswell, E. A., Antigenic properties of chemically induced tumors, *Ann. N.Y. Acad. Sci.,* 101, 80, 1962.

64. Hellström, I., Sjögren, H. O., Warner, G. A., and Hellström, K. E., Blocking of cell-mediated tumor immunity by sera from patients with growing neoplasms, *Int. J. Cancer,* 7, 226, 1971.

65. Currie, G. A. and Basham, C., Serum mediated inhibition of the immunological reactions of the patient to his own tumour: a possible role for circulating antigen, *Br. J. Cancer,* 26, 427, 1972.

66. Baldwin, R. W. and Robins, R. A., Factors interfering with immunological rejection of tumours, *Br. Med. Bull.,* 32, 118, 1976.

67. Rossen, R. D., Reisberg, M. A., Hersh, E. M., and Gutterman, J. U., The C1q binding test for soluble immune complexes: clinical correlations obtained in patients with cancer, *J. Natl. Cancer Inst.,* 58, 1205, 1977.

68. Kamo, I. and Friedman, H., Immunosuppression and the role of suppressive factors in cancer, *Adv. Cancer Res.*, 25, 271, 1977.
69. Nyholm, R. E. and Currie, G. A., Monocytes and macrophages in malignant melanoma. II. Lysis of antibody-coated human erythrocytes as an assay of monocyte function, *Br. J. Cancer*, 37, 337, 1978.
70. Hersh, E. M., Gutterman, J. U., Mavligit, G. M., Mountain, C. W., McBride, C. M., Burgess, M. A., Lurie, P. M., Zelen, M., Takita, H., and Vincent, R. G., Immunocompetence, immunodeficiency and prognosis in cancer, *Ann. N.Y. Acad. Sci.*, 276, 386, 1976.
71. Wybran, J. and Fudenberg, H. H., T-cell rosettes in human cancer, in *Clinical Tumor Immunology*, Wybran, J. and Staquet, M. J., Eds., Pergamon Press, New York, 1976, 31.
72. Gershon, R. K., Suppressor T cells: classes of activity in *Immune Depression and Cancer*, Siskind, G. W., Christian, C. L., and Litwin, S. D., Eds., Grune & Stratton, New York, 1975, 1.
73. Mikulski, S. M. and Muggia, F. M., The suppressor mechanisms and their significance in tumor immunology, *Cancer Immunol. Immunother.*, 4, 139, 1978.
74. Zembala, M., Mytar, B., Popiela, T., and Asherson, G. L., Depressed in vitro peripheral blood lymphocyte response to mitogens in cancer patients: the role of suppressor cells, *Int J. Cancer*, 19, 605, 1977.
75. Twomey, J. J., Laughter, A. H., Farrow, S., and Douglas, C. C., Hodgkin's disease, an immuno-depleting and immunosuppressive disorder, *J. Clin. Invest.*, 56, 467, 1975.
76. Broder, S., Humphrey, R., Durm, M., Blackman, M., Meade, B., Goldman, C., Strober, W., and Waldman, T., Impaired synthesis of polyclonal (non-paraprotein) immunoglobulins by circulating lymphocytes from patients with multiple myeloma, role of suppressor cells, *N. Engl. J. Med.*, 293, 887, 1975.
77. Yu, A., Watts, H., Jaffe, N., and Parkman, R., Concomitant presence of tumor-specific cytotoxic and inhibitor lymphocytes in patients with osteogenic sarcoma, *N. Engl. J. Med.*, 297, 121, 1977.
78. Cooperband, S. R., Glasgow, A. H., and Mannick, J. A., Natural immunosuppressive factors, in *Immune Depression and Cancer*, Siskind, G. W., Christian, C. L., and Litwin, S. D., Eds., Grune & Stratton, New York, 1975, 135.
79. Ashikawa, K., Inoue, K., Shimizu, T., and Ishibashi, Y., An increase of serum alpha-globulin in tumor-bearing hosts and its immunological significance, *Jpn. J. Exp. Med.*, 41, 339, 1971.
80. Nimberg, R. B., Glasgow, A. H., Menzoian, J. O., Constantian, M. B., Cooperband, S. R., Mannick, J. A., and Schmid, K., Isolation of an immunosuppressive peptide fraction from the serum of cancer patients, *Cancer Res.*, 35, 1489, 1975.
81. Uete, T., Ogi, K., Fukazawa, S., and Takeuchi, Y., Clinical observation on the origin of C-reactive protein in blood, *Clin. Biochem.*, 4, 9, 1971.
82. Claus, D. R., Osmand, A. P., and Gewurz, H., Radioimmunoassay of human C-reactive protein and levels in normal sera, *J. Lab. Clin. Med.*, 87, 120, 1976.
83. Mortensen, R. F., Braun, D., and Gewurz, H., Effects of C-reactive protein on lymphocyte functions. III. Inhibition of antigen-induced lymphocyte stimulation and lymphokine production, *Cell. Immunol.*, 28, 59, 1977.
84. McFarlane, H., Ngu, V. A., Udeozo, I. O. K., Osunkoya, B. O., Luzzatto, L., and Mottram, F. C., Some acute phase proteins in Burkitt lymphoma in Nigerians, *Clin. Chim. Acta*, 17, 325, 1967.
85. Carpenter, C. M., Heiskell, C. L., and Aldrich, H., The significance of abnormal serum proteins in cancer detection, *Rocky Mount. Med. J.*, 63(6), 59, 1966.
86. Robins, R. A. and Baldwin, R. W., Immune complexes in cancer, *Cancer Immunol. Immunother.*, 4, 1, 1978.
87. Fisher, B., The changing role of surgery in the treatment of cancer, in *Cancer, A Comprehensive Treatise*, Vol. 6, Becker, F., Ed., Plenum Press, New York, 1977, 401.
88. Watkins, S. M., The effects of surgery on lymphocyte transformation in patients with cancer, *Clin. Exp. Immunol.*, 14, 69, 1973.
89. Cochran, A. J., Spilg, W. G. S., Mackie, R. M., and Thomas, C. E., Postoperative depression of tumour-directed cell-mediated immunity in patients with malignant disease, *Br. Med. J.*, 4, 67, 1972.
90. Goh, K.-O., Radiation, cell-mediated immunity and cancer, in *The Handbook of Cancer Immunology*, Vol. 1, Waters, H., Ed., Garland STPM Press, New York, 1978, 307.
91. Ghossein, N. A. and Bosworth, J. L., Immunocompetence in radiation therapy patients, in *The Handbook of Cancer Immunology*, Vol. 4, Waters, H., Ed., Garland STPM Press, New York, 1978, 161.
92. Kallman, R. F. and Rockwell, S., Effects of radiation on animal tumor models, in *Cancer. A Comprehensive Treatise*, Vol. 6, Becker, F., Ed., Plenum Press, New York, 1977, 225.
93. O'Toole, C., Perlmann, P., Unsgaard, B., Moberger, G., and Edsmyr, F., Cellular immunity to human urinary bladder carcinoma. I. Correlation to clinical stage and radiotherapy, *Int. J. Cancer*, 10, 77, 1972.
94. Cochran, A. J., *Man, Cancer and Immunity*, Academic Press, New York, 1978, 136.

95. Stjernsward, J., Immunological changes after radiotherapy for mammary carcinoma, *Ann. Inst. Pasteur, Paris*, 122, 883, 1972.
96. Blomgren, H., Wasserman, J., and Littbrand, B., Blood lymphocytes after radiation therapy of carcinoma of prostate and urinary bladder, *Acta Radiol. Ther.*, 13, 357, 1974.
97. Blomgren, H., Berg, R., Wasserman, J., and Glas, U., Effect of radiotherapy on blood lymphocyte population in mammary carcinoma, *Int. J. Radiat. Oncol. Biol. Phys.*, 1, 177, 1976.
98. Blomgren, H., Glas, U., Melén, B., and Wasserman, J., Blood lymphocytes after radiation therapy of mammary carcinoma, *Acta Radiol. Ther.*, 13, 185, 1974.
99. Chaskes, S., Kingdon, G. C., and Balish, E., Serum immunoglobulin level in humans exposed to therapeutic total-body gamma irradiation, *Radiat. Res.*, 62, 145, 1975.
100. Muggia, F. M., Ghossein, N. A., and Wohl, H., Eosinophilia following radiation therapy, *Oncology*, 27, 118, 1973.
101. Ghossein, N. A., Bosworth, J. L., Stacey, P., Muggia, F. M., and Krishnaswamy, V., Radiation-related eosinophilia, correlation with delayed hypersensitivity, lymphocyte count, and survival in patients treated by curative radiotherapy, *Radiology*, 117, 413, 1975.
102. Kennealey, G. T. and Mitchell, M., Factors that influence the therapeutic response, in *Cancer. A Comprehensive Treatise*, Vol. 5, Becker, F., Ed., Plenum Press, New York, 1977, 3.
103. Allen, J. C., Infection complicating neoplastic disease and cytotoxic therapy, in *Infection and the Compromised Host*, Allen, J. C., Ed., Williams & Wilkins, Baltimore, 1976, 151.
104. Harris, C. C., The carcinogenicity of anticancer drugs, a hazard in man, *Cancer (Philadelphia)*, 37, 1014, 1976.
105. Campbell, A. C., Hersey, P., Mac Lennan, I. C. M., Kay, H. E. M., Pike, M. C., and the Medical Research Councils' Working Party on Leukaemia in Childhood, Immunosuppressive consequences of radiotherapy and chemotherapy in patients with acute lymphoblastic leukaemia, *Br. Med. J.*, 2, 385, 1973.
106. Leventhal, B. G., Cohen, P., and Triem, S. C., Effect of chemotherapy on the immune response in acute leukemia, a review, in *Immunological Parameters of Host-Tumor Relationships*, Vol. 3, Weiss, D., Ed., Academic Press, New York, 1974, 52.
107. Mitchell, M. S., Evaluation of immunosuppressive agents, in *Antineoplastic and Immunosuppressive Agents*, Vol. 1, Sartorelli, A. C. and Johns, D. G., Eds., Springer-Verlag, New York, 1974, 555.
108. Hersh, E. M., Immunosuppressive agents, in *Antineoplastic and Immunosuppressive Agents*, Vol. 1, Sartorelli, A. C. and Johns, D. G., Eds., Springer-Verlag, New York, 1974, 577.
109. Gutterman, J. U., Chemoimmunotherapy of human cancer: the need for a unified drug development program, *Cancer Immunol. Immunother.*, 3, 153, 1978.
110. Hersh, E. M., Gutterman, J. U., Mavligit, G. M., Granatek, C. H., Rossen, R. D., Rios, A., Goldstein, A. L., Patt, Y. Z., Rivera, E., Richman, S. P., Bottino, J. C., Farquhar, D., Morris, D., and Ezaki, K., Clinical rationale for immunotherapy and its role in cancer treatment, in *Immunotherapy of Human Cancer*, M. D. Anderson Hospital and Tumor Institute 22nd Annual Clinical Conference on Cancer, University of Texas System Cancer Center, Raven Press, New York, 1978, 83.
111. Woodruff, M. F. A., Clunie, G. J. A., McBride, W. H., McCormack, R. J. M., Walbaum, P. R., and James, K., The effect of intravenous and intramuscular injection of *Corynebacterium parvum*, in *Corynebacterium parvum. Applications in Experimental and Clinical Oncology*, Halpern, B., Ed., Plenum Press, New York, 1975, 383.
112. McCormick, K. J., Stehlin, J. S., de Ipolyi, P. D., Giovanella, B. C., Ruzich, J. V., and Anderson, R. F., Monocyte function during systemic hyperthermia induced by immunochemotherapy with *Corynebacterium parvum*, in *Proc. Am. Assoc. Cancer Res.*, Vol. 20, Weinhouse, S., Ed., Waverly Press, Baltimore, 1979, 155.
113. Hersh, E. M., Murphy, S., Gutterman, J., Quesada, J., Gschwind, C., and Morgan, J., Some host defense modifying effects of intravenous microbial adjuvants, in *Proc. Am. Assoc. Cancer Res.*, Vol. 20, Weinhouse, S., Ed., Waverly Press, Baltimore, 1979, 144.
114. Israel, L., Edelstein, R., and Samak, R., Some new approaches to cancer immunotherapy in man, in *Immunotherapy of Human Cancer*, M. D. Anderson Hospital and Tumor Institute 22nd Annual Clinical Conference on Cancer, University of Texas System Cancer Center, Raven Press, New York, 1978, 363.
115. Wybran, J. and Staquet, M. J., Eds., *Clinical Tumor Immunology*, Pergamon Press, New York, 1976.
116. Hager, J. C. and Heppner, G. H., Evaluation of specific immune reactivity in human patients with solid cancers, in *The Handbook of Cancer Immunology*, Vol. 4, Waters, H., Ed., Garland STPM Press, New York, 1978, 195.
117. Rose, N. R. and Friedman, H., Eds., *Manual of Clinical Immunology*, American Society for Microbiology, Washington, D.C., 1976.

118. **Wang, A.-C.**, The structure of immunoglobulins, in *Basic & Clinical Immunology*, Fudenberg, H. H., Stites, D. P., Caldwell, J. L., and Wells, J. V., Eds., Lange Medical Publ., Los Altos, CA, 1976, chap. 2.

119. **Cochran, A. J., Mackie, R. M., Grant, R. M., Ross, C. E., Connell, M. D., Sandilands, G., Whaley, K., Hoyle, D. E., and Jackson, A. M.**, An examination of the immunology of cancer patients, *Int. J. Cancer*, 18, 298, 1976.

120. **Smith, R. T.**, Possibilities and problems of immunologic intervention in cancer, *N. Engl. J. Med.*, 287, 439, 1972.

121. **Davis, N. C. and Ho, M.**, Quantitation of immunoglobulins, in *Manual of Clinical Immunology*, Rose, N. R. and Friedman, H., Eds., American Society for Microbiology, Washington, D.C., 1976, chap. 2.

122. **Gewurz, H. and Suyehira, L. A.**, Complement, in *Manual of Clinical Immunology*, Rose, N. R. and Friedman, H., Eds., American Society for Microbiology, Washington, D.C., 1976, chap. 4.

123. **Oppenheim, J. J. and Schecter, B.**, Lymphocyte transformation, in *Manual of Clinical Immunology*, Rose, N. R. and Friedman, H., Eds., American Society for Microbiology, Washington, D.C., 1976, chap. 9.

124. **Winchester, R. J. and Ross, G.**, Methods for enumerating lymphocyte populations, in *Manual of Clinical Immunology*, Rose, N. R. and Friedman, H., Eds., American Society for Microbiology, Washington, D.C., 1976, chap. 7.

125. **Williams, R. C. and Messner, R. P.**, Alterations in T- and B-cells in human disease states, *Ann. Rev. Med.*, 26, 181, 1975.

126. **Wybran, J. and Fudenberg, H. H.**, Thymus-derived rosette-forming cells in various human disease states: cancer, lymphoma, bacterial and viral infections, and other diseases, *J. Clin. Invest.*, 52, 1026, 1973.

127. **Chao, W. and Yokoyama, M. M.**, Determination of B lymphocyte populations using antibody-coated polyacrylamide beads, *Clin. Chim. Acta*, 78, 79, 1977.

128. **Gupta, S., Good, R. A., and Siegel, F. P.**, Rosette-formation with mouse erythrocytes. II. A marker for human B and non-T lymphocytes, *Clin. Exp. Immunol.*, 25, 319, 1976.

129. **Koski, I. R., Poplack, D. G., and Blaese, R. M.**, A nonspecific esterase stain for the identification of monocytes and macrophages, in *In Vitro Methods in Cell-mediated and Tumor Immunity*, Bloom, B. R. and David, J. R., Eds., Academic Press, New York, 1976, 359.

130. **Douglas, S. D.**, Cells involved in immune responses, in *Basic & Clinical Immunology*, Fudenberg, H. H., Stites, D. P., Caldwell, J. L., and Wells, J. V., Eds., Lange Medical Publ., Los Altos, CA, 1976, 81.

131. **Pauly, J. L., Sokal, J. E., and Han, T.**, Whole-blood culture technique for functional studies of lymphocyte reactivity to mitogens, antigens, and homologous lymphocytes, *J. Lab. Clin. Med.*, 82, 500, 1973.

132. **O'Leary, J., Reinsmoen, N., and Yanis, E. J.**, Mixed lymphocyte reaction, in *Manual of Clinical Immunology*, Rose, N. R. and Friedman, H., Eds., American Society for Microbiology, Washington, D.C., 1976, chap. 109.

133. **Mac Lennan, I. C. M., Campbell, A. C., and Gale, D. G. L.**, Quantitation of K cells, in *In Vitro Methods in Cell-Mediated and Tumor Immunity*, Bloom, B. R. and David, J. R., Eds., Academic Press, New York, 1976, 511.

134. **Cohen, S., David, J., Feldmann, M., Glade, P. R., Mayer, M., Oppenheim, J. J., Papermaster, B. W., Pick, E., Pierce, C. W., Rosentreich, D. L., and Waksman, B. H.**, Current state of studies of mediators of cellular immunity: a progress report, *Cell. Immunol.*, 33, 233, 1977.

135. **Territo, M. C., Golde, D. W., and Cline, M. J.**, Macrophage activation and function, in *Manual of Clinical Immunology*, Rose, N. R. and Friedman, H., Eds., American Society for Microbiology, Washington, D.C., 1976, chap. 16.

136. **Currie, G. A. and Eccles, S. A.**, Serum lysozyme as a marker of host resistance. I. Production by macrophages resident in rat sarcomata, *Br. J. Cancer*, 33, 51, 1976.

137. **Lieberman, R. and Fudenberg, H. H.**, Effects of BCG on lysozyme and "active" T cells in patients with malignant melanoma: a preliminary study, *Clin. Immunol. Immunopathol.*, 12, 191, 1979.

138. **Stossel, T. P. and Taylor, M.**, Phagocytosis in *Manual of Clinical Immunology*, Rose, N. R. and Friedman, H., Eds., American Society for Microbiology, Washington, D.C., 1976, chap. 17.

139. **Vose, B. M. and Moore, M.**, Reactivity of peripheral blood leukocytes against human foetal cells. II. Cytotoxic potential of preparations enriched or depleted of different leukocyte populations, *Int. J. Cancer*, 19, 34, 1977.

140. **Eilber, F. R. and Morton, D. L.**, Impaired immunologic reactivity and recurrence following cancer surgery, *Cancer (Philadelphia)*, 25, 362, 1970.

141. **Spitler, L. E.**, Delayed hypersensitivity skin testing, in *Manual of Clinical Immunology*, Rose, N. R. and Friedman, H., Eds., American Society for Microbiology, Washington, D.C., 1976, chap. 6.

142. **Sever, J. L.**, Application of a microtechnique to viral serological investigations, *J. Immunol.*, 88, 320, 1962.

143. McCormick, K. J., Van Hoosier, G. L., Jr., and Trentin, J. J., Attempts to find human adenovirus type-12 tumor antigens in human tumors, *J. Natl. Cancer Inst.,* 40, 255, 1968.

144. McCormick, N. K., McCormick, K. J., and Trentin, J. J., Microtechnique for indirect immunofluorescence, *Appl. Microbiol.,* 26, 1015, 1973.

145. Hanks, J. H. and Wallace, J. H., Determination of cell viability, *Proc. Soc. Exp. Biol. Med.,* 98, 188, 1958.

146. Twomey, J. J., Rossen, R. D., Lewis, V. M., Morgan, A. C., and McCormick, K. J., Rheumatoid factor positive plasma and humoral cytotoxicity to malignant melanoma, *Cancer (Philadelphia),* 41, 1307, 1978.

147. Sung, J. S., Shizuya, H., Black, D. D., and Mumford, D. M., A radiomicroassay for cytotoxic antibody to human spermatozoa. Quantification by tritiated actinomycin D, *Clin. Exp. Immunol.,* 27, 469, 1977.

148. Lewis, M. G., Possible immunological factors in human malignant melanoma in Uganda, *Lancet,* 2, 921, 1967.

149. Crowle, A. J., *Immunodiffusion,* 2nd ed., Academic Press, New York, 1973.

150. Gupta, R. K., Golub, S. H., and Morton, D. L., Correlation between tumor burden and anticomplementary activity in sera from cancer patients, *Cancer Immunol. Immunother.,* 6, 63, 1979.

151. Theofilopoulos, A. N. and Dixon, F. J., Immune complexes in human sera detected by the Raji cell radioimmune assay, in *In Vitro Methods in Cell-Mediated and Tumor Immunology,* Bloom, B. R. and David, J. R., Eds., Academic Press, NewYork, 1976, 555.

152. Zubler, R. H. and Lambert, P.-H., The ^{125}I-Clq binding test for the detection of soluble immune complexes, in *In Vitro Methods in Cell-Mediated and Tumor Immunology,* Bloom, B. R. and David, J. R., Eds., Academic Press, New York, 1976, 565.

153. Kyle, R. A., Diagnosis of monoclonal gammopathies, in *Manual of Clinical Immunology,* Rose, N. R. and Friedman, H., Eds., American Society for Microbiology, Washington, D.C., 1976, chap. 98.

154. McIntire, K. R. and Waldmann, T. A., Alpha-fetoprotein in *Manual of Clinical Immunology,* Rose, N. R. and Friedman, H., Eds., American Society for Microbiology, Washington, D.C., 1976, chap. 100.

155. Zamcheck, N. and Kupchik, H. Z., Summary of clinical use and limitations of the carcinoembryonic antigen assay and some methodological considerations, in *Manual of Clinical Immunology,* Rose, N. R. and Friedman, H., Eds., American Society for Microbiology, Washington, D.C., 1976, chap. 99.

156. Savel, H., Effect of autologous tumor extracts on cultured human peripheral blood lymphocytes, *Cancer (Philadelphia),* 24, 56, 1969.

157. Gutterman, J. U., Mavligit, G. M., Hunter, C. Y., and Hersh, E. M., Lymphocyte transformation against human tumor antigens, in *In Vitro Methods in Cell-Mediated and Tumor Immunity,* Bloom, B. R. and David, J. R., Eds., Academic Press, New York, 1976, 587.

158. Vanky, F. and Stjernsward, J., Lymphocyte stimulation test for detection of tumor-specific reactivity in humans, in *In Vitro Methods in Cell-Mediated and Tumor Immunity,* Bloom, B. R. and David, J. R., Eds., Academic Press, New York, 1976, 597.

159. Bean, M. A., Bloom, B. R., Cerottini, J. -C., David, J. A., Herberman, R. B., Lawrence, H. S., Mac Lennen, I. C. M., Perlmann, P., and Stutman, O., Evaluation of *in vitro* methods for assaying tumor immunity, in *In Vitro Methods in Cell-Mediated and Tumor Immunity,* Bloom, B. R. and David J. R., Eds., Academic Press, New York, 1976, 27.

160. Takasugi, M. and Klein, E., A microassay for cell-mediated immunity, *Transplantation,* 9, 219, 1970.

161. McCoy, J. L., Dean, J. H., Cannon, G. B., Maurer, B. A., Oldham, R. K., and Herberman, R. B., Detection of cell-mediated immunity against tumor-associated antigens of human breast carcinoma by migration inhibition and lymphocyte-stimulation assays, in *Clinical Tumor Immunology,* Wybran, J. and Staquet, M. J., Eds., Pergamon Press, New York, 1976, 77.

162. Powell, A., Sloss, A. M., Smith, R. N., and Murrell, H., Antigenic specificity and cellular mechanisms in leukocyte adherence inhibition analysis of immunity to simple proteins and hapten-protein conjugates, *Cancer Res.,* 39, 570, 1979.

163. Goldrosen, M. H. and Howell, J. H., Eds., International Workshop on Leukocyte Adherence Inhibition, *Cancer Res.,* 39, No. 2, Part 2, 1979.

164. Weese, J. L., Herberman, R. B., Hollinshead, A. C., Cannon, G. B., Keels, M., Kibrite, A., Morales, A., Char, D. H., and Oldham, R. K., Specificity of delayed cutaneous hypersensitivity reactions to extracts of human tumor cells, *J. Natl. Cancer Inst.,* 60, 255, 1978.

165. Black, M. M. and Leis, H. P., Jr., Cellular responses to autologous breast cancer tissue, sequential observations, *Cancer (Philadelphia),* 32, 384, 1973.

166. McCormick, K. J., Stehlin, J. S., Jr., Giovanella, B. C., de Ipolyi, P. D., and Clark, C. A., unpublished observations, 1979.

Chapter 3

IMMUNOCOMPETENCE IN HEAD AND NECK CANCER PATIENTS UNDERGOING RADIOTHERAPY

Vernon K. Jenkins

TABLE OF CONTENTS

I. INTRODUCTION

Immunity in man relates to a process involving several mechanisms to protect an intact host from invasion by matter that is recognized as foreign. Man has, in general, inherited nonspecific or innate immune capacities which include inflammatory and antimicrobial reactions from invertebrate ancestors. Specific or adaptive immunity, on the other hand, involves cell-mediated and humoral processes which are largely evolutionary refinements. Adaptive immunity in man is derived from lymphoid tissue.

This chapter will address several aspects of specific and nonspecific immunity in patients with neoplasms of the head and neck and the effects of radiotherapeutic procedures on the capacities of such patients to respond immunologically. Radiotherapists have long been aware of the lymphopenia that ensues in patients treated locally with radiation and indeed routinely monitor levels of lymphocytes in patients under treatment to avoid severe depletion of peripheral blood lymphocytes. Only in recent years, however, have innovative techniques become available to assess numbers and function of subpopulations of lymphocytes. The newer methods of assessment of immunocompetence as well as standard techniques for measuring delayed hypersensitivity are varied and involve both in vitro measurements of lymphocyte reactivity and in vivo measurements of cell-mediated immunity. A discussion of the different methods of assessment of immunocompetence is made in Chapter 2.

II. SIGNIFICANCE OF IMMUNOCOMPETENCE

Evidence continues to accumulate indicating that the cells of most human tumors are recognized as foreign and that the host has the capacity to react immunologically against neoplastic cells. Therefore, immunological recognition and reaction to malignant cells by the cancer host may play an important role in the control of oncogenesis.[1-3] Clinical demonstration of the importance of the role of immunity in cancer development was the observation that noncancer patients who were immunosuppressed for organ transplantation or patients with primary immunodeficiency disease developed a much higher incidence of cancer than did the normal population.[4]

Furthermore, an increasing amount of data suggests that immunological competence plays an important role in the response of patients to cancer therapy. Depressed cellular immunity has been correlated with a poor clinical course for some cancer patients despite aggressive treatment.[5-10] On the other hand, near normal cellular immunity and recovery of immune reactivity shortly after treatment have been correlated with a superior clinical course.[9-13] Observations of untoward consequences of immunodeficiency in cancer patients have focused attention on the effect of cancer treatments on host immunity. Of general concern is whether chemotherapy, radiotherapy, surgery, or a combination of these modalities is immunosuppressive and may facilitate growth of residual or metastatic foci thus negating benefits of the therapy.[14-19] Both acute and delayed effects of therapy on host immunity may be relevant to this concern. Of particular interest in this chapter is the correlation of immunocompetence, before and after radiation therapy, in patients with neoplasms of the head and neck with clinical outcome for the patients.

III. IMMUNODEFICIENCY IN UNTREATED PATIENTS

Patients with cancerous lesions of the head and neck usually have normal numbers or only slightly depressed numbers of lymphocytes in their peripheral blood before therapy.[13,20-24] Since, however, the total pool of lymphocytes is comprised of a heterogeneous population of cells with differing functions, it is conceivable that patients

Table 1
PERCENTAGES AND NUMBERS OF PERIPHERAL BLOOD T CELLS IN HEAD AND NECK CANCER PATIENTS

%T Rosettes		T Cells/mm³		
Normal controls	Untreated patients	Normal controls	Untreated patients	Ref.
71.5	62.5	1478	1126	8
63.2	52.0	1745	888	9
74.9	52.4	1460	861	26
55.0	50.5	—	—	21
—	—	1875	1283	27

Table 2
DNCB REACTIONS IN PATIENTS WITH HEAD AND NECK CANCER

Normal control	Untreated patients			
%Positive	Status of lesion	No. patients tested	%Positive	Ref.
95	Localized	86	64	6
	Locally advanced or disseminated	34	15	
		120	50	
—	Localized (T_{1-2})	24	67	28
	(T_{3-4})	6	17	
	Locally advanced (N_{1-3})	30	50	
	Disseminated	3	33	
		63	52	
95	Localized (T_{1-2})	47	70	27
	(T_3)	19	32	
	Locally advanced (N_{1-3})	67	54	
	Disseminated	4	50	
		137	56	
96.5	Localized and with one node	8	75	9
	Locally advanced	16	44	
		24	54	

may be deficient in levels of one or more of the subpopulations of lymphocytes and indeed have suppressed immune responsiveness. Further, subpopulations may be present in normal or near normal numbers, but a given number of cells may be deficient in capacity to respond immunologically. The question of numbers of (or levels of) subpopulations of lymphocytes is usually approached by evaluation of peripheral blood lymphocytes forming rosettes with sensitized or unsensitized sheep red blood cells.[8,9,26] Although the numbers determined for these rosette-forming cells (RFC) are dependent on function (rosette forming ability), they are thought to represent thymus-derived lymphocytes (T cells) and bone marrow-derived lymphocytes (B cells), and their levels have been correlated with host immunocompetence.[19,25] The percentage of

T cell rosettes is consistently less in patients with head and neck lesions than in the normal control population (Table 1). Likewise, the numbers of T cells/mm³ for the patients are depressed by one third to one half compared to the numbers in the normal control population,[9,20,26] a deficit that may become greater during clinical progression of the disease.[27] There is also some evidence that B cell levels are less by about one half in patients with head and neck lesions than in normal controls.[9,27] Other evidence, presented as percentage of B cells, does not indicate a B cell deficiency.[20]

The question of impairment of immunological reactivity of lymphocyte subpopulations is approached by both in vivo and in vitro assays. In vivo measurement of delayed hypersensitivity has usually been determined by the patient's response to common microbial skin-test antigens and to application of de novo antigens such as dinitrochlorobenzene (DNCB). In vitro lymphocyte transformation tests with the mitogens phytohemagglutinin (PHA) and concanavalin A (ConA) have been used by several investigators to measure function of T lymphocytes and the response to pokeweed mitogen (PWM) to assess the function of B lymphocytes.

Whereas about 95% of persons in normal health react positively to application of DNCB, only 50 to 56% of patients with head and neck lesions are reactive (Table 2). The deficit appears to be related to the extent of the disease in that about two thirds of the patients with small localized lesions are reactive, but only about one third or less of patients with bulky lesions are reactive.[6,27,28] That about one half of the patients with head and neck lesions are deficient in cell-mediated responses as indicated by DNCB skin reactions is not clearly supported by studies involving sensitivity to application of recall antigens. Although Eilber et al.[6] using a battery of skin-test antigens found that only two thirds of patients with malignancies of the head and neck were responsive to one or more recall antigens, the rate was not significantly less than the 85% reaction rate of normal controls. Other investigators also found reactivity to one or more microbial antigens in patients to range from 69 to 89%.[9,22,28,29] It should be noted that positive reactions to these tests require not only the viability of immunologically reactive cells but also prior exposure to the antigen, or immunologic memory. Failure to react to a single antigen in the battery of commonly encountered antigens is strong evidence of immunologic anergy.[30] Although the incidence of anergy in the total group of patients which includes patients in all clinical stages was not significantly increased, there is some evidence, although not incontrovertible, to indicate that patients with advanced disease are more likely to be anergic. Stefani et al.[9] found that all of 12 patients with localized lesions or only one positive lymph node reacted to two or more recall antigens and, in contrast, only 7 of 16 (44%) patients with two or more involved lymph nodes reacted to two or more antigens. Similarly, Clement and Kramer[29] also presented data showing that 8 of 10 patients with localized lesions had positive reactions to two or more recall antigens, but only 3 of 8 patients with advanced lesions had positive reactions to two or more antigens. On the other hand, Eilber et al.[6] did not find a difference in skin-test reactions between patients with small localized lesions and patients with advanced disease.

There is strong evidence to indicate that the capacity of circulating lymphocytes to undergo blastogenic transformation in vitro in response to T cell mitogens is depressed in patients with head and neck lesions (Table 3). Wanebo et al.[27] showed that the response to PHA for purified lymphocytes from patients was only about 56% and ConA response was about 66% of the responses of lymphocytes from controls. Several other investigators using PHA or ConA to stimulate lymphocytes in vitro have also shown patients to have a deficit in T cell responses with values ranging from 48 to 75% of control values.[10,13,20,21,27,31,32] Whether the degree of suppression of responsiveness to T cell mitogens is related to clinical progression is equivocal, Silverman et al.[31] found that the mean PHA response for patients with clinical Stage I lesions of the

Table 3
LYMPHOCYTE RESPONSES TO T CELL MITOGENS FOR PATIENTS WITH HEAD AND NECK CANCER

Mean Response in Vitro of Peripheral Blood
Lymphocytes

Expressed as Percent of Control Response

PHA		ConA		
No. patients	% of Control	No. patients	% of Control	Ref.
48	$\simeq 56$	31	66	27
11	56	—	—	21
9	57	9	48	20
24	64	—	—	10
106	73	106	50	13[a]
44	75	—	—	31

[a] Whole-blood cultures.

larynx were not less than the control response, but for patients with Stages II to IV laryngeal lesions the PHA response was only 71% of the control response. Patients with Stages I and II oral and oropharynx lesions were equally depressed to about 72% of control response. Wanebo et al.[27] present the strongest evidence to indicate that degree of suppression relates to clinical progression. The investigators found that mean PHA and ConA responses for patients with small squamous cell tumors, no lymph node involvement and no metastases ($T_1N_0M_0$) were 1 SD below the responses in the control group and patients with larger tumors ($T_3N_0M_0$) had PHA and ConA responses that were more than 1 SD below values for patients with T_1 lesions. In contradistinction, the authors also found that patients with one lymph node involved ($T_{1-4}N_1M_0$) had mean mitogenic responses that were comparable to patients with T_1 lesions. Patients with N_2 lesions, however, had the greatest suppression in response of lymphocytes to the mitogens. Jenkins et al.[33] using PHA and ConA in whole-blood cultures did not find a relationship between mitogenic responsiveness and neoplastic progression.

In contrast to a deficit in T cell reactivity it appears that in vitro responses of lymphocytes to PWM are not suppressed pretreatment for patients with cancer of the head and neck.[13,27]

Speculation as to the cause of the T cell deficiency in head and neck cancer patients as indicated by reduced T cell levels, suppressed responses in vitro of lymphocytes to T cell mitogens, and a reduced DNCB reactivity involves several influences such as tumor burden, a factor(s) in the serum of patients that may interfere with immune response, and the general condition of the patient. Patients with head and neck cancer have a high incidence of history of alcohol consumption and cigarette smoking.[28,31] Lundy et al.[34] have shown that patients with acute alcoholism have marked depression of lymphocyte stimulation by PHA and ConA but not by PWM. Straus et al.[35] have shown that the incidence of DNCB anergy in patients with Laenner's cirrhosis is greater than 30%. Although alcohol consumption may be contributory, detailed studies of the effects of rate of alcohol consumption on cellular immunity in head and neck cancer patients have not been reported. Chronic cigarette smoking is also implicated by studies in experimental animals that show depressed PHA responsiveness of peripheral blood lymphocytes after chronic exposure to cigarette smoke.[36] However, preliminary reports on in vitro lymphocyte responses show no difference between smokers and nonsmokers.[37,38] Alcohol and cigarette smoking may both contribute to malnourishment which in turn produces debilitation. Severely debilitated patients may have lymphopenia and reduced lymphocyte responses in vivo and in vitro.[39]

Another possible mechanism for reduced responsiveness of lymphocytes is that some inhibitory factor is present in the sera of these patients and interferes with lymphocyte response. Catalona et al.[1] and Whittaker et al.[40] have described such factors in the sera of patients with other types of neoplasms. Support for such a mechanism is derived from studies in which serum or plasma from patients with head and neck lesions was placed in cultures of normal lymphocytes and a decrease in responses of the normal cells to PHA and ConA was noted. Twomey et al.[41] found that serum from patients with squamous cell carcinomas of the head and neck significantly inhibited normal lymphocyte reactivity to PHA. Similarly, Jenkins et al.[42] found that plasma from head and neck cancer patients significantly suppressed responses of normal lymphocytes to PHA and ConA, but not to PWM. Characterization of the factor(s) that may be inhibitory have not been made. The concept that alpha globulins may have an "immuno-regulatory" function combined with evidence by Hughes[43] and Mandel et al.[44] that show elevated IgA levels in patients with head and neck lesions, make alpha globulins reasonable candidates for inhibitory factors in the serum.

IV. RADIOTHERAPY AND THE IMMUNE RESPONSE

Radiation therapy, administered as a single modality or in combination with surgery or chemotherapy, plays a vital role in the treatment of patients with cancer of the head and neck. The therapeutic effectiveness of radiation therapy depends on the destructive effects of the radiation on the cancer cell, but also on the damage of the normal cells within the volume of tissue through which ionizing radiation passes.

Early and late sequelae of irradiation on immunity probably depends on several factors including total dosage, rapidity of treatment, the volume of lymphoid tissue in the treatment fields, recovery capacity of lymphoid tissue involved, age and condition of the patient, and individual tolerance to this therapeutic modality. Several of these factors are taken into consideration when clinical stage is considered. For example, patients with advanced lesions have more bulky tumors and are treated to a greater volume, including a greater volume of lymphoid tissue, than are patients with small localized lesions. The rate of delivery of the treatment and total dosage are about the same for the total group of patients.

Radiation therapy for head and neck cancer results in an acute decrease in numbers of circulating lymphocytes to about 50 to 75% of pretreatment numbers followed by a gradual recovery (Table 4). The degree of depression and the rate of recovery are related to several factors one of which may be the volume of tissue that was exposed to radiation. Since the time of the first reports of lymphopenia following postoperative radiation therapy for breast carcinoma, several possible causes of the depression have been proposed to explain the effects of radiotherapy on the immune system. Many of the explanations implicated irradiation of the thymus gland and subsequent deficiency in cellular immunity. However, several authors[7,45-47] have reported lymphopenia and decreased in vitro lymphocyte responses in patients following irradiation to fields that did not include the thymus gland. Their data indicate that irradiation to a localized area that does not include the thymus can have a profound effect on the number of lymphocytes circulating in the blood, probably as a direct result of radiation interaction with lymphocytes that reside in or circulate through the volume of tissue exposed. That the degree of lymphopenia in patients with head and neck cancer is related to

Table 4
EFFECTS OF RADIOTHERAPY ON NUMBERS
OF PERIPHERAL BLOOD LYMPHOCYTES

Mean number of lymphocytes/mm^3
(No. of patients)

Untreated patients	Time after treatment	Treated patients	Percent change	Ref.
2140 (106)	End of treat	1125 (90)	↓48	13
	1 Month	1380 (45)	↓36	
	2—3 Months	1500 (48)	↓30	
	7—12 Months	1500 (64)	↓30	
	19—24 Months	1600 (15)	↓25	
	> 24 Months	1950 (35)	↓9	
2046 (13)	End of treat	1558 (13)	↓24	22
	2 Weeks	1671 (13)	↓18	
	2 Months	1719 (13)	↓16	
	6 Months	2120 (13)	↑4	
2747 (11)	End of treat	2089 (10)	↓24	23
	3 Months	— (9)	↓ ≃ 24	
	6—9 Months	— (4)	↓ ≃ 24	
1714 (11)	1 Month	683 (11)	↓60	21

Table 5
EFFECTS OF RADIATION THERAPY ON T AND B CELL LEVELS IN
PATIENTS WITH HEAD AND NECK CANCER

Numbers/mm^3 and Percent of Rosette Forming Cells (RFC)

	Pretreat	End of treat	1-2 Mos. post	3 Mos. post	6-9 Mos. post	> 48 Mos. post	> 60 Mos. post	Ref.
T-RFC	888		419	503	398			9
	52.0%		42.6%	44.8%	46.9%			
T-RFC	≃ 1911	≃ 1523		≃ 1370	≃ 1128			23
	69.6%	72.9%		65.6%	54.0%			
T-RFC	907		305					21
	50.5%		43.2%					
T-RFC	861		≃ 1080					26
	52.4%		59.8%					
T-RFC						1001		24
						55.8%		
T-RFC	1126						970	8
	62.5%						58.2%	
B-RFC	193		124	144	115			9
	11.7%		12.1%	12.7%	13.6%			
B-RFC	≃ 1083	≃ 985		≃ 965	≃ 940			23
	39.4%	47.2%		46.2%	45.0%			

volume of tissue treated is supported by studies of Jenkins et al.[33] who showed that during radiation treatment patients with localized lesions who received radiation to relatively smaller bilateral fields of the face and neck experienced only a 35% decrease in lymphocyte count, but patients with advanced lesions and radiation to larger fields that included the supraclavicular area experienced a 67% decrease in lymphocyte count.

Both T and B cells are reportedly affected by radiation therapy in patients with several histological types of tumors located at various anatomical sites.[19,47,48] Few reports have been made on percentages and numbers of T and B cells in the blood of patients after radiation treatment for head and neck cancer, but most of the studies that have been done showed a further decrease in the level of T cells after radiation up to 6 to 9 months (Table 5). An exception is the study by Olkowski and Wilkins[26] who showed a significant increase in the percentages and levels of T cells in patients 4 to 8 weeks after radiotherapy. T cell levels and percentages in patients who lived beyond 4 years and who were considered cured of their disease were not decreased compared with values for patients tested before radiation therapy.[8,24] B cell percentages and levels were not significantly reduced by the radiation treatment for patients who were followed up to 6 to 9 months after treatment.[9,20,23] The data that indicate that the B cell levels are not decreased in head and neck cancer patients are in contrast to a report by Blomgren et al.[49] who found that lymphopenia in patients with mammary gland carcinoma involved rather the B cell population as reflected by B cell rosettes.

Numbers of lymphocytes and numbers and percentages of T and B cells after radiation treatment may be significant, but an important question is whether the treatment further compromises the capacity of the patients to function immunologically. A number of studies in patients with solid tumors at other anatomical sites indicate that although T or B cell numbers recover in radiation-treated patients the lymphocytes may be abnormal in their function.

In a study of 45 patients, 6 of whom were patients with head and neck lesions, Gross et al.[50] concluded that cancericidal Cobalt-60 radiation did not affect the rate of DNCB response. In contrast, Stefani et al.[9] using a larger number of head and neck cancer patients found that their rate of DNCB reactivity was decreased for up to 6 months after radiotherapy (Table 6). Cell-mediated immunity as indicated by in vivo reactions to common skin-test antigens did not appear to be altered during or up to 1 month after radiation treatment, but was suppressed at 3 and 6 months after radiotherapy (Table 6). Although the evidence is not incontrovertible, it appears that fewer patients were able to mount delayed hypersensitivity reactions 3 to 6 months after radiation therapy for head and neck lesions than were capable of reactions before radiotherapy. A question remains as to whether the decrease in hypersensitivity is due to radiation, due to normal progression of the malignancy or both. The relatively short interval between radiation and decrease in rate of patients that react positively suggests that radiation is contributory.

Pursuant to the question of effects of radiotherapy on functional immunity in head and neck cancer patients, several investigators have tested in vitro responses of peripheral blood lymphocytes to T cell and B cell mitogens (Table 7). Jenkins et al.[13] using whole-blood cultures and several other investigators[10,21-24,31,32] using purified lymphocytes in culture have found that by the end of radiation treatment the in vitro responses of lymphocytes to PHA and ConA are reduced to 50 to 76% of values for patients before treatment. Such deficits are attributed to effects of radiation on lymphoid cells within the irradiated volume and indicate reduced T cell capacity in the patients. There was little or no recovery in lymphocyte responses to T cell mitogens for the patients within 30 days after treatment. Several investigators[10,13,22,23] found an increase in T cell responses about 6 months after treatment, but Stefani and Kerman,[10] Jenkins et al.,[13] and Tarpley et al.[24] found deficits extending to about 1 year, more than 2 years and more than 4 years, respectively. Silverman et al.,[31] on the other hand, found that the mean PHA response for 33 patients who were tested more than 48 months after radiation treatment and who were cured of their head and neck carcinoma was comparable to the PHA response for patients before therapy. Responses to PWM were also suppressed during treatment to 40% or 55% of pretreatment values.[13,22] Jenkins et al.[13] found the depression to remain for more than 24 months after treatment in patients tested at about 3-month intervals, but Slater et al.[22] found that the PWM responses were increased 6 months post-treatment to 176% of pretreatment response.

Table 6
EFFECTS OF RADIATION THERAPY ON DELAYED
HYPERSENSITIVITY IN HEAD AND NECK CANCER PATIENTS

Numbers of patients and percent positive reactions to DNCB		Numbers of patients and percent positive reaction to one or more recall antigens		
Pretreat	Post-treat	Pretreat	Post-treat	Ref.
5/6 (83%)	≥2 Months, 4/6 (67%) ≥8 Months, 4/5 (80%)			50
		16/18 (89%)	End of treat. 17/18 (94%)	29
14/23 (61%)	1 Month, 9/21 (43%) 3 Months, 7/14 (50%) 6 Months, 6/13 (46%)	21/29 (72)	1 Month, 18/22 (82%) 3 Months, 9/17 (53%) 6 Months, 9/15 (60%)	9[a]
		9/13 (69%)	During treat. 10/13 (77%) 2 Weeks, 9/13 (69%) 2 Months, 8/13 (62%) 6 Months, 6/12 (50%)	22

Patients with positive reactive to two or more antigens.

The data demonstrate that cellular immunity, as indicated by in vitro mitogenic responses, is further suppressed by radiation therapy in patients with head and neck lesions, many of whom are already immunologically deficit. Suppressed immunity may still be present for more than 4 years, but some reports indicate at least a partial recovery at 6 months and one report indicates a recovery after 48 months. The apparent disparity in the time of recovery of responses may be related to stage of neoplastic progression at the time of treatment and therefore to the volume of tissue treated. It should also be borne in mind that during the first 12 months after treatment the patient population includes those patients who will show no evidence of disease and become 5-year and 10-year cures, but also contains the population who will succumb to their disease within 12 to 18 months. Data by Jenkins et al.[13] show that although a total group of 66 patients tested 7 to 12 months after treatment had a mean PHA response that was suppressed to about 60% of the mean response for 106 patients tested before treatment, the response for 27 patients tested 7 to 12 months after treatment who had no evidence of disease and who became long-term survivors had a mean response to PHA that was 80% of pretreatment values. It is possible, therefore, that the recovery in mitogenic responses noted at about 6 months after treatment (Table 7) was in patients who also had a good clinical response. The recovery noted may have been only temporary, however, because most of the patients tested about 12 months or more after treatment were again deficient in their mitogenic responses (Table 7).

V. IMMUNOCOMPETENCE IN PREDICTING CLINICAL COURSE

Patients with carcinoma of the head and neck frequently have fewer T cells in their peripheral blood which may in part account for their decreased delayed hypersensitivity reactions to DNCB and for patients in advanced stages to a decreased response to recall antigens. Further, in vitro lymphocyte transformation tests with PHA or ConA demonstrate that lymphocyte responsiveness is depressed in untreated patients with carcinoma of the head and neck. Therapeutic irradiation depresses immunity further as indicated by decreases in T cell levels, reduction in percentage of patients with delayed hypersensitivity reactions, and suppressed in vitro responses of lymphocytes to T cell mitogens.

Table 7

EFFECTS OF RADIOTHERAPY ON IN VITRO LYMPHOCYTE RESPONSE TO MITOGENS IN HEAD AND NECK CANCER PATIENTS

Percent of Pretreatment Responses at Times after Treatment

Mitogen	End of treat	≤ 1 Mo.	2-3 Mos.	3-6 Mos.	6-9 Mos.	9-12 Mos.	12-24 Mos.	> 24 Mos.	> 48 Mos.	Ref.
PHA	50	49	48	52	60	60	44	44		13
ConA	52	52	52	52	50	50	37	44		
PWM	40	53	36	48	48	48	60	67		
PHA	62	68	67	79						22
ConA	59	62	78	102						
PWM	55	48	58	176						
PHA	55		78		71					23
ConA	76		97		96					
PHA		58	85	108		58				10
PHA		47								21
PHA									74	24
PHA									102	31

Table 8
RELATION OF PATIENT SURVIVAL AND PHA RESPONSE BEFORE RADIOTHERAPY FOR HEAD AND NECK CANCER PATIENTS

Method of testing	Relative values of response	No. patients alive/total no. at risk %	Time	Ref.
PHA Response in cultures of isolated lymphocytes	< Median for total groups of patients	6/12 (50%)[a]	1 Year	10
	> Median for total group of patients	11/12 (92%)	1 Year	
PHA Response in whole-blood cultures	< Mean for total group of patients	10/33 (30%)	18 Months	13
	> Mean for total group of patients	28/44 (64%)	18 Months	

One patient had persistent disease.

The most convincing evidence that such immunological measurements can be related to prognosis is data showing that patients who have a poor lymphocyte response to PHA prior to radiation therapy are at a much greater risk of succumbing to their disease than are patients who have a good response to PHA (Table 8). Stefani and Kerman[10] found that only 5 of 12 patients (42%) who had responses to PHA below the median for a total group of 24 patients were alive and free of disease at 1 year after treatment, whereas 11 of 12 (92%) with PHA responses above the median were alive and free of disease at 1 year. Similarly, Jenkins et al.[13] studying a larger group of patients found that only 10 of 33 patients with less than the mean PHA response for the total group of 77 patients lived beyond 18 months, but 28 of 44 patients with greater than the mean response were alive and free of disease at 18 months. Delayed hypersensitivity reactions before radiation treatment have also been correlated with rate of survival. Stefani et al.[9] found that the estimated survival rate for eight patients who failed to react to two or more skin-test antigens was about 45% at 7 months after radiotherapy, whereas the rate for 21 patients who reacted positively to two or more antigens was greater than 90% at 7 months and nearly 80% at 1 year after treatment.

A prognostic significance of post-treatment measurements of immunity for patients with head and neck lesions has not been established. Jenkins et al.[13] have shown that PHA responses before, during, and for up to 12 months after treatment for patients who had a good clinical course were significantly greater than PHA responses for patients who died from their disease within 18 months. The data appear to relate only to the "current" or "ongoing" immune status of the patients and do not indicate a change or depression in immunity prior to development of metastases or death. The inability to relate to change in responsiveness to metastases and death is evidenced by the test results on the patients who died within 18 months. All patients experienced depression of PHA responses at the end of radiation treatment to about 40% of pre-treatment responses and their values remained low until death. In order to correlate immune responses after treatment to clinical condition or prognosis, tests will have to be made on larger groups of patients and at more frequent intervals.

The question of whether further depression of immunity in head and neck cancer patients by radiation therapy compromises the patients and contributes to a poor clinical outcome has not been satisfactorily answered. The critical question may not be whether radiation treatment further suppresses immunity, but rather what is the net effect on the cancer of a modality that is immunosuppressive, but at the same time an effective tumoricidal treatment. A number of patients who had severely depressed immune responses after treatment were also successfully treated by the radiation. Another major question is how much residual immunity is required after definitive treatment. Numerous prospective studies appear warranted to determine the relative effects of radiation therapy on immunity, local tumor control, and on development of systemic metastases. Information on immunocompetence before and soon after radiation therapy may be of value to both physician and patient because it offers prospects of early evaluation of the results of treatment, points out the likelihood of occult metastases, and assists in selection of modalities for subsequent management of the disease.

REFERENCES

1. Catalona, W. J., Sample, W. F., and Chretien, P. B., Lymphocyte reactivity in cancer patients: correlation with tumor histology and clinical stage, *Cancer,* 31, 65, 1973.
2. Harris, J. and Copeland, D., Impaired immunoresponsiveness in tumor patients, *Ann. N. Y. Acad. Sci.,* 230, 56, 1974.
3. Hellstrom, I., Hellstrom, K. E., Sjorgren, H. O., and Warner, G. A., Demonstration of cell-mediated immunity to human neoplasms of various histological types, *Int. J. Cancer,* 7, 1, 1971.
4. Penn, I. and Starzl, T., Malignant tumors arising *de novo* in immunosuppressed organ transplant recipients, *Transplantation,* 14, 407, 1972.
5. Chretien, P. B., Crowder, W. L., and Gertner, H. R., Correlation of preoperative lymphocyte reactivity with the clinical course of cancer patients, *Surg. Gynecol. Obstet.,* 136, 380, 1973.
6. Eilber, F. R., Morton, D. L., and Ketcham, A. S., Immunologic abnormalities in head and neck cancer, *Am. J. Surg.,* 128, 534, 1974.
7. O'Toole, C., Perlmann, P., Unsgaard, B., Almgard, L. E., Johansson, B., Moberger, G., and Edsmyr, F., Cellular immunity to human urinary bladder carcinoma. I. Correlation to clinical stage and radiotherapy, *Int. J. Cancer,* 10, 77, 1972.
8. Potvin, C., Tarpley, J. L., and Chretien, B., Thymus-derived lymphocytes in patients with solid malignancies, *Clin. Immunol. Immunopathol.,* 3, 476, 1975.
9. Stefani, S., Kerman, R., and Abbate, J., Serial studies of immunocompetence in head and neck cancer patients undergoing radiation therapy, *Am. J. Roentgenol. Radium Ther. Nucl. Med.,* 126(4), 880, 1976.
10. Stefani, S. and Kerman, R., Lymphocyte response to phytohaemagglutinin before and after radiation therapy in patients with carcinomas of the head and neck, *J. Otolaryngol.,* 91(7), 605, 1977.
11. Dellon, A. L., Potvin, C., and Chretien, P. B., Thymus-dependent lymphocyte levels during radiation therapy for bronchogenic and esophageal carcinoma: correlations with clinical course in responders and non-responders, *Am. J. Roentgenol. Radium Ther. Nucl. Med.,* 123, 500, 1975.
12. Hersh, E. M., Whitecar, J. P., Jr., McCredie, K. B., Bodey, G. P., and Freireich, E. J., Chemotherapy, immunocompetence, immunosuppression and prognosis in acute leukemia, *N. Engl. J. Med.,* 285, 1211, 1971.
13. Jenkins, V. K., Griffiths, C. M., Ray, P., Perry, R. R., and Olson, M. H., Radiotherapy and head and neck cancer — role of lymphocyte response and clinical stage, *Arch. Otolaryngol.,* 106, 414, 1980.
14. Campbell, A. C., Hersey, P., MacLennan, I. C. M., Kay, H. E. M., Pike, M. C., and the Medical Research Council's Working Party on Leukemia in Childhood, Immunosuppressive consequences of radiotherapy and chemotherapy in patients with acute lymphoblastic leukaemia, *Br. Med. J.,* 2, 385, 1973.
15. Dao, T. L. and Kovaric, J., Incidence of pulmonary and skin metastases in women with breast cancer who received postoperative irradiation, *Surgery,* 52, 203, 1962.
16. Deodhar, S. D., Crile, G., Jr., and Esselstyn, C. B., Jr., Study of the tumor cell-lymphocyte interaction in patients with breast cancer, *Cancer,* 29, 1321, 1972.
17. Fisher, B., Slack, N. H., Cavanaugh, P. J., Gardner, B., and Ravdin, R. G., Post-operative radiotherapy in treatment of breast cancer; results of the NSABP clinical trial, *Ann. Surg.,* 172, 711, 1970.
18. Meyer, K. K., Radiation-induced lymphocyte-immune deficiency: a factor in the increased visceral metastases and decreased hormonal responsiveness of breast cancer, *Arch. Surg.,* 101, 114, 1970.
19. Stjernsward, J., Jondal, M., Vanky, F., Wigzell, H., and Sealy, R., Lymphopenia and change in distribution of human B and T lymphocytes in peripheral blood induced by irradiation for mammary carcinoma, *Lancet,* 1, 1352, 1972.

20. Lamelin, J. P., Ellouz, R., De-The, G., and Revillard, J. P., Lymphocyte subpopulations and mitogenic responses in nasopharyngeal carcinoma, prior to and after radiotherapy, *Int. J. Cancer*, 20, 723, 1977.

21. Wara, W. M., Phillips, T. L., Wara, D. W., Ammann, A. J., and Smith, V., Immunosuppression following radiation therapy for carcinoma of the nasopharynx, *Am. J. Roentgenol.*, 123, 482, 1975.

22. Slater, J. M., Ngo, E., and Lau, B. H. S., Effect of therapeutic irradiation on the immune responses, *Am. J. Roentgenol.*, 126, 313, 1976.

23. Nordman, E. and Toivanen, A., Effects of irradiation on the immune function in patients with mammary, pulmonary or head and neck carcinoma, *Acta Radiol. Oncol. Radiat. Phys. Biol.*, 17, 3, 1978.

24. Tarpley, J. L., Potvin, C., and Chretien, P. B., Prolonged depression of cellular immunity in cured laryngopharyngeal cancer patients treated with radiation therapy, *Cancer*, 35, 638, 1975.

25. Wybran, J. and Fudenberg, H. H., How clinically useful is T and B cell quantitation? *Ann. Intern. Med.*, 80, 765, 1974.

26. Olkowski, Z. L. and Wilkins, S. A., Jr., T-lymphocyte levels in the peripheral blood of patients with cancer of the head and neck, *Am. J. Surg.*, 130, 440, 1975.

27. Wanebo, H. J., Jun, M. Y., Strong, E. W., and Oettgen, H., T-cell deficiency in patients with squamous cell cancer of the head and neck, *Am. J. Surg.*, 130, 445, 1975.

28. Lundy, J., Wanebo, H., Pinsky, C., Strong, E., and Oettgen, H., Delayed hypersensitivity reactions in patients with squamous cell cancer of the head and neck, *Am. J. Surg.*, 128, 530, 1974.

29. Clement, J. A. and Kramer, S., Immunocompetence in patients with solid tumors undergoing Cobalt-60 irradiation, *Cancer*, 34, 193, 1974.

30. Southam, C. M., The immunologic status of patients with non-lymphomatous cancer, *Cancer Res.*, 28, 1435, 1968.

31. Silverman, N. A., Alexander, J. C., Jr., Hollinshead, A. C., and Chretien, P. B., Correlation of tumor burden with *in vitro* lymphocyte reactivity and antibodies to herpesvirus tumor-associated antigens in head and neck squamous carcinoma, *Cancer*, 37, 135, 1976.

32. Rafla, S., Yang, S. J., and Meleka, F., Changes in cell-mediated immunity in patients undergoing radiotherapy, *Cancer*, 41, 1076, 1978.

33. Jenkins, V. K., Ray, P., Ellis, H. N., Griffiths, C. M., Perry, R. R., and Olson, M. H., Lymphocyte response in patients with head and neck cancer — effect of clinical stage and radiotherapy, *Arch. Otolaryngol.*, 102, 596, 1976.

34. Lundy, J., Raaf, J. H., Deakins, S., Jacobs, D. A., Tsung-dao, L., Jacobowitz, D., Spear, C., Wanebo, H., and Old, L. J., Acute and chronic effects of alcohol on the immune system, *Surg. Gynecol. Obstet.*, 141, 212, 1975.

35. Straus, B., Berenyi, M. R., Huan, J., and Straus, E., Delayed hypersensitivity in alcoholic cirrhosis, *Am. J. Dig. Dis.*, 16, 509, 1971.

36. Thomas, W. R., Holt, P. G., and Keast, D., Cellular immunity in mice chronically exposed to fresh cigarette smoke, *Arch. Environ. Health*, 27, 372, 1973.

37. Suciu-Foca, N., Molinaro, A., Buda, J., and Reemtsma, K., Cellular immune responsiveness in cigarette smokers, *Lancet*, 1, 1062, 1974.

38. Whitehead, R. H., Hooper, B. E., Grunshaw, D. A., and Hughes, L. E., Cellular immune responsiveness in cigarette smokers, *Lancet*, 1, 1232, 1974.

39. Law, D. K., Dudrick, S. J., and Abdou, N. I., Immunocompetence of patients with protein-caloric malnutrition, *Ann. Intern. Med.*, 79, 545, 1973.

40. Whittaker, M. G., Rees, K., and Clark, C. G., Reduced lymphocyte transformation in breast cancer, *Lancet*, 1, 892, 1971.

41. Twomey, P. L., Catalona, W. J., and Chretien, P. B., Cellular immunity in cured cancer patients, *Cancer*, 33, 435, 1974.

42. Jenkins, V. K., Dillard, E. A., Jr., Griffiths, C. M., and Olson, M. H., Depressed lymphocyte responses in blood cultures from healthy individuals grown in plasma from cancer patients, *Res. J. Reticuloendothel. Soc. Abstr. Suppl.*, 22, 21, 1977.

43. Hughes, N. R., Serum concentrations of γG, γA, and γM immunoglobulins in patients with carcinoma, melanoma, and sarcoma, *J. Natl. Cancer Inst.*, 46, 1015, 1971.

44. Mandel, M. A., Dvorak, K., and DeCosse, J. J., Salivary immunoglobulins in patients with oropharyngeal and brochopulmonary carcinoma, *Cancer*, 31, 1408, 1973.

45. Chee, C. A., Illbery, P. L. T., and Rickinson, A. B., Depression of lymphocyte replicating ability in radiotherapy patients, *Br. J. Radiol.*, 47, 37, 1974.

46. Jenkins, V. K., Olson, M. H., Ellis, H. N., and Dillard, E. A., Jr., *In vitro* lymphocyte response of patients with uterine cancer as related to clinical stage and radiotherapy, *Gynecol. Oncol.*, 3, 191, 1975.

47. Byfield, P. E., Stratton, J. A., and Small, R., Lymphocyte response after radiotherapy, *Lancet*, 1, 309, 1974.

48. Stratton, J. A., Byfield, P. E., Byfield, J. E., Small, R. C., Benfield, J., and Pilch, Y., A comparison of the acute effects of radiation therapy, including or excluding the thymus, on the lymphocyte sub-populations of cancer patients, *J. Clin. Invest.*, 56, 88, 1975.
49. Blomgren, H., Glas, U., Melen, B., and Wasserman, J., Blood lymphocytes after radiation therapy of mammary carcinoma, *Acta Radiol. Ther. Phys. Biol.*, 13, 185, 1974.
50. Gross, L., Manfredi, O. L., and Protos, A. A., Effect of Cobalt-60 irradiation upon cell-mediated immunity, *Radiology*, 106, 653, 1973.

Chapter 4

EFFECT OF RADIATION ON IMMUNOLOGY IN BRONCHOGENIC CARCINOMA

Stefano S. Stefani, Donthamsetti S. Rao, and Julianne Souchek

Numerous tests are available to assess immunocompetence, such as in vivo tests of primary and delayed hypersensitivity and in vitro quantitation of lymphocyte blastogenesis. Are the results of these tests impaired by radiotherapy in patients with bronchogenic carcinoma? And if so, how much? The purpose of this review is to try to answer these two questions. In assessing the effect of radiation, we will always keep in mind the well-known observations of impaired immune reaction in untreated carcinoma of the lung and the additional depressing effect of poor nutrition and progression of the disease on the same immunologic profile.

Although there is now a large amount of information on the immunologic status in lung cancer, the literature is still relatively modest on the impact of radiation on immunology in the same patients. For this review, together with the contribution from other investigators, we will rely as well on our personal unpublished work.* Therapeutic doses of irradiation do not adversely affect cell-mediated immunity as gauged by the delayed hypersensitivity response to multiple skin-test antigens.[6,8,19,20] This conclusion is based on three studies in which patients were tested to multiple recall antigens before and immediately after a course of radiotherapy: the first study[6] consisted of 48 patients with solid tumors, including 9 lung cancer, the second[8] of 28 patients with bronchogenic carcinoma. Our data (Figure 1) support and extend the above observations up to 12 months post-therapy: we found no significant weakening in the skin-test responses although the mean at any time post-therapy was somewhat below the pretherapy levels.

Cell-mediated immunity as determined by a newly presented (primary) antigen, dinitrochlorobenzene (DNCB), is also not affected by cancericidal doses of Cobalt 60 radiation. Gross et al.[9] in 45 cancer patients, 9 with primary in the lung, whom he tested before, and 3 and 9 months after radiation, observed post-therapy the same response as pretherapy in 64.5%, a gain in about 20% and a loss in 15.5% of these patients.

Lymphopenia is a constant effect of radiotherapy.[2,10,11,17] Jenkins et al.[10] found a significant reduction already after doses in the order of 2000 to 2600 rad delivered with a Cobalt 60 through an anterior and posterior opposed lung fields. At the end of therapy (4000 to 5000 rad) the blood lymphocytes had decreased to 26% of the pre-

---

* Our data has been obtained from a group of 39 patients with locally advanced bronchogenic carcinoma who were randomized to receive curative radiotherapy only in a study investigating the effectiveness of concomitant BCG therapy with radiotherapy. The standard radiotherapy protocol called for daily doses of 200 rad to a total dose of 6000 rad in 6 weeks from a supervoltage source. The irradiation was delivered to the primary tumor and mediastinal lymphnodes; in rare instances the supraclavicular area was also part of the irradiation target. Before and for 1 year at various monthly intervals after the initial radiation treatment, these patients were tested with various assays to measure their cellular and humoral immunity. We computed for each immunologic assay the changes in values from pre therapy to 3, 4 to 5, 6, 9, and 12 months after initial radiation treatment (post-therapy). The pretherapy value was subtracted from each post-therapy value to give the differences (d). The mean of the difference or change (d) and the 95% confidence interval about the mean are shown in Figures 1 to 8. If the confidence interval contains zero then the change is not different at the 5% significance level from zero (= pretherapy value) at that point in time. This is equivalent to a t-test comparing the mean value of the assay at two points in time (pretherapy and post-therapy). The numbers in parantheses in each graph indicate the number of patients tested at that particular point in time. All patients had pretherapy values, and the majority had 2 to 3 tests post-therapy.

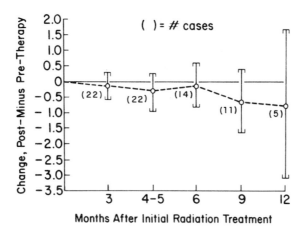

FIGURE 1.   Change in number of positive skin tests — mean and 95% confidence intervals — as a function of time postradiotherapy.

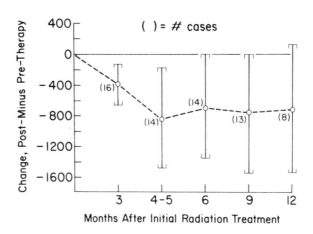

FIGURE 2.   Change in the absolute lymphocyte count — mean and 95% confidence intervals — as a function of time postradiotherapy.

therapy values. Quite similar observations were made by Prasad et al.[16a] after cumulative doses of 2025 and 4050 rad. In our study (Figure 2) the peak depression is noted at 4 to 5 months after the initial radiation treatment. From that point on, and up to 12 months, there is no discernable recovery in the lymphocyte count.

If cellular-mediated immunity, when tested in vivo, does not seem to be affected by radiation, the opposite is true when in vitro tests are used. Thus several reports[11,14,15,19] indicate that the number of total T rosette forming cells (T-RFC) — already impaired in untreated lung cancer patients — is further depressed during and immediately following radiotherapy. This depressed status persists for 12 months, the entire period of our study (Figure 3) and the difference with the pretherapy values is statistically significant for almost all points in time evaluated. The changes in the level of T cells, post-

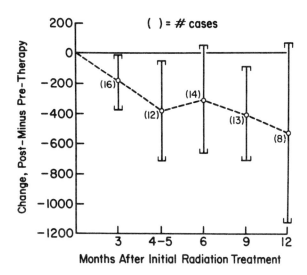

FIGURE 3. Change in the absolute number of total T lymphocytes — mean and 95% confidence intervals — as a function of time postradiotherapy.

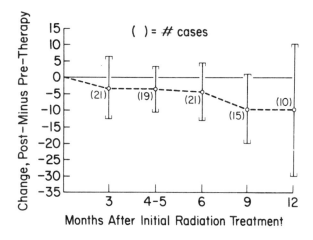

FIGURE 4. Change in the percent of total T lymphocytes — mean and 95% confidence intervals — as a function of time postradiotherapy.

therapy, parallel the changes observed in the absolute lymphocyte count. Moreover, Potvin et al.,[15] dividing his patients in two groups: the responders (i.e., patients who were tumor-free at an average of 8.3 months after therapy) and nonresponders (i.e., patients who developed metastases within an average of 3.6 months after therapy), observed that the T cell levels increased abruptly at 1 month after therapy in the *responders* but declined or failed to increase in the *nonresponders*. A subsequent paper by the same authors[7] confirmed this observation. We did not analyze our data in this way, thus we are unable to specify whether and how much of our observed post-therapy depression in the T cell values is due simply to the effect of progression of the disease and to the ensuing deterioration of patient's general condition. The percent of

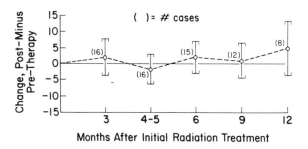

FIGURE 5.   Change in the percent of B lymphocytes — mean and 95% confidence intervals — as a function of time postradiotherapy.

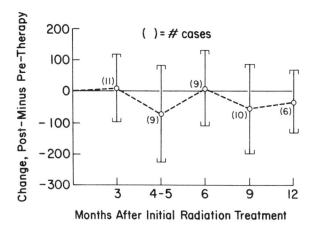

FIGURE 6.   Change in the absolute number of B lymphocytes — mean and 95% confidence intervals — as a function of time postradiotherapy.

total T cells is also depressed;[1,11] up to 12 months postradiation according to our study (Figure 4), although the difference with pretherapy values never reached statistical significance. This postradiation pattern is quite different from that of the percent B cells, which, with one exception, is characterized by mean percentages always higher than the pretherapy levels (Figure 5). This observation is similar to that of Olkowski et al.[14] Paired analysis of the levels of circulating B cells showed normal values at 3 and 6 months post initial treatment; and some depression at other times, up to 12 months, although never to a significant level (Figure 6). By contrast, Olkowski et al.[14] found, at completion of radiation therapy, B cells levels significantly lower than the preradiotherapy levels; 8 weeks later they had returned approximately half-way toward the pretherapy values.

From our observation, it appears then that in patients with bronchogenic carcinoma the T cells are selectively depleted by irradiation, either because they are intrinsically more radiosensitive or because, although destroyed at the same rate as the B cells, they are replaced more slowly. The specific elimination of T cells by radiotherapy, and a

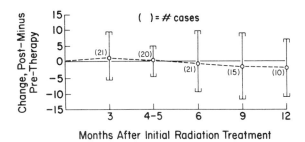

FIGURE 7. Change in the percent of active T lymphocytes — mean and 95% confidence intervals — as a function of time postradiotherapy.

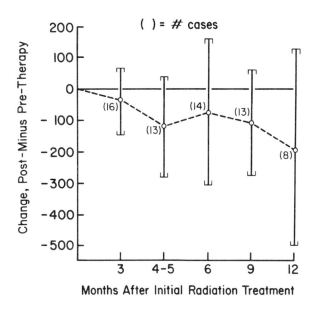

FIGURE 8. Change in the absolute number of active T lymphocytes — mean and 95% confidence intervals — as a function of time postradiotherapy.

shift in the B/T cells ratio, has been reported already by Stjernsward et al.[21] in patients with carcinoma of the breast. A similar conclusion was reached by Braeman[2] in lung cancer patients, using the in vitro PHA and pokeweed mitogen tests. According to Raben et al.,[17] Stratton et al.,[22] and Wara et al.[24] the drop in the T cells postradiation is accompanied by an increase in the proportion of "null cells" (lymphocytes with neither T nor B cell surface markers). Following radiation, we did not find any change in the percent of active T (Figure 7), the subgroup of T cells described by Wybran et al.[25] However, when these cells were expressed in absolute numbers, there was a persistent, although never significant, drop in the cell count up to 1 year post-therapy (Figure 8). These results would indicate that within the radiosensitive population of E rosette forming T lymphocytes, there is a relatively radio-resistant subpopulation, the "active" T cells. Raben et al.[17] came to the same conclusion studying a group of 20 patients with breast or pelvic malignancies.

The lymphocyte response to PHA stimulation is significantly depressed in patients with bronchogenic carcinoma.[5,12,18] It is further and markedly depressed during and after a radical course of radiotherapy:[5,8,12,16,18] from an average of 45.7% transformation before treatment to 65.9% of its original response at the end of treatment.[5] The patient response recovers to the original levels within 6 weeks, according to Gropp and Havemann,[8] within 6 months, according to Kerman and Stefani,[12] while for Braeman and Deeley,[5] the response is impaired for at least 18 months — the entire period of their study — although there is some indication of recovery starting from the third month after the first treatment.

Of interest are two additional observations made by Braeman and Deeley:[5] (1) that the greater the proportional drop during treatment, the longer is the survival of the patient after treatment (p = 0.004); and (2) that there is no correlation between the radiation dose and the drop in the PHA response. These authors advance the stimulating hypothesis that the fall in PHA response during treatment is the result of tumor breakdowns present in the circulating blood, tumor breakdowns which will inhibit the lymphocyte transformation.[5] In other words, the larger the amount of radiation-induced (?) tumor breakdown, the lower the PHA response and the longer the survival.

Alternative explanation to the postradiotherapy drop in the lymphocytes response to PHA stimulation is advanced by Merz et al.:[13] that this reduced transformation may reflect a delayed response of the lymphocytes, due to radiation-induced delay in DNA synthesis and cell division, rather than a truly depressed immune response. Data gathered on 37 patients with lung cancer tested before and after radiation therapy give strong support to this hypothesis.[13]

Radiation has also a depressing effect on the in vitro lymphocyte transformation to PPD stimulation.[4,8] Five of eleven patients tested showed a positive response before radiotherapy: all became negative responders at the end of therapy and remained such during the 18 months follow-up.[4] Gropp and Havemann[8] found, already 6 weeks after the end of X-ray therapy, the lymphocyte reaction to be as high as before treatment, regardless of the in vitro PPD concentration used. In contrast to PHA and PPD, the average response of the lymphocytes to pokeweed mitogen (P.W.M.) is not affected by a dose of 3200 rad in 8 fractions, given twice weekly over 4 weeks, according to Braeman.[2] These conclusions were based on data obtained from 48 patients with carcinoma of the bronchus.[2] In contrast, Olkowski et al.[14] found a significant (p < 0.05) drop in counts per minutes in suspensions of lymphocytes stimulated with P.W.M. at the end of a full course of radiotherapy. The response to P.W.M. remained depressed up to 28 weeks after therapy, although the difference was not any longer statistically significant. Lymphocyte cytotoxicity against two human tumor targets was tested by Olkowski et al.,[14] before and after radiotherapy. When compared to the pretherapy values, more patients showed an increase in their lymphocyte cytotoxicity only at 8 weeks after radiotherapy.

In conclusion, cell-mediated immunity does not seem to be affected by radiation, when in vivo tests are employed. By contrast, in vitro tests indicate a definite, marked, and prolonged depression of the cellular, but not humoral, immunity. We do not have a valid explanation for these contradictory observations.

REFERENCES

1. Anthony, H. M., Kirk, J. A., Madsen, K. E., Mason, M. K., and Templeman, G. H., E and EAC rosetting lymphocytes in patients with carcinoma of bronchus, *Clin. Exp. Immunol.*, 20, 41, 1975.
2. Braeman, J., Lymphocyte response after radiotherapy, *Lancet*, 2, 683, 1973.
3. Braeman, J. and Deeley, T. J., Immunologic studies in irradiation of lung cancer, *Ann. Clin. Res.*, 4, 355, 1972.
4. Braeman, J. and Deeley, T. J., Radiotherapy and immune response in cancer of the lung, *Br. J. Radiol.*, 46, 446, 1973.
5. Braeman, J. and Deeley, T. J., The lymphocyte response and prognosis in cancer of the lung, *Br. J. Radiol.*, 48, 668, 1975.
6. Clement, J. A. and Kramer, S., Immunocompetence in patients with solid tumors undergoing Cobalt 60 irradiation, *Cancer*, 34, 193, 1974.
7. Dellon, A. L., Potvin, C., and Chretien, P. B., Thymus dependent lymphocyte levels during radiation therapy for bronchogenic and esophageal carcinoma: correlations with clinical course in responders and nonresponders, *Am. J. Roentgenol.*, 123, 500, 1975.
8. Gropp, C. and Havemann, K., Cellular immune reactions in patients with bronchogenic carcinoma before and after radio-, chemo-, and immunotherapy, *Z. Immunol. Forsch.*, 153, 236, 1977.
9. Gross, L., Manfredi, O. L., and Protos, A. A., Effect of cobalt-60 irradiation upon cell-mediated immunity, *Radiology*, 105, 653, 1973.
10. Jenkins, V. K., Olson, M. H., and Ellis, H. N., In vitro methods of assessing lymphocyte transformation in patients undergoing radiotherapy for bronchogenic cancer, *Texas Rep. Biol. Med.*, 31, 19, 1973.
11. Kenady, D. E., Chretien, P. B., Potvin, C., Simon, R. M., Alexander, J. C., and Goldstein, A. L., Effect of thymosin in vitro and T cell levels during radiation therapy. Correlations with radiation portal and initial T cell levels, *Cancer*, 39, 642, 1977.
12. Kerman, R. and Stefani, S., Phytohemagglutinin stimulation of lymphocytes in lung cancer patients, *Oncology*, 34, 10, 1977.
13. Merz, T., Hazra, T., Ross, M., and Ciborowski, L., Transformation delay of lymphocytes in patients undergoing radiation therapy, *Am. J. Roentgenol.*, 127, 337, 1976.
14. Olkowski, Z. L., McLaren, J. R., and Skeen, M. J., Effects of combined immunotherapy with levamisole and bacillus Calmette — Guerin on immunocompetence of patients with squamous cell carcinoma of the cervix, head and neck and lung undergoing radiation therapy, *Cancer Treat. Rep.*, 62, 1651, 1978.
15. Potvin, C., Dellon, A. L., and Chretien, P. B., T-cell levels in bronchogenic carcinoma: correlations with tumor stage and clinical course, *Surg. Forum*, 25, 96, 1974.
16. Prasad, R., Prasad, N., Harrell, J. E., Thornby, J., Liem, J. H., Hudgins, P. T., and Tsuang, J., Arylhydrocarbon hydroxylase inducibility and lymphoblast formation in lung cancer patients, *Int. J. Cancer*, 23, 316, 1979.
16a. Prasad, N., Prasad, R., Thornby, J., Harrell, J. E., and Hudgins, P. T., Lymphocyte replication in lung cancer patients undergoing radiotherapy, *Oncology*, 37, 107, 1980.
17. Raben, M., Walach, N., Galili, U., and Schlesinger, M., The effect of radiation therapy on lymphocyte subpopulations in cancer patients, *Cancer*, 37, 1417, 1976.
18. Rafla, S., Yang, S. J., and Meleka, F., Changes in cell-mediated immunity in patients undergoing radiotherapy, *Cancer*, 41, 1976, 1978.
19. Stefani, S., Kerman, R., and Abbate, J., Immune evaluation of lung cancer patients undergoing radiation therapy, *Cancer*, 37, 2792, 1976.
20. Stefani, S., Menon, M., and Soucheck, J., unpublished data, 1980.
21. Stjernsward, J., Jondal, M., Vanky, F., Wigzell, H., and Sealy, R., Lymphopenia and change in distribution of human B and T lymphocytes in peripheral blood induced by irradiation for mammary carcinoma, *Lancet*, 1, 1352, 1972.
22. Stratton, J. A., Byfield, P. E., Byfield, J. E., Small, R. C., Benfield, J., and Pilch, Y., A comparison of the acute effects of radiation therapy, including or excluding the thymus, on the lymphocyte subpopulations of cancer patients, *J. Clin. Invest.*, 56, 88, 1975.
23. Thomas, J., Coy, P., Lewis, H., and Yuen, A., Effect of therapeutic irradiation on lymphocyte transformation in lung cancer, *Cancer*, 27, 1046, 1971.
24. Wara, W., Phillips, T., Wara, D., and Ammann, A., Immunosuppression after radiation therapy for carcinoma of the nasopharynx, *Am. J. Roentgenol.*, 123, 482, 1975.
25. Wybran, J., Carr, M. F., and Fudenberg, H. H., The human rosette forming cells in various human diseases states: cancer, lymphoma, bacterial and viral infections and other diseases, *J. Clin. Invest.*, 52, 1026, 1973.

Chapter 5

RADIOTHERAPY AND IMMUNE RESPONSE IN MALIGNANT LYMPHOMAS

Sameer Rafla and Shung-Jun Yang

TABLE OF CONTENTS

I. INTRODUCTION

The relation between the immune response and Hodgkin lymphoma was appreciated as far back as the early 1930s when skin anergy to tuberculin was noted in patients with Hodgkin's disease sometimes even in the presence of active tuberculosis.[1,2] However, it was Schier who is credited with the demonstration that patients with Hodgkin's disease are anergic to a host of antigens including tuberculin, mumps, candida, and Trichophyton antigens.[3] Since then, immunologic reactions have been studied extensively in patients with Hodgkin's disease and to a lesser extent in those with non-Hodgkin lymphomas. It has been established that Hodgkin's disease is characterized by a defect primarily in cell-mediated immunity resulting in delayed homograft rejection, defective lymphocyte function, and diminished delayed hypersensitivity. Humoral immunity appears to be intact until very late in the course of the disease. In contrast to Hodgkin's disease, non-Hodgkin lymphomas present no uniform picture: some appear normal in host immunity, others may show impairment of humoral or cellular immunity.

Congenital immunodeficiencies such as ataxia telangiectasia and Wiscott-Aldrich syndrome have been associated with increased incidence of lymphomas[4] as well as other malignancies.[5,6] Patients suffering from immunoinflammatory diseases such as autoimmune hemolytic anemia, Sjogren syndrome, and lupus erythematosis are more prone to develop malignant lymphomas, irrespective of whether immune suppressive drugs were used in their treatment.[7] Among transplant recipients, Hoover[8] in a survey of 6297 cases reported 44 neoplasms — with malignant lymphomas occurring in 56.8% of the cases — a risk increase of 350- and 700-fold for male and female patients, respectively.

The disproportionate number of lymphomas in immunologically abnormal populations has provided the basis for speculation about their pathogenesis (i.e., of lymphomas). The theory of immune surveillance was proposed. It denotes that the immune function of seeking and destroying clinically unrecognized *in situ* tumors has failed allowing clinically undetected lymphomas to become evident. Once the tumor is established in the host, the subsequent immune response of a patient in the presence of this growing tumor is further impaired as seen frequently in newly diagnosed patients prior to any treatment.

Radiation effect on the immune system has been extensively studied in experimental tumors. It is known that lymphoid cells are extremely sensitive to radiation injury and that immune suppression occurs early after small doses of radiation. However, work with animal tumors usually involves whole body irradiation by a single exposure. Many of the conclusions drawn from such studies may not apply in clinical radiotherapy which commonly employs protracted irradiation to a limited region (for whole body irradiation in humans, see Chapter 6).

However, results from murine experiments[9] suggest that clinical radiotherapy may cause systemic immune suppression by repeatedly damaging small fractions of the circulating lymphocytes which are passing through the irradiated area during each of the multiple exposures.

Studies of the effect of radiation on immune response in patients suffering from malignant lymphoma (Hodgkin and non-Hodgkin) is complicated by the lack of matching controls, the limited size of samples studied, and the limited sensitivity of present day methods of testing. Since the ideal setting of a large population of patients with adequately staged disease and matched controls examined serially with a full battery of in vivo and in vitro standardized immunologic testing is not available, we will address the subject separately in its two aspects: immune status of patients untreated and immune status of patients treated.

II. IMMUNE STATUS EVALUATED IN VIVO

Tests commonly used to evaluate immune status in vivo depend on skin reactions, mainly delayed hypersensitivity and graft rejection.

Impaired ability to reject homograft of the skin was known for a long time in patients with malignant lymphomas.[10-12] Its invasive nature prohibited wide use of the phenomenon for large scale studies. As a result, the bulk of data about in vivo patient's reaction evolved mainly through skin testing for delayed-type cutaneous hypersensitivity. Early work depended on reactions to frequently encountered microbial antigens[13-16] to which most normal controls have been exposed and are reactive. Failure of patients to react to these common recall antigens constituted anergy or alternatively lack of previous exposure. The difficulty in distinguishing these two causes was circumvented by the technical advances in skin testing, namely the development of chemical allergens. While the great majority of normal individuals can be sensitized to some chemical allergens such as 2, 4-dintrochlorobenzene (DNCB), patients with Hodgkin's disease frequently showed depressed reactions upon challenge.[17,18] Sensitization to DNCB has since served as a standard in vivo test along with reactions to common antigens for hypersensitivity studies.

A. Findings in Untreated Patients

Among 50 untreated patients of Hodgkin's disease tested with both intradermal antigens and DNCB, Brown et al.[19] found anergy only in advanced diseases. Similarly, Young et al.[20] in a study of 103 untreated Hodgkin's disease patients reported no difference in the incidence of DNCB positive reactivity between Stage I patients and the normal controls, but noted that the frequency of anergy increased with advancing stages as well as the presence of symptoms and unfavorable histological disease types. Since the results were somewhat variant among different antigens, mumps antigen was favored for detection of anergy from a selection of five tested (mumps, candida albicans, histoplasmin, PPD, and coccidiodin). These findings are not unanimously accepted, however. Other authors disclaim the presence of significant correlation between skin reactivity and advanced stages, although patients as a group were invariably depressed as compared with controls.[15,21-23]

These seemingly contradictory results could be attributed to the antigen dose used. By lowering the sensitizing dose of DNCB from 2% to 0.5% (500 μg), Eltringham and Kaplan[21] found significantly higher incidence of anergy in 154 untreated patients with Hodgkin's disease including Stage I. In a similar vein they found increased responsiveness to streptokinase-streptodornase when 50 instead of 5 units of the test antigen were used. Thus, it was demonstrated that the depression in skin response is a quantitative rather than an all-or-none defect of immunity. This finding provides credence to the view that immunological deficiency might play a primary role in the pathogenesis of Hodgkin's disease, rather than being a secondary effect to the presence of the disease.

The prognostic significance of skin reactivity is still a controversial subject. Anergy was found to be more pronounced when disease was complicated with lymphopenia, systemic symptoms, and unfavorable histology.[19,20] Correlation with constitutional symptoms appeared to depend on the sensitizing dose of DNCB.[21,24]

Correlation appeared to exist between initial skin reaction at diagnosis and clinical response to treatment, with more positive reactions noted in patients that responded to therapy (radiotherapy for the majority of the patients) as compared to nonresponders.[25] Correlation between skin reactivity and survival is unclear. Young[20] reported a slight difference in early death rate between anergic patients and those that were reactive to an antigen or DNCB.

In contrast with Hodgkin's disease, untreated patients with non-Hodgkin lymphoma frequently demonstrate positive skin reaction[26,27] but anergy was reported among some patients with unfavorable histology[28] or late stage of disease.[29] It is of interest to note that various degrees of anergy exist also in patients suffering from solid tumors, especially melanomas and sarcomas with some correlation between skin reactivity, and stage of disease and survival of patients.[30-32]

B. Irradiated Patients

Conversion from anergic to reactive status has been associated with tumor control in some solid tumors treated by radiotherapy[33] or surgery.[34] In Hodgkin's disease, Van Rijswijk and colleagues[35] tested skin reactions to PPD, Candida, Varidase, and Trichophyton within 1 month after completing radiotherapy and found further depression as compared to the status before treatment or diagnostic laparotomy (including splenectomy). Splenectomy per se appears to have no immunosuppressive effect.[35,36] However, the total proportion of patients capable of reacting to recall antigens or DNCB challenge may not change after radiotherapy.[37] It may even become somewhat higher[38] if longer time elapses between treatment and retesting. Kun and Johnson[37] retested their patients after 5 years of disease-free survival and found 87% of them to be reactive — an incidence similar to that prior to radiotherapy (90%). They also observed the presence of conversions of several patients from negative to positive or the reverse. Fuks and associates[38] confirmed the occurrence of this bidirectional "conversion" phenomenon after radiotherapy. In their series, patients demonstrating positive sensitization to DNCB at presentation frequently became anergic (88% of patients) immediately after completion of radiotherapy with slow recovery occurring over a period of months, considerably reducing the proportion of nonreactive patients by year-end. It was uncertain whether sufficient recovery would continue and eventually raise the response rate to initial pretreatment levels.

III. IMMUNE STATUS EVALUATED BY LABORATORY MEASUREMENTS

A. Lymphocyte Function In Vitro

Since in vitro studies of immune status revolve mainly around lymphocyte function, this was widely investigated utilizing in vitro stimulation of the cells with a battery of mitogens such as phytohemagglutinin (PHA), Concanavalin A (ConA), and pokeweed mitogen (PWM) or specific antigens of chemical, microbial, or tumor origin, or allogeneic cells.

1. Untreated Patients

In *untreated patients* who present with any of the histological types of malignant lymphoma, impaired responses are generally encountered with advanced disease.[22,23,39-41] However, other authors claim the defect to be present in all stages of Hodgkin's disease,[15,16,42-44] disseminated lymphocytic lymphoma,[26,27] and reticulum cell sarcomas.[45,46] Faquet[43] claimed that untreated patients with Hodgkin's disease fall into three groups; each with a different pattern of dose-response: normal, consists of 26% of patients, and two groups of abnormals, one insensitive to submaximal concentrations of PHA (57% of patients) and the other insensitive to all concentrations (17% of patients). This interesting concept has not been confirmed by others, however.

Technical refinement of early methods of testing helped reveal minor deficiencies otherwise unnoticed by the conventional techniques. The use of wide spectrum of mitogen concentrations[43,44,47] and culture termination times[48,49] revealed otherwise undetected differences between controls and patients with early Hodgkin's disease. The assay of PHA stimulated protein synthesis in 20-hr cultures, instead of the commonly

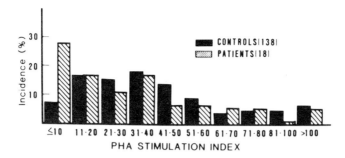

FIGURE 1. Frequency distribution of patients and controls according to responses to PHA.

measured DNA synthesis or morphologically identified blast formation in 3 to 7 day cultures enabled incubation of cells to be carried out in medium free of serum, thus eliminating an undesirable source of variation.[47] Furthermore, the necessity of concomitant study of patients and controls was demonstrated by Tan et al.[44] in their work on untreated children with Hodgkin's disease. The "time controls" help to hold in check some of the unavoidable experimental variations, thereby making comparisons more meaningful between measurements obtained during different periods in time. The same purpose was served by the use of "relative proliferation index" (as used by Dean and associates[50] in breast and lung cancer) which required three normal individuals to be tested on the day that any patient is studied. Future investigations will no doubt take into consideration the phenomena revealed by these technical modifications, especially since variations related to dose-response, time-response, serum, and type of controls may account at least in part for discrepancies noted in different publications. For instance, response to PHA as a correlate to certain clinical manifestations of the disease was claimed by some investigators[15,22,40,45,47,49] and questioned by others.[41,42,51] Similarly the correlation between results of in vivo and in vitro tests was confirmed by some[22,24,43,52] and discounted by others.[38,53]

In this department PHA reactivity test was used to evaluate immune status in 19 patients before treatment. Nine patients suffered from Hodgkin's disease and 10 from non-Hodgkin lymphoma. The methods were described elsewhere.[54] The mean stimulation index and standard error was 32.39 ± 6.85 for the patient group, considerably lower than 44.0 ± 2.80 of healthy controls. A graphic representation of these results is seen in Figure 1.

2. Treated Patients

Work with patients irradiated for treatment of malignant lymphoma has yielded varying results. Some authors reported recovery of previously depressed lymphocyte reactivity while others found further depression occurs immediately following radiotherapy.[35] Recovery is initiated soon after. The proportion of patients that ultimately convert back to pretreatment levels is dependent upon the length of the observation period (higher percentage after longer periods) and a continuing status of freedom from disease. Jackson and associates[40] compared lymphocyte transformation in patients in remission for periods less or exceeding 6 months following radiotherapy for Hodgkin's disease. The former group showed depressed reactivity whereas the latter was similar to healthy controls. Data from Papac[45] on lymphocyte response to PHA in 38 patients, (19 with lymphosarcomas or reticulum cell sarcomas and 19 with Hodgkin's disease) demonstrated similar findings (controls were subjects with chronic diseases).

The correlation between tumor regression and lymphocyte function was highlighted

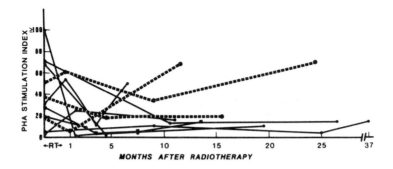

FIGURE 2.   Changes in PHA reactivity following radiotherapy. Solid lines, Hodgkin's disease, dotted lines, non-Hodgkin's disease.

by Hersh and Irwin[39] who used cell survival in culture, PHA-induced blastogenesis, and mitotic index in 33 patients (26 H.D. and 7 reticulum cell sarcoma) treated by radiotherapy to show that a return to normal function of lymphocytes may occur after radiation-induced remission. Such claims are by no means unanimously accepted. Winkelstein[15] reported depressed PHA simulation in a group of 22 patients (presenting with recurrent H.D.) who were treated by radiotherapy or its combination with chemotherapy (with disease regression). No details were given as to the time elapsed before retesting. King and associates[55] also reported impaired responses to mitogens (PHA, ConA, and PWM) in patients in remission induced by curative doses of radiation (or its combination with chemotherapy) for Hodgkin's disease or lymphosarcoma. Faguet[43] indicated that whereas the overall incidence of depressed lymphocyte responses had not changed after irradiation (74% before and 76% after radiation), the incidence of severe depression increased considerably (17% before and 47% after radiation), while that of mild abnormality decreased (57% and 29%, respectively).

Hancock et al.[25] analyzed leukocyte migration inhibition which is a measure of the soluble factor MIF released by transformed lymphocyte. Higher incidence of immunocompetence indicated by this assay was seen among patients in remission treated mainly by radiation as compared to those not responding to therapy. Fuks and colleagues[38] monitored protein synthesis in lymphocytes stimulated by a wide range of mitogen concentrations. Patients with Hodgkin's disease in long-term remission for 1 to 10 years showed stimulation ratios lower for all PHA concentrations than that of untreated patients and much lower than that of healthy controls. In addition patients treated 8 to 10 years earlier demonstrated no better lymphocyte response to PHA as compared to those who completed radiotherapy only a year earlier. On the other hand, the same authors reported that although responses to allogenic lymphocytes (another indicator of T cell function) were reduced from the nearly normal responding capacities found in untreated patients, a continued improvement was observed after 2 years post-treatment, reaching normal levels in patients in continuous remission for 5 years or more.

Of the 18 untreated patients in this study, PHA reactivity was repeated in 11 patients (8 H.D. and 3 non-H.D.) treated by radiotherapy or by radiotherapy and chemotherapy. Results are plotted on Figure 2. Of nine patients (6 H.D. and 3 non-H.D.) studied within 6 months postirradiation, six had lower than their corresponding preirradiation PHA stimulation indices while three showed an improved response. Two of the three initial increases were followed by subsequent fluctuations, although all three were above pretreatment levels at final testing 11 to 24 months postirradiation. Some improvement in PHA reactivity subsequent to the initial decreases was observed in all patients. However, substantial recoveries were not frequent. The remaining 2 of the

11 patients were not available for testing until 9 and 11½ months post-treatment. One showed considerable suppression and remained so 16 months later, the other showed fluctuations around the pre irradiation value with an eventual rise detected by the 37th month.

The above discussion indicates that the length of interval between completion of radiotherapy and retesting is an important factor in deciding the outcome of the test. Repeated assays after treatment would likely show immediate suppression followed by a certain degree of recovery within the first year or so after treatment. Lymphocyte function may vary according to patients' clinical responses with more impairment occurring among the nonresponders as compared to the responders. Patients enjoying longer disease-free periods are likely to show lesser impairment. However, even long-term remissions do not guarantee a fully recovered lymphocyte response.

B. Peripheral Blood Lymphocyte Counts

The absolute number of lymphocytes has long been considered a general prognostic factor in lymphomatous diseases.[56] In untreated patients with Hodgkin's disease lymphocyte counts tend to be at the lower end of the normal range or slightly below the lower limit. Low lymphocyte counts are commonly encountered in disseminated disease,[21,22,43] unfavorable histology types (such as lymphocyte depletion types), negative skin tests for delayed hypersensitivity, shorter mean survival time,[20] or diminished PHA response.[22,45] In untreated patients with non-Hodgkin lymphomas, abnormal numbers of lymphocytes may also occur and may be associated with abnormal percentage (and/or numbers) of T or B lymphocytes with poor survival.[27] Successfully *treated patients* of Hodgkin's disease and lymphosarcoma may show normal lymphocyte counts,[37,55,57] whereas patients in relapse or who failed to respond to radiotherapy may have a lower mean number of lymphocytes.[25] Lymphopenia is commonly observed in treated patients immediately following completion of radiotherapy, slowly returning to higher levels in time. However, despite the frequently encountered recoveries, it is not uncommon to find lymphopenia among cured patients of long standing. Furthermore, there appears to be no association between the pretreatment lymphocyte count and that observed 1 to 10 years later. Patients who presented with lymphopenia may have lymphocyte counts within normal range after radiotherapy and those with normal pretreatment counts may have deficient numbers of lymphocyte during long periods of complete remission.[38] However, claims to the presence of correlation between normal lymphocyte counts and disease remission under radiotherapy do exist[37,55] with some authors believing that a low-mean number of lymphocytes is consistent with persistent disease.[25]

C. T and B Lymphocyte Counts

The nature and origin of the neoplastic cell in malignant lymphomas have been much discussed in recent years. In Hodgkin's disease, the origin of the proliferating cells has been suggested to be T lymphocytes,[58,59] B lymphocytes,[60,61] or monocytes.[62] Several types of non-Hodgkin lymphomas are claimed to be of B cell origin such as Waldenstrom's macroglobulinemia,[63] Burkitt's lymphoma,[64,65] and varying percentage of almost every other type.[26,66-69] Jaffe and associates[70] claimed that childhood lymphomas are nevertheless of T cell origin.[71-73] Moreover, it has been possible to identify T cell subpopulations responsible for lymphoblastic lymphomas, mycosis fungoides, and Sezary's syndrome.[74] Continuing studies of cell markers will lead to better understanding of the immumology, pathogenesis, prognosis, and classification of these diseases.

The relative and absolute numbers of T and B lymphocytes in the circulating blood, lymph nodes, spleen, or other disease tissues have been examined with a view to relate findings to stage, disease activity, and prognosis. T lymphocytes are usually identified by their ability to form spontaneous rosettes with sheep erythrocytes (E-rosette). They have also been assayed by the use of antithymocyte serum in cytotoxicity test or immunofluorescent stains. B lymphocytes can be enumerated by the presence of surface immunoglobulins or receptors for Fc-portion of the immunoglobulin molecule and for the third component of complement, C3.

1. Untreated Patients

In untreated Hodgkin's disease the percentage of spontaneous rosetting cells may[53,75] or may not[76,77] differ from controls of healthy volunteers or patients with non-neoplastic disease. The absolute number of T cells is often reduced due to either reduced percentage of T cell, lymphopenia, or both.[16,53,75-78] Furthermore, the absolute number of T cells as well as B cells has been reported to fall progressively with advancing disease.[23] A predominance of T lymphocytes has been reported in disease involved lymph nodes[76,79] and spleens[80] as compared with noninvolved organs. The percentage of B cells has been variably reported as normal[16,77,78,81] or decreased.[23,82] It is not clear whether correlation exists between the percentage (and/or number) of T cells or B cells and lymphocyte function as reflected in skin reaction in vivo and stimulated transformation in vitro. While Case[23] failed to establish a relation between the T or B cells in patients with Hodgkin's disease and lymphocyte function (such as DNCB sensitization, mitogen stimulation, and immunoglobulin levels), Bobrove[53] demonstrated correlations between E-rosette forming T cells and PHA response, and a similar relation between presence of constitutional symptoms and reduced absolute T and B lymphocyte counts.

In non-Hodgkin lymphoma the situation is somewhat different. In untreated patients suffering from lesions of unfavorable histology a reduction in T cell percentage in peripheral blood has been reported.[28] Gajl-Peczalska[27] reported frequent T cell deficiency in the circulating blood of patients suffering from poorly differentiated lymphocyte lymphoma, a finding usually associated with lymphopenia. Changes in B cells were variable but more often than not their percentage (and/or absolute number) was increased, often with demonstrable monoclonal expansion. There was no correlation between T or B cell numbers and delayed hypersensitivity. Abnormal proportions of T and B cells were found to be a poor prognostic sign.

Bloomfield and colleagues[83] reported that patients suffering from diffuse lymphomas with B cell markers survive longer than those with null cell lymphomas. Poor survival was also associated with T cell predominance as claimed by Stathopoulos[84] in a study of 34 patients with non-Hodgkin lymphomas.

Our own data on 16 untreated patients showed lower mean T cell percentages in seven patients presenting with Hodgkin's disease, 56.29 ± 5.06 (standard error of mean), as compared to controls (60.0 ± 0.86). Findings in nine patients with non-Hodgkin lymphoma, 60.11 ± 5.29, were normal. Similarly, the means and standard errors of total T cell number per cubic millimeter of blood were 1439 ± 350 in seven Hodgkin's disease patients and 1598 ± 300 in eight non-Hodgkin's disease patients as compared to 1768 ± 83 in 118 controls. Figure 3 presents frequency distribution of patients and controls among various T cell percentage groups. There is a relative abundance of patients in the group having less than 50% T cells and fewer in the groups having more than 70% T cells. No correlation was observed between T cell percentage and PHA stimulation.

2. Treated Patients

Radiation has been reported to induce lymphopenia and alterations in the relative and absolute numbers of both B and T lymphocytes when used in the treatment of cancer in various anatomic sites.[85-88] Some investigators showed more pronounced ef-

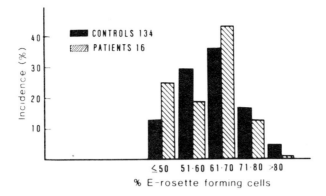

FIGURE 3. Frequency distribution of patients and controls according to percentages of T cells.

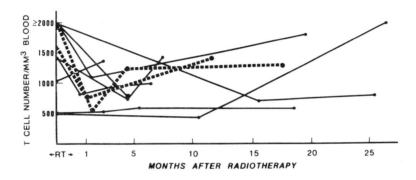

FIGURE 4. Changes of T cell number following radiotherapy. Solid lines, Hodgkin's disease, dotted lines, non-Hodgkin's disease.

fect on T cells as compared to B cells[89,90] and others observed that depression is not specific to either.[91-93] Extended field irradiation or total lymphoid irradiation when applied in cases of malignant lymphomas has been shown to affect T and B cell numbers. Hunter and associates[77] found a decrease of T cell number 1 to 4 months following radiotherapy for Hodgkin's disease from pretreatment levels. Fuks and colleagues[38] noted T and B lymphocytopenia immediately upon completion of radiotherapy for Hodgkin's disease. Patients in continuous remission for 12 to 111 months after radiation showed a certain degree of recovery with an elevated percentage and absolute number of B lymphocytes over that of the untreated patients and normal donors. Earlier, Engeset and colleagues[81] reported increased number of B cells in patients radiated for Hodgkin's disease 5 to 36 months prior to testing. This was due mainly to an increase in the proportion of B cells from a mean of 10% in the untreated patients to 34% in the treated group. These findings were further substantiated by Steele and Han[57] who showed that recovery after radiotherapy resulted in a higher percentage of B cells as compared to T cells. They studied 36 patients, 23 with Hodgkin's disease, and 13 with non-Hodgkin lymphomas. All patients had received radiotherapy, some also received chemotherapy for 6 months. All had been in complete remission for at least two years and off therapy. The number of T cells were lower and B cells higher than that of healthy controls.

Figure 4 shows our data on serial changes of T cell number following radiotherapy or its combination with chemotherapy. Of 10 patients (8 Hodgkin's disease, 2 non-Hodgkin lymphomas) retested, 8 (6 Hodgkin's disease, 2 non-Hodgkin lymphomas) showed an initial drop of total T cell number followed by a subsequent recovery to varying extent. The decrease was frequently due to lymphopenia as distinctive declines in percent in E-rosettes were not common among these patients.

D. Serum Immunoglobins and Mononuclear Phagocytes

Although Hodgkin's disease is associated primarily with defects in cell-mediated immunity, patients may also show impaired humoral immune response. Decreased serum immunoglobulin levels generally occur with advancing disease and its therapy,[94-96] although a small number (10 to 20%) of patients in all stages may be hypogammaglobulinemic.[23] Analysis of specific classes of immunoglobulin shows occasional cases of elevated IgG[26,97] and normal or moderately reduced IgA and IgM levels.[97] In non-Hodgkin lymphomas, hypogammaglobulinemia has been frequently demonstrated.[98,99] Lapes[29] reported reductions in at least two of the three Ig classes (IgG, IgA, IgM), with a significantly greater incidence in Stage IV patients. Gajl-Pecjalska[26] found immunoglobulin abnormalities, frequently associated with monoclonal B cell proliferation.

Radiotherapy appears to exert no long lasting effect on serum immunoglobulin levels in malignant lymphoma. While IgG and IgM levels may be reduced in some patients in remission at one year following treatment,[25] immunoglobulin scores are generally within normal ranges in long-term survivors after radical radiotherapy.[37,57]

The status of monocytes and macrophages in malignant lymphomas is essentially unexplored. Phagocytic activity has been sporadically reported as increased,[100,101] normal,[102,103] or decreased.[46,55] In view of the complex relationship among various mononuclear cell types in carrying out different aspects of the immunological function, the mononuclear phagocytes in malignant lymphomas will have to be carefully studied in order to reach a thorough understanding of the defect in these malignancies.

IV. SERUM FACTORS

Sera from cancer patients capable of blocking tumor-specific cell-mediated immunity against autologous tumor was first demonstrated by Hellstrom and colleagues[104] and later shown by others using various methods.[105-108] Sjogren and colleagues[109] showed that these blocking factors consisted mainly of circulating immune complexes (CIC) and that the antigen probably originated from tumor tissue. The presence of serum blocking factors in breast cancer[108] and other solid tumors[110] was reported to correlate with tumor burden and poor prognosis. In malignant lymphomas, patients' plasma or sera were shown to inhibit lymphocyte transformation upon stimulation by mitogens or antigens.[111,112] The presence of CIC in lymphoproliferative disorders was associated with unfavorable prognosis.[113,114] Among untreated patients, CIC was present in 22% of 50 patients with Hodgkin's disease and 36% of 78 patients with non-Hodgkin's malignant lymphoma, with prevalence in the groups of patients with disseminated disease.[115] However, the significance of this finding is not clear since there was no difference between the CIC positive and negative groups of patients as far as their response to treatment is concerned.

Sera from cancer patients were also shown to inhibit E-rosette formation.[116,117] Recently, protein extracts from spleens of patients with Hodgkin's disease[118] were demonstrated to contain an immunosuppressive factor which did the same to cells from normal controls. Furthermore, E-rosette formation and PHA stimulation of lymphocytes from untreated patients with Hodgkin's disease could be restored to normal levels by extensive washing of the cells or by incubating the cells in fetal calf or fetal human sera. These cells, however, remain susceptible to the immunosuppressive effect of the spleen extracts and sera from patients with Hodgkin's disease but not extracts from other neoplasma or normal subjects.[38,119]

The effect of radiotherapy on these serum factors is still largely unexplored. It would be interesting to find out whether successful tumor ablation by radiation would affect these factors quantitatively or qualitatively and whether such incidence carries a prognostic significance.

V. CLINICAL IMPLICATION OF LONG-TERM DISTURBANCE OF THE IMMUNE SYSTEM

Two other aspects that may be linked to disease or radiation-induced immunosuppression deserve detailed consideration namely infection and development of second malignancies.

A. Infection

The relation between infection (such as T.B.) and Hodgkin's disease is one of the early indicators of abnormalities in the immune response associated with the disease.[120,121] The incidence of Herpes and varicella infections (HZ-V) in Hodgkin's was reported to be 8%[122] versus less than 0.5% in general population.[123] *Pneumocystis carinii* and fungal infections were also notably prevalent among patients with Hodgkin's disease.[124,125] The association between Hodgkin's disease and viral infection is particularly interesting since the latter is also linked to deficiency in cell-mediated immunity.[13]

Non-Hodgkin lymphoma on the other hand is associated with a different class of infections, particularly bacterial of the encapsulated variety such as pneumococcus, staphylococcus, and hemophilus[125] which are related to globulin deficiency and derangements of antibody immune complex.

Infection in untreated patients may result from granulocytopenia, impaired granulocyte function, monocytopenia, impaired monocyte function, hypogammaglobulinemia, or impaired cellular immunity.[125]

The incidence of viral infection, particularly *Herpes zoster*, has increased greatly recently to values from 34%[126] to as high as 52%,[127-129] a fact strongly related to increased aggressive treatment by chemotherapy and radiotherapy. Reboul and colleagues in 1978 reported this to be 24% in patients treated by extensive field radiotherapy.[126] The incidence seems to be reduced when smaller volumes are treated, 11% only after limited field irradiation. Since the incidence of herpes is strongly linked to suppression of cell-mediated immunity, the implication that radiotherapy contributes to this suppression is clear. Moreover, the incidence of herpes as well as immune suppression related to radiotherapy peaks in the first post-radiation year. Strong claims also exist to relate herpes to incidence of lymphopenia and skin anergy that occur after radiotherapy.[128] No satisfactory evidence exists to suggest that the incidence of herpes is dose related. Similar immunosuppressive effect was attributed to chemotherapy. In a randomized trial carried by Cancer and Leukemia Group B, Rafla and his colleagues[130] reported the incidence of *Herpes zoster* to be 14% after 6 courses of chemotherapy (none severe) and 11% after 12 courses of the same chemotherapy (Table 1) with a much higher incidence of the severe forms (7%). Patient population was similar in both cases — all suffered from Stage IV Hodgkin's disease and all were previously untreated. The chemotherapy was identical in all instances and consisted of CCNU, VElban, procarbazine in addition to prednisone given every fourth cycle.

The incidence of herpes seems to be substantially increased especially in its severe disseminated forms when aggressive chemotherapy and radiotherapy are combined, occurring in 24% of patients (severe forms in 16%) treated with both modalities in sequence within a short interval.[130]

Even when a diseased spleen is removed, splenectomy seems to increase the vulner-

Table 1
INCIDENCE OF HERPES IN A CONTROLLED RANDOMIZED TRIAL (CALGB)

Treatment	To-tal	% Mild	% Moderate	% Severe	% Life threaten-ing
6-CVPP	39	8	6	0	0
12-CVPP	44	2	2	7	0
6-CVPP + RT	43	0	2	2	0
3-CVPP + RT + 3-CVPP	42	3	5	16	0

Table 2
RELATION BETWEEN SPLENECTOMY AND INCIDENCE OF HERPES (CALGB)

Treatment	Total pa-tients	% Herpes toxicity	Patients splenec-tomy	% Herpes toxicity
6 CVPP	39	14%	13[d]	15%
12 CVPP	44	11%[a]	14[e]	57%
6 CVPP + RT	43	4%[b]	14[f]	35%
3 CVPP + RT + CVPP	42	24%[c]	15[g]	47%

[a] 2/3 cases: severe
[b] 1/2 cases: severe
[c] 2/3 cases: severe
[d] One pt. had itching only
[e] 4 pts. off study or early
[f] 2 pts. had rash only and one lost
[g] 2 pts. had rash only and one early loss

ability of patients to *Herpes zoster*, especially when this is followed by aggressive combined therapy. Table 2 shows the effect of splenectomy on the incidence of herpes, as well as other infections, in the same group of patients. Radiotherapy in this case was limited to treatment of regions where disease volume was substantial at presentation. It is clear that splenectomy under these conditions has a deleterious effect on patients immune response, whether cell mediated (causing an almost 47% phenomenal incidence of herpes in the sandwich therapy arm) or the antibody complex mechanism (resulting in a markedly increased incidence of bacterial infection). These findings however are not in agreement with those of Reboul and colleagues[126] in their study of 80 children who claimed that splenectomy has no influence on incidence of *Herpes zoster*.

B. Development of Second Malignancies

The relation between immunosuppression and *incidence of second* malignancy is unclear and rather tenuous. The long lapse between treatment and incidence of second malignancy argues against immunosuppression since recovery of immune status seems to escalate with passage of time. However, such recovery is by no means universal and our present tests are too crude to detect possible minor deficiencies. It is conceivable that the mutagenic effect of therapy is accentuated by its immunosuppression.

The incidence of second malignancies in patients with untreated Hodgkin and non-Hodgkin lymphoma is rare since it entails concomitant discovery of the two malignancies. In a group of 526 patients suffering from multiple malignancies which were analyzed, only 10 cases were found where malignant lymphoma was either the first primary or one of two malignancies discovered simultaneously. Six cases formed the first group and four were found in the second group. Simultaneous incidence does not seem to be of particular significance. The question which has led to much interest in recent literature is whether radiotherapy or chemotherapy play a role in the induction of second malignancy by virtue of immunosuppression. Louie et al.[7] collected from the literature 109 examples of neoplasms in patients receiving azathioprine, cyclophospha- mide, or other cytotoxic drugs. Some also received corticosteroid and radiotherapy. The majority of patients who suffered a second malignancy developed either leukemias or malignant lymphomas.

In a controlled trial reported by Harris and collaborators[131] azathiaprine was asso- ciated with incidence of malignant lymphoma in 3 of 27 patients given the drug versus none in patients who did not receive the drug. The carcinogenic effect of radiotherapy was well-documented in patients treated by radiation for benign disease such as anky- losing spondylitis and thymic lesions in children.

However, the incidence of second malignancies in long survivors after successful therapy for Hodgkin's and non-Hodgkin's lymphomas continue to be controversial. Historically, Hodgkin's disease was reported not to be associated with a significant incidence of second malignancies during a period of 15 years (1948 to 1962) that pre- ceded the wide use of intensive chemotherapy.[132] This risk has increased substantially nowadays especially for leukemias. Rosenberg[133] from Stanford University reported recently that the incidence of acute myeloid leukemia (as a second malignancy) in Hodgkin's patients is significantly higher in patients treated by radiotherapy as com- pared to those treated by intensive chemotherapy and radiotherapy. He also noted an increased incidence of non-Hodgkin's lymphoma in this group of patients.

Glicksman and colleagues[134] reviewed the findings in 1325 patients treated by differ- ent combinations of radiotherapy and chemotherapy (cancer and leukemia group B studies) and concluded that there is an increased incidence of acute myeloid leukemia which seems to be linked to maintenance chemotherapy, especially chlorambucil. Ra- diotherapy was judged not to be a contributing factor to the incidence of second ma- lignancy. Long follow-up periods in a large group of cured patients is necessary for accurate evaluation of the incidence of second malignancy since they tend to appear after a latent period averaging more than 10 years.

VI. PROSPECTS FOR IMMUNE MANIPULATIONS

As can be discerned from the above discussion, lymphoproliferative neoplasms are likely to co-exist with immunological deficit, commonly detected through nonspecific immune reactions. The defect varies in extent with disease activity, treatment, and prognosis. Moreover, tumor-associated antigens exist in malignant lymphomas. These findings provide the rationale for attempts to manipulate the immune system as part of the treatment. There is reason to believe that immunological approaches can be taken to promote nonspecific immunocompetence which may lead to a general upswing of immune reactions and to potentiate specific immunity against the patients' cancer cells. Encouraging results on the use of BCG as maintenance therapy in malignant lymphoma have been reported.[135,136] In a controlled trial Hoerni[137] was able to dem- onstrate a beneficial effect of BCG (by scarification) given to lymphoma patients in remission. Sokel and associates[138] studied the effect of intradermal BCG injections in 50 tuberculin-negative patients (both Hodgkin's and non-Hodgkin's) and was able to demonstrate that BCG induced delay of recurrences. Kimura[139] noted prolongation of remission period in patients with Hodgkin's disease who received immunotherapy OK- 432 (the streptococcal preparation) and chemotherapy over those receiving no immu- notherapy. The anthelmintic drug, levamisole, was reported to convert negative skin reaction in Hodgkin's disease to positives (mainly in response to mumps and candida) and to raise E-rosette number to normals.[140] The drug appeared to interfere with the inhibiting effect of serum from patients with Hodgkin's disease on T cell function.[141]

Future trials of various manipulations of immune system will no doubt continue to add to knowledge in this field.

REFERENCES

1. Parker, F., Jr., Jackson, H., Jr., Fitzhugh, G., and Spies, T. D., Studies of diseases of the lymphoid and myeloid tissues. IV. Skin reaction to human and avian tuberculin, *J. Immunol.*, 22, 277, 1932.
2. Steiner, P. E., Etiology of Hodgkin's disease; skin reactions to avian and human tuberculin proteins in Hodgkin's disease, *Arch. Int. Med.*, 54, 11, 1934.
3. Schier, W. W., Cutaneous anergy and Hodgkin's disease, *N. Engl. J. Med.*, 250, 353, 1954.
4. Kersey, J. H., Spector, B. D., and Good, R. A., Primary immunodeficiency disease and cancer: the immunodeficiency cancer registry, *Int. J. Cancer*, 12, 333, 1973.
5. Boder, E., Ataxia-telangiectasia: recent clinical and pathological observations, in *Proc. of the 2nd Int. Workshop on Immunodeficiency Diseases in Man*, Bergsma, D. and Good, R. A., Eds., New York National Foundation, March of Dimes, 1975.
6. Melief, C. J. M. and Schwartz, R. S., Immunocompetence and malignancy, in *Cancer: A Comprehensive Treatise*, Vol. 1, Becker, F. F., Ed., Plenum Press, New York, 1975, 121.
7. Louie, S. and Schwartz, R. S., Immunodeficiency and the pathogenesis of lymphoma and leukemia, *Semin. Hematol.*, 2, 117, 1978.
8. Hoover, F., and Fraumeni, J. F., Jr., Risk of cancer in renal-transplant recipients, *Lancet*, 2, 55, 1973.
9. Eltringham, J. R. and Weissman, I., Regional lymph node irradiation: effect on immune response, *Radiology*, 94, 438, 1970.
10. Kelly, W. D., Lamb, D. L., Varco, R. L., and Good, R. A., An investigation of Hodgkin's disease with respect to the problem of hemotransplantation, *Ann. N.Y. Acad. Sci.*, 87, 187, 1960.
11. Green, I. and Corso, P. F., A study of skin homografting in patients with lymphomas, *Blood*, 14, 235, 1959.
12. Miller, D. G., Lizardo, J. G., and Synderman, R. A., Homologous and heterologous skin transplantation in patients with lymphomatous disease, *J. Natl. Cancer Inst.*, 26, 569, 1961.
13. Schier, W. W., Roth, A., Ostroff, G. J., and Schrift, M. H., Hodgkin's disease and immunity, *Am. J. Med.*, 20, 94, 1956.
14. Sokal, J. E. and Primikiros, N., Delayed skin test response in Hodgkin's disease and lymphosarcoma: effect of disease activity, *Cancer*, 14, 597, 1961.
15. Winkelstein, A., Mikulla, J. M., Sartiano, G. P., and Ellis, L. D., Cellular immunity in Hodgkin's disease: comparison of cutaneous reactivity and lymphoproliferative responses to phytohemagglutinin, *Cancer*, 34, 549, 1974.
16. Holm, G., Mellstedt, H., Bjorkholm, M., Johansson, B., Killander, D., Sundblad, R., and Soderberg, G., Lymphocyte abnormalities in untreated patients with Hodgkin's disease, *Cancer*, 37, 751, 1976.
17. Good, R. A., Kelly, W. D., Rotstein, J., and Varco, R. L., Immunological deficiency disease. III. Hodgkin's disease and other lymphomas, *Allergy*, 6, 275, 1962.
18. Aisenberg, A. C., Studies on delayed hypersensitivity in Hodgkin's disease, *J. Clin. Invest.*, 41, 1964, 1962.
19. Brown, R. S., Haynes, H. A., Foley, H. T., Goodwin, H. A., Berard, C. W., and Carbone, P. P., Hodgkin's disease: immunologic, clinical and histologic features of 50 untreated patients, *Ann. Intern. Med.*, 67, 291, 1967.
20. Young, R. C., Corder, M. P., Haynes, H. A., and DeVita, V. T., Delayed hypersensitivity in Hodgkin's disease, *Am. J. Med.*, 52, 63, 1972.
21. Eltringham, J. R. and Kaplan, H. S., Impaired delayed-hypersensitivity responses in 154 patients with untreated Hodgkin's disease, *Natl. Cancer Inst. Monogr.*, 36, 107, 1973.
22. Ziegler, J. B., Hansen, P., and Penny, R., Intrinsic lymphocyte defect in Hodgkin's disease: analysis of the phytohemagglutinin dose-response, *Clin. Immunol. Immunopathol.*, 3, 451, 1975.
23. Case, D. C., Hansen, J. A., Corrales, E., Young, C. W., Dupont, B., Pinsky, C. M., and Good, R. A., Comparison of multiple in vivo and in vitro parameters in untreated patients with Hodgkin's disease, *Cancer*, 38, 1807, 1976.

24. Advani, S. H., D'Silva, H., Gothoskar, B. P., Dinshaw, K. A., Nair, C. N., Gopalkrishna, R., Talwalkar, G. V., and Desai, P. B., Cellular immunity in Hodgkin's disease, Cancer, 43, 492, 1979.

25. Hancock, B. W., Bruce, L., Dunsmore, I. R., Ward, A. M., and Richmond, J., Follow-up studies on the immune status of patients with Hodgkin's disease after splenectomy and treatment in relapse and remission, Br. J. Cancer, 36, 347, 1977.

26. Gajl-Peczalska, K. J., Hansen, J. A., Bloomfield, C. D., and Good, R. A., B lymphocytes in untreated patients with malignant lymphoma and Hodgkin's disease, J. Clin. Invest., 52, 3064, 1973.

27. Gajl-Peczalska, K. J., Bloomfield, C. D., Coccia, P. F., Sosin, H., Brunning, R. D., and Kersey, J. H., B and T cell lymphomas — analysis of blood and lymph nodes in 87 patients, Am. J. Med., 59, 674, 1975.

28. Thatcher, N., Gasiunas, N., Crowther, D., and Potter, M. R., Lymphocyte function in the blood of patients with untreated non-Hodgkin lymphoma: influence of stage and pathology, Med. Ped. Oncol., 3, 311, 1977.

29. Lapes, M., Rozenzweig, M., Barbieri, B., Joseph, R. R., and Smalley, R. V., Cellular and humoral immunity in non-Hodgkin's lymphoma; correlation of immunodeficiencies with clinicopathologic factors, Am. J. Clin. Pathol., 67, 347, 1977.

30. Eilber, F. R. and Morton, D. L., Impaired immunologic reactivity and recurrence following cancer surgery, Cancer, 25, 362, 1970.

31. Maisel, R. H. and Ogara, J. H., Abnormal dinitrochlorobenzene skin sensitization — a prognostic sign of survival in head and neck squamous cell carcinoma, Laryngoscope, 84, 2012, 1974.

32. Pinsky, C. M., Wanebo, H., Mike, V., and Oettgen, H., Delayed cutaneous hypersensitivity reactions and prognosis in patients with cancer, Ann. N.Y. Acad. Sci., 276, 407, 1976.

33. Ghossein, N. A., Bosworth, J. L., and Bases, R. E., The effect of radical radiotherapy on delayed hypersensitivity and the inflammatory response, Cancer, 35, 1616, 1975.

34. Eilber, F. R., Nizze, J. A., and Morton, D. L., Sequential evaluation of general immune competence in cancer patients: correlation with clinical course, Cancer, 35, 660, 1975.

35. Van Rijswijk, R. E. N., Sybesma, J. Ph. H. B., Kuipers, J. T., Zegers, B. J. M., and Borst-Eilers, E., The influence of splenectomy, radiotherapy and chemotherapy on the immune response in Hodgkin's disease, Neth. J. Med., 19, 201, 1976.

36. Wagener, D. J. T., Gestman, E., and Wessels, H. M. C., The influence of splenectomy on the in vitro lymphocyte response to phytohemagglutinin and pokeweed mitogen in Hodgkin's disease, Cancer, 36, 194, 1975.

37. Kun, L. E. and Johnson, R. E., Hematologic and immunologic status in Hodgkin's disease 5 years after radical radiotherapy, Cancer, 36, 1912, 1975.

38. Fuks, Z., Strober, S., Bobrove, A. M., Sasazuki, T., McMichael, A., and Kaplan, H. S., Long-term effect of radiation on T and B lymphocytes in peripheral blood of patients with Hodgkin's disease, J. Clin. Invest., 58, 803, 1976.

39. Hersh, E. M. and Irvin, W. S., Blastogenic responses of lymphocytes from patients with untreated and treated lymphomas, Lymphology, 2, 150, 1969.

40. Jackson, S. M., Garrett, J. V., and Craig, A. W., Lymphocyte transformation changes during the clinical course of Hodgkin's disease, Cancer, 25, 843, 1970.

41. Corder, M. P., Young, R. C., Brown, R. S., and DeVita, V. T., Phytohemagglutinin-induced lymphocyte transformation: the relationship to prognosis of Hodgkin's disease, Blood, 39, 595, 1972.

42. Young, R. C., Corder, M. P., Berard, C. W., and DeVita, V. T., Immune alterations in Hodgkin's disease, Arch. Intern. Med., 131, 446, 1973.

43. Faguet, G. B., Quantitation of immunocompetence in Hodgkin's disease, J. Clin. Invest., 56, 951, 1975.

44. Tan, C. T. C., de Sousa, M., Tan, R., Hansen, J. A., and Good, R. A., In vitro responses of peripheral blood and spleen lymphoid cells to mitogens and antigens in childhood Hodgkin's disease, Cancer Res., 38, 886, 1978.

45. Papac, R. J., Lymphocyte transformation in malignant lymphomas, Cancer, 26, 279, 1970.

46. Twomey, J. J. and Douglass, C. C., An in vitro study of lymphocyte and macrophage function with lymphoproliferative neoplasms, Cancer, 33, 1034, 1974.

47. Levy, R. and Kaplan, H. S., Impaired lymphocyte function in untreated Hodgkin's disease, N. Engl. J. Med., 290, 181, 1974.

48. Benezra, D. and Hochman, A., In vitro activation of lymphocytes from patients with malignant disease. I. Kinetics and difference in magnitude of response, Isr. J. Med. Sci., 7, 553, 1971.

49. Matchett, K. M., Huang, A. T., and Kremer, W. B., Impaired lymphocyte transformation in Hodgkin's disease; evidence for depletion of circulating T-lymphocytes, J. Clin. Invest., 52, 1908, 1973.

50. Dean, J. H., Herberman, R. B., Silva, J., McCoy, J. L., and Oldham, R. K., The relative proliferative index as a more sensitive parameter for evaluating lymphoproliferative responses of cancer patients to mitogens and alloantigens, Int. J. Cancer, 20, 359, 1977.

51. Braeman, J. and Cottam, P., The PHA response in Hodgkin's disease, *Eur. J. Cancer,* 11, 879, 1975.
52. Grace, P. R., Perlin, E., and Royston, I., In vitro lymphocyte dysfunction in Hodgkin's disease, *J. Natl. Cancer Inst.,* 56, 239, 1976.
53. Bobrove, A. M., Fuks, Z., Strober, S., and Kaplan, H. S., Quantitation of T and B lymphocytes and cellular immune function in Hodgkin's disease, *Cancer,* 36, 169, 1975.
54. Rafla, S., Yang, S. J., and Meleka, F., Changes in cell-mediated immunity in patients undergoing radiotherapy, *Cancer,* 41, 1076, 1978.
55. King, G. W., Yanes, B., Hurtubise, P. E., Balcerzak, S., and LoBuglio, A. F., Immune function of successfully treated lymphoma patients, *J. Clin. Invest.,* 57, 1451, 1976.
56. Aisenberg, A. C., Lymphocytopenia in Hodgkin's disease, *Blood,* 25, 1037, 1965.
57. Steele, R. and Han, T., Effects of radiochemotherapy and splenectomy on cellular immunity in long-term survivors of Hodgkin's disease and non-Hodgkin's lymphoma, *Cancer,* 42, 133, 1978.
58. Order, S. E. and Hellman, S., Pathogenesis of Hodgkin's disease, *Lancet,* 1, 571, 1972.
59. Biniaminov, M. and Ramot, B., Possible T-lymphocyte origin of Reed-Sternberg cells, *Lancet,* 1, 368, 1974.
60. Garvin, A. J., Spicer, S. S., Parmley, R. T., and Munster, A. M., Immunohistochemical demonstration of IgG in Reed-Sternberg and other cells in Hodgkin's disease, *J. Exp. Med.,* 139, 1077, 1974.
61. Boecker, W. R., Hossfeld, D. K., Gallmeier, W. M., and Schmidt, C. G., Clonal growth of Hodgkin cells, *Nature (London),* 258, 235, 1975.
62. Long, J. C., Zamecnik, P. C., Aisenberg, A. C., and Atkins, J., Tissue culture studies in Hodgkin's disease. Morphologic, cytogenetic cell surface and enzymatic properties of cultures derived from splenic tumors, *J. Exp. Med.,* 145, 1484, 1977.
63. Hansen, J. A. and Good, R. A., Malignant disease of the lymphoid system in immunological perspective, *Human Pathol.,* 5, 567, 1974.
64. Klein, E., Klein, G., Nadkarni, J. S., Nadkarni, J. J., Wigzell, H., and Clifford, P., Surface IgM Kappa specificity on a Burkitt lymphoma cell in vivo and in derived culture lines, *Cancer Res.,* 28, 1300, 1968.
65. Shevach, E. M., Herberman, R., Frank, M. L., and Green, I., Receptors for complement and immunoglobulin on human leukemic cells and human lymphoblastoid cell lines, *J. Clin. Invest.,* 51, 1933, 1972.
66. Stein, H., Lennert, K., and Parwaresch, M. R., Malignant lymphoma of B-cell type, *Lancet,* 2, 855, 1972.
67. Aisenberg, A. C. and Long, J., Lymphocyte surface characteristics in malignant lymphoma, *Am. J. Med.,* 58, 300, 1975.
68. Brouet, J. C., Labaume, S., and Seligmann, M., Evaluation of T and B lymphocyte membrane markers in human non-Hodgkin malignant lymphomata, *Br. J. Cancer,* 31(Suppl. 2), 1211, 1975.
69. Payne, S. V., Smith, J. L., Jones, D. B., and Wright, D. H., Lymphocyte markers in non-Hodgkin's lymphomas, *Br. J. Cancer,* 36, 57, 1977.
70. Jaffe, E. S., Shevach, E. M., Frank, M. M., Berard, C. W., and Green, I., Nodular lymphoma — evidence for origin from follicular B lymphocytes, *N. Engl. J. Med.,* 290, 813, 1974.
71. Smith, J. L., Clein, G. P., Barker, C. R., and Collins, R. D., Characterization of malignant mediastinal lymphoid neoplasm (Sternbergsarcoma) as thymic in origin, *Lancet,* 1, 74, 1973.
72. Kersey, J. J., Nesbit, M. E., Luckasen, J. R., Hallgren, H. M., Sabad, A., Yunis, E. J., and Gajl-Peczalska, K. J., Acute lymphoblastic leukemia and lymphoma cells with thymus derived (T) markers, *Mayo Clin. Proc.,* 49, 584, 1974.
73. Kaplan, J., Mastrangelo, R., and Peterson, W. D., Childhood lymphoblastic lymphoma, A cancer of thymus-derived lymphocytes, *Cancer Res.,* 34, 521, 1974.
74. Berard, C. W., Jaffe, E. S., Braylan, R. C., Mann, R. B., and Nanba, K., Immunologic markers of non-Hodgkin's lymphomas, *Recent Results Cancer Res.,* 64, 138, 1978.
75. Anderson, E., Depletion of thymus dependent lymphocytes in Hodgkin's disease, *Scand. J. Haematol.,* 12, 263, 1974.
76. Bukowski, R. M., Noguchi, S., Hewlett, J. S., and Deodhar, S., Lymphocyte subpopulations in Hodgkin's disease, *Am. J. Clin. Pathol.,* 65, 31, 1976.
77. Hunter, C. P., Tannenbaum, H., Churchill, W. H., Moloney, W. C., and Schur, P. H., Immunologic abnormalities in patients with malignant lymphoproliferative disease, *J. Natl. Cancer Inst.,* 58, 1185, 1977.
78. Heier, H. E., Klepp, R., Gundersen, S., Godal, T., and Normann, T., Blood B and T lymphocytes and in vitro cellular immune reactivity in untreated human malignant lymphomas and other malignant tumors, *Scand. J. Haematol.,* 18, 137, 1977.
79. Stathopoulos, G., Papmichail, M., Peckham, M. J., Davies, A. J. S., and Holborow, E. J., The T and B lymphocyte content of lymph nodes and spleen in Hodgkin's disease, *Br. J. Exp. Pathol.,* 58, 712, 1977.

80. Hunter, C. P., Pinkus, G., Woodward, L., Moloney, W. C., and Churchill, W. H., Increased T lymphocytes and IgMEA-Receptor lymphocytes in Hodgkin's disease spleens, *Cell. Immunol.*, 31, 193, 1977.

81. Engeset, A., Froland, S. S., Bremer, K., and Host, H., Blood lymphocytes in Hodgkin's disease — increase of B-lymphocytes following extended field irradiation, *Scand. J. Haematol.*, 11, 195, 1973.

82. Han, T. and Minowada, J., Impairment of cell-mediated immunity in patients with untreated Hodgkin's disease: evaluated by skin test, lymphocyte stimulation tests and T and B lymphocyte counts, *N.Y. State J. Med.*, 78, 216, 1978.

83. Bloomfield, C. D., Kersey, J. H., Brunning, R. D., and Gajl-Peczalska, K. J., Prognostic significance of lymphocyte surface markers in adult non-Hodgkin's malignant lymphoma, *Lancet*, 2, 1330, 1976.

84. Stathopoulos, G., Kay, H. E. M., Hamlin, I. M. E., and McKay, A. M., Surface characteristics of lymphoma cells in relation to treatment, response and survival, *Eur. J. Cancer*, 14, 479, 1978.

85. Stjernsward, J., Jondal, M., Vanky, F., Wigzell, H., and Sealy, R., Lymphopenia and change in distribution of human B and T lymphocytes in peripheral blood induced by irradiation for mammary carcinoma, *Lancet*, 1, 1352, 1972.

86. Blomgren, J., Berg, R., Wasserman, J., and Glas, U., Effect of radiotherapy on blood lymphocyte population in mammary carcinoma, *Int. J. Rad. Oncol. Biol. Phys.*, 1, 177, 1976.

87. Catalona, W. J., Potvin, C., and Chretien, P. B., Effect of radiation therapy for urologic cancer on circulating thymus-derived lymphocytes, *J. Urol.*, 112, 261, 1974.

88. Dellon, A. L., Potvin, C., and Chretien, P. B., Thymus-dependent lymphocyte levels during radiation therapy for bronchogenic and esophageal carcinoma: correlations with clinical course in responders and nonresponders, *Am. J. Roentgenol. Radium Ther. Nucl. Med.*, 123, 500, 1975.

89. Heier, H. E., Christensen, I., Froland, S. S. and Engest, A., Early and late effects of irradiation for seminoma testis on the number of blood lymphocytes and their B and T subpopulations, *Lymphology*, 8, 69, 1975.

90. Kohorn, E. I., Mitchell, M. S., Dwyer, J. M., Knowlton, A. H., and Klein-Angerer, S., Effect of radiation on cell-mediated cytotoxicity and lymphocytic subpopulations in patients with ovarian carcinoma, *Cancer*, 41, 1040, 1978.

91. Campbell, A. A., Wiernick, G., Wood, J., Hersey, C. A., Waller, I. C., and MacLennan, M., Characteristics of the lymphopenia induced by radiotherapy, *Clin. Exp. Immunol.*, 23, 200, 1976.

92. Hoppe, T. T., Fuks, Z. Y., Strober, S., and Kaplan, H. S., The long term effects of radiation on T and B lymphocytes in the peripheral blood after regional irradiation, *Cancer*, 40, 2071, 1977.

93. Rand, R. J., Jenkins, D. M., and Bulmer, R., T- and B-lymphocyte subpopulations following radiotherapy for invasive squamous cell carcinoma of the uterine cervix, *Clin. Exp. Immunol.*, 33, 159, 1978.

94. Arends, T., Coonrad, E. V., and Rundles, R. W., Serum proteins in Hodgkin's disease and malignant lymphomas, *Am. J. Med.*, 16, 833, 1954.

95. Aisenberg, A. C. and Leskowitz, S., Antibody formation in Hodgkin's disease, *N. Engl. J. Med.*, 268, 1269, 1963.

96. Ultman, J. E., Cunningham, J. K., and Gellhorn, A., The clinical picture of Hodgkin's disease, *Cancer Res.*, 26, 1047, 1966.

97. McCormick, D. P., Ammann, A. J., Ishizaka, K., Miller, D. G., and Hong, R., A study of allergy in patients with malignant lymphoma and chronic lymphocytic leukemia, *Cancer*, 27, 93, 1971.

98. Ultmann, J. E., Fish, W., Osserman, E., and Gellhorn, A., The clinical implications of hypogammaglobulinemia and lymphocytic lymphosarcoma, *Ann. Intern. Med.*, 51, 501, 1959.

99. Miller, D. G., Patterns of immunological deficiency in lymphomas and leukemias, *Ann. Intern. Med.*, 57, 703, 1962.

100. Sheagren, J. N., Block, J. B., and Wolff, S. M., Reticuloendothelial system phagocyte formation in patients with Hodgkin's disease, *J. Clin. Invest.*, 46, 855, 1976.

101. Cline, M. J., Bactericidal activity of human macrophages: analysis of factors influencing the killing of listeria monocytogens, *Infect. Immunol.*, 2, 156, 1970.

102. Blaese, R. M., Oppenheim, J. J., Seeger, R., and Waldmann, T. A., In vitro lymphocyte transformation: the restoration of purified lymphocyte responses by allogenic macrophages from normal and anergic patients, *Clin. Res.*, 18, 422, 1970.

103. Dorner, M., Lenhard, V., Manke, H. G., Rapp, W., Resch, K., Rother, U., Schopf, E., and Seelig, P., Cell and hormonal immunity in patients with Hodgkin's disease (Investigation to study the influence of therapy), *Inn. Med.*, 4, 112, 1977.

104. Hellstrom, I., Sjogren, H. O., Warner, G., and Hellstrom, K. E., Blocking of cell-mediated tumor immunity by sera from patients with growing neoplasms, *Int. J. Cancer*, 7, 226, 1971.

105. Jose, D. G. and Seshadri, R., Circulating immune complexes in human neuroblastoma: direct assay and role in blocking specific cellular immunity, *Int. J. Cancer*, 13, 824, 1974.

106. **Halliday, W. J., Maluish, A., and Isbister, W. H.,** Detection of antitumor cell-mediated immunity and serum blocking factors in cancer patients by leukocyte adherence inhibition test, *Br. J. Cancer,* 29, 31, 1974.
107. **Vanky, F., Klein, E., Stjernsward, J., and Nilsonne, U.,** Cellular immunity against tumor-associated antigens in humans: lymphocyte stimulation and skin reaction, *Int. J. Cancer,* 14, 277, 1974.
108. **Yonemoto, R. H., Eugisawa, T., and Waldman, S. R.,** Effect of serum blocking factors on leukocyte adherence inhibition in breast cancer patients, *Cancer,* 41, 1289, 1978.
109. **Sjogren, H. O., Hellstrom, I., Bansal, S. C., Warner, G. A., and Hellstrom, K. E.,** Elution of "blocking factors" from human tumors, capable of abrogating tumor-cell destruction by specifically immune lymphocytes, *Int. J. Cancer,* 9, 274, 1972.
110. **Rossen, R. D., Reisberg, M., Hersh, E. M., and Gutterman, J. U.,** The Clq binding test for soluble immune complexes: clinical correlation obtained in patients with cancer, *J. Natl. Cancer Inst.,* 58, 1205, 1977.
111. **Trubowitz, S., Mascek, B., and Rosario, A. D.,** Lymphocyte response to phytohemagglutinin in Hodgkin's disease, lymphatic leukemia and lymphosarcoma, *Cancer,* 19, 2019, 1966.
112. **Gaines, J. D., Gilmer, M. A., and Remington, J. S.,** Deficiency of lymphocyte antigen recognition in Hodgkin's disease, *Natl. Cancer Inst. Monogr.,* 36, 117, 1973.
113. **Amlot, P. L., Pussell, B., Slaney, J. M., and Williams, B. D.,** Correlation between immune complexes and prognostic factors in Hodgkin's disease, *Clin. Exp. Immunol.,* 31, 166, 1978.
114. **Brown, C. A., Hall, C. L., Long, J. C., Carey, K., Witzmann, S. A., and Aisenberg, A. C.,** Circulating immune complexes in Hodgkin's disease, *Am. J. Med.,* 64, 289, 1978.
115. **Heier, H. E., Landaas, T. O., and Marton, P. F.,** Circulating immune complexes and prognosis in human malignant lymphoma: a prospective study, *Int. J. Cancer,* 23, 292, 1979.
116. **Chisari, F. V. and Edgington, T. S.,** Lymphocyte E rosette inhibitory factor: a regulatory serum lipoprotein, *J. Exp. Med.,* 142, 1092, 1975.
117. **Whitehead, R. H., Roberts, G. P., Thatcher, J., Teasdale, C., and Hughes, L. E.,** Masking for receptors and sheep erythrocytes on human T-lymphocytes by sera from breast cancer patients, *J. Natl. Cancer Inst.,* 58, 1573, 1977.
118. **Bieber, M. M., Fuks, Z., and Kaplan, H. S.,** E-rosette inhibiting substance in Hodgkin's disease spleen extracts, *Clin. Exp. Immunol.,* 29, 369, 1977.
119. **Fuks, Z., Strober, S., and Kaplan, H. S.,** Interaction between serum factors and T lymphocytes in Hodgkin's disease, *N. Engl. J. Med.,* 295, 1273, 1976.
120. **Hersh, E. M., Bodey, G. P., Nies, B. A., and Freireich, E. J.,** Causes of death in acute leukemia, *JAMA,* 193, 105, 1965.
121. **Casazza, A. R., Duvall, C. P., and Carbone, P. P.,** Summary of infectious complications occurring in patients with Hodgkin's disease, *Cancer Res.,* 26, 1290, 1966.
122. **Sokal, J. E. and Firat, D.,** Varicella-zoster infection in Hodgkin's disease, clinical and epidermiological aspects, *Am. J. Med.,* 39, 452, 1965.
123. **McGregor, R. M.,** Herpes zoster, chicken pox and cancer with general practice, *Br. Med. J.,* 1, 84, 1957.
124. **Ruskin, J. and Reington, J. S.,** Pneumoncytis carini injection in the immunosuppressed host. Antimicrobial agents, *Chemotherapy,* 70, 76, 1967.
125. **Hersh, E. M., Gutterman, J. U., and Mavligit, G. M.,** Effect of hematological malignancies and their treatment on host defense factors, *Clin. Hematol.,* 5, 425, 1976.
126. **Reboul, F., Donaldson, S., and Kaplan, H. S.,** Herpes zoster and varicella infections in children with Hodgkin's disease — an analysis of contributing factors, *Cancer,* 41, 95, 1978.
127. **Goffinet, D. R., Glatstein, E. J., and Merigan, T. C.,** Herpes zoster-varicella infections and lymphoma, *Ann. Int. Med.,* 76, 235, 1972.
128. **Wilson, J. F., Marsa, G. W., and Johnson, R. E.,** Herpes zoster in Hodgkin's disease. Clinical, histologic and immunologic correlations, *Cancer,* 29, 461, 1972.
129. **Feldman, S., Hughes, W. T., and Kim, H. Y.,** Herpes zoster in children with cancer, *Am. J. Dis. Child.,* 126, 178, 1973.
130. **Rafla, S., Coleman, M., Pajak, T., and Vinciguerra, V.,** Toxicity and preliminary results of combined radiation and chemotherapy in the treatment of Hodgkin's disease (a randomized study of C.A.L.G.B.), *Int. J. Radiat. Oncol. Biol. Phys.,* 5(Suppl. 2), 140, 1979.
131. **Harris, J., Jessop, J. D., and de Santiago, D. M. C.,** Further experience with azathioprine in rheumatoid arthritis, *Br. Med. J.,* 4, 463, 1971.
132. **Berg, J. W.,** The incidence of multiple primary cancers. I. Development of further cancers in patients with lymphomas, leukemias and myelomas, *J. Natl. Cancer Inst.,* 38, 741, 1967.
133. **Rosenberg, S. A.,** Hodgkin's disease keynote address, *Int. J. Radiat. Oncol. Biol. Phys.,* 5(Suppl. 2), 19, 1979.
134. **Glicksman, A. S., Pajak, T., Stutzman, L., Nissen, N., and Cooper, R.,** Second malignancies in patients successfully treated for Hodgkin's disease, *Int. J. Radiat. Oncol. Biol. Phys.,* 5(Suppl. 2), 135, 1979.

135. Thomas, J. W., Plenderleith, I. H., Landi, S., and Clements, D. V., BCG as maintenance therapy in non-Hodgkin's lymphoma, in *BCG Immunotherapy,* Vol. 1, Lamoureux, G., Turcotte, R., and Portelance, V., Eds., Grune & Stratton, New York, 1976, 297.
136. Hoerni, B., Chauvergne, J., Hoerni-Simon, G., Durand, M., and Lagarde, C., BCG-immunotherapy of malignant lymphomas. Current results of a controlled trial, *Cancer Immunol. Immunother.,* 19, 57, 1977.
137. Hoerni, B., Durand, M., Richaud, P., DeMascarel, A., Hoerni-Simon, G., Chauvergne, J., and Lagarde, C., Successful maintenance immunotherapy by BCG of non-Hodgkin's malignant lymphomas: results of a controlled trial, *Br. J. Haematol.,* 42, 507, 1979.
138. Sokal, J. E., Aungst, C. W., and Synderman, M., Delay in progression of malignant lymphoma after BCG vaccination, *N. Engl. J. Med.,* 291, 1226, 1974.
139. Kimura, I., Clinical and experimental studies on immunotherapy in malignant lymphoma, *Acta Haematol. Jap.,* 41, 1142, 1978.
140. Ramot, B. and Biniaminov, M., Effect of levamisole on lymphocytes of Hodgkin's disease patients in vivo and in vitro, *Progr. Cancer Res. Ther.,* 2, 239, 1977.
141. Del Giacco, G. S., Tognella, S., Leone, A. L., Locci, F., Cornaglia, P., Sangiuolo, A., and Grifoni, V., Interference of levamisole with inhibition of E-rosette formation by Hodgkin's disease and systemic lupus erythematosus cytoxic sera, *Blood,* 53, 1002, 1979.

Chapter 6

LEUKEMIA: WHOLE BODY IRRADIATION AND RECONSTITUTION

Eva Lotzová

TABLE OF CONTENTS

I. LEUKEMIAS AND THEIR TYPES

Leukemias represent an extremely heterogeneous complex group of diseases of hemopoietic-lymphoid compartment. Moreover, the leukemic cells present in bone marrow, peripheral blood, or other organs of individual patients portray a largely heterogeneous population with regard to their aggressiveness, size, morphology, biochemistry, reproductive kinetic characteristics, sensitivity to neoplastic agents, and other types of therapy, etc. The etiology of this disease, although being actively studied, is still largely unknown. It is indicated from various studies that patients with the hematopoietic disorders, independently if congenital or acquired, often develop leukemia. The examples of such disorders are represented by Down's syndrome, Fanconi's anemia, Bloom's syndrome, and paroxysmal nocturnal hemoglobinuria.[1-7] Patients with congenital and acquired immunodeficiency diseases were also reported to be prone to leukemic disease;[8] in the latter group of patients the impaired immune system is most likely to be responsible for susceptibility to leukemia.

Bone marrow injury, displayed by anemia, thrombocytopenia, or leukopenia has been well-established to result from chronic exposure to chemicals. A significant number of individuals have been observed to develop leukemia after such drug-induced blood dyscrasias.[9] Presently, benzene is the only well-confirmed chemical leukemogen; more than 100 cases of acute leukemia have been ascribed to chronic exposure to benzene.[10-13] In some of the individuals exposed for a long time period to benzene, acute leukemia occurred while they were still under exposure, although in others leukemia presented itself with a latent period of 15 years, long after recovery from bone marrow aplasia.[11,14,15] In all instances of benzene-associated leukemia in which chromosomal analysis was performed, the chromosomal abnormalities were detected.[11] Chloramphenicol has been reported to be another chemical leukemogen,[16-19] although the relation between chemical-associated marrow aplasia and acute leukemia is not as clear for this agent as it is for benzene. In individuals subjected to chloramphenicol the time elapse between chloramphenicol administration and leukemia development ranged broadly, from 7 months to 12 years. Chromosomal bone marrow analysis were done in two chloramphenicol-treated patients and abnormalities were detected in both cases.[18,20] Association between leukemia development and phenylbutazone ingestion has been observed in some individuals.[20-25] Oxyphenbutazone, a chemical analogue of phenylbutazone, has also been implicated in leukemia induction.[21,22,26] In fact, it has been suggested that any agent with bone marrow injury potential may induce leukemia.

Radiation exposure has also been implicated as a causative leukemic factor. This is evidenced by high leukemia incidence within radiologists, victims of radiation accidents, atomic bomb survivors, and patients that were subjected to radiation for various disorders.[27] The genetic involvement in the control of leukemia is suggested by an increase of leukemia incidence in the families of leukemic patients. In addition, the fact that a monozygotic twin of a leukemic sibling often develops the same disease[28] indicates strongly the hereditary nature of leukemia.

Involvement of viruses in induction of leukemia was suggested on the basis of their known leukemogenic effect in experimental animals and also by the presence of reverse transcriptase, (an RNA-directed DNA polymerase — the enzyme associated with RNA tumor viruses in animals) in cells of patients with acute leukemia.[29] Moreover, by electron microscopy studies virus-like particles were detected in blast cells of patients with acute leukemia.[30] Despite these indications and in contrast to animal leukemias where viruses were demonstrated as causative agents, the role of viruses in human leukemia remains to be established.

There are two major forms of leukemia, chronic and acute. Such division is based on morphological studies and natural history of the disease. Chronic leukemias can

Table 1
CLASSIFICATION OF LEUKEMIAS

Chronic Leukemias

Chronic myelocytic leukemia (CML)
Chronic myelomonocytic leukemia (CMML)
Chronic lymphocytic leukemia (CLL)

Acute Leukemias

Myelocytic
    Acute myeloblastic leukemia (AML)
    Acute promyelocytic leukemia (APML)
    Acute myelomonocytic leukemia (AMML)
    Acute monocytic leukemia
    Erythroleukemia

Nonmyelocytic
    Acute lymphoblastic leukemia (ALL)
    Acute undifferentiated leukemia (AUL)

be grouped into chronic myelocytic leukemia (abbreviated CML), chronic myelomonocytic leukemia (abbreviated CMML), and chronic lymphocytic leukemia (abbreviated CLL).

The acute leukemias can be subdivided into two groups, myelocytic and nonmyelocytic. Acute myelocytic leukemias are represented by the following categories, according to the predominant cell type involved in the disease:[31,32] (1) acute myeloblastic leukemia (abbreviated AML), which displays maturation to or beyond the promyelocytic level; AML is the most common form of myelocytic leukemia with dominancy of myeloblast like cells in the bone marrow; (2) acute promyelocytic leukemia (abbreviated APML); it is an uncommon form of leukemia which expresses features similar to AML with regard to its maturation stage, and/or could exhibit hypergranular promyelocytes with plenteous Auer rods (abnormal primary granules) which are not present in AML; (3) acute myelomonocytic leukemia (abbreviated AMML), the type which shows myelomonocytic characteristics; this type represents a rather heterogeneous form of leukemia; (4) acute monocytic leukemia, representing a relatively pure monocytic form; and (5) erythroleukemia, which exhibits main involvement of immature erythroid precursors.

Nonmyelocytic leukemias are represented by two types, i.e., acute lymphoblastic leukemia (ALL) and acute undifferentiated leukemia (AUL). The latter form shows no maturation and is predominantly myeloblastic. AUL is considered by some as a form of myelogenous leukemia[31,32] and by others more like ALL.[33,34] The latter classification is based on in vitro growth characteristics of AUL.[33,34] The classification of leukemias is summarized in Table 1.

Despite the considerable progress made in therapy of leukemia, contributed especially to the discovery of new chemotherapeutic agents, leukemia is still an often fatal disease. The major problem appears to be connected with recurrence of leukemia. For example, in the case of adult acute myelogenous leukemia, the majority of patients die of recurrence of leukemia within 2 years of onset of the disease.[35] Even though the antileukemia effective chemotherapeutic agents are available, their use is limited because of their tenacious myeloid toxicity. For this reason their prolonged use at high (i.e., effective) doses is not realistic. The same limitations are confined to radiotherapy of leukemia since dosages of irradiation, effective in destroying most of the leukemic cells, are highly myelosuppressive, due to the sensitivity of hemopoietic system, especially bone marrow tissue, to radiation. However, the picture is not all so black since the hemopoietic toxicity caused by irradiation or high doses of drugs can be repaired by bone marrow transplantation, and as a consequence effective treatment of leukemia may become plausible.

II. BONE MARROW TRANSPLANTATION

A. Hemopoietic Cells — Important Components of Bone Marrow Transplants

The foundation for clinical bone marrow transplantation was established almost three decades ago by the experiment of Jacobson, demonstrating that mice could be protected from lethal effects of irradiation by shielding of the spleen.[36] Several years elapsed before it had been finally proven that the radiation-protective effect, achieved by shielding of the spleen, was due to the presence of hemopoietic stem cells in this organ. Later, several laboratories showed in rodents that i.v. injection of bone marrow cells (or spleen cells) could protect lethally irradiated animals from radiation-caused death, by restoring the host's hemopoiesis.[37-42] Subsequently, based on chromosomal analysis, it was determined that the protective effect of bone marrow transplantation was due to the repopulation of the host's radiation-damaged hemopoietic compartment by the donor's hemopoietic cells.[38]

In the 1960s, Till and McCulloch demonstrated experimentally that murine bone marrow cells, when injected intravenously into heavily irradiated recipients, form macroscopic nodules of hemopoietic cells in the spleens of transplanted animals 8 to 10 days after transplantation.[43] Such hemopoietic nodules were found to be composed of erythroid, granulocytic, megakaryocytic, and undifferentiated cells either as pure populations or mixtures. These nodules were designated spleen colonies, and the cells that formed them were called colony forming units — spleen (abbreviated CFU-S). Colonies of hemopoietic cells were found also in bone marrow upon transplantation, however, these could be detected only by microscopic examination. When comparisons between the morphological type of spleen and bone marrow colonies were made, it was found that the hemopoietic colonies formed in the spleen display a distinctive differentiation pattern than the colonies formed in the bone marrow, the former being predominantly of erythroid, whereas the latter primarily of granulocytic nature.[44,45] The clonality of hemopoietic colonies was indicated by the linear relationship between the number of bone marrow cells transplanted and the number of colonies formed, and also by radiation survival experiments.[43] The direct proof for the clonal nature of hemopoietic colonies came from the experiments employing chromosomal marker analysis.[46,47]

Further experimentation on splenic colonies, using the murine system, led to the observation that a single cell residing in bone marrow has a multipotent colony-forming potential upon bone marrow transplantation. In addition, the same cell was found to possess capability to undergo self-renewal.[48,49] Bone marrow cells with these characteristics were designated hemopoietic stem cells and for obvious reasons, these cells represent the most critical components in bone marrow transplant. In man as well as in experimental animals, these cells reside in hemopoietic tissues. In contrast to most of the other tissues, hemopoietic tissues retain the capacity for proliferation, formation of blood-composing elements, and self-renewal (thus, their designation hemopoietic — "poietic" meaning formation and "hemo" — denoting relationship to blood). It is due to these cells that bone marrow tissue exhibit radiation-protection upon transplantation. As has been indicated earlier, most of the cell components residing in bone are unable to initiate hemopoiesis, in fact, murine hemopoietic stem cells are relatively rare (1 in 1000 of total number of bone marrow cells). Via their proliferation and differentiation potential into myeloid, erythroid, megakaryocytic, and lymphoid series, hemopoietic stem cells generate various progenitor cell populations.[50-52]

Table 2

TYPES OF HEMOPOIETIC STEM CELLS AND THEIR
PROGENY

Type of hemopoietic cells	Type of colonies formed	Stimuli required
Hemopoietic stem cell (HSC)	All types	Microenvironmental regulatory factors
Committed stem cells (progenitors)		
Granulocyte (neutrophil) & macrophage progenitors (GM-CFC)	Monocytes-macrophages & neutrophils	GM-CSF
Peritoneal macrophage progenitors (M-CFC)	Macrophages	GM-CSF
Eosinophil progenitors (EO-CFC)	Eosinophils	EO-CSF
Megakaryocyte progenitors (MEG-CFC)	Megakaryocytes	MEG-CSF (thrombopoietin?)
Erythropoietic progenitors (E-CFC)	Erythrocytes	E-CSF (erythropoietin?)
B Lymphocyte progenitors (BL-CFC)	B Lymphocytes	?
T Lymphocyte progenitors (TL-CFC)	T Lymphocytes	?

Note: CFC — colony-forming cells; CSF — colony-stimulating factor.

Types of hemopoietic stem cells and their progeny and stimuli required are illustrated in Table 2. Progenitor cells are thought to possess some, although limited degree of self-replication, and differ from stem cells with regard to their restriction to follow specific pathway of hemopoiesis, e.g., erythropoiesis, granulopoiesis, or other. Specific stimuli are required for progenitor cell's differentiation along certain differentiation pathway.[53] Descendants of progenitor cells can be categorized for the first time morphologically to belong to a certain hemopoietic cell population, for instance, erythroblast, myeloblast, etc. The progeny of the latter hemopoietic cell population is represented by mature hemopoietic cells present in the peripheral blood and other organs. The mature hemopoietic cells have a limited life span and fail to renew themselves.[53]

The topic whether pluripotent hemopoietic stem cell is the progenitor of erythrocytes, polymorphs, monocytes, macrophages, eosinophils, platelets, and lymphocytes, or whether various unipotent stem cells for each cell line exist, has been subjected to intense debate for several years.[54,55] Presently, there is substantial evidence for the existence of both pluripotent and unipotent stem cell classes. In the murine system, both types of stem cells were identified.[43,56,57] Even though in humans only the unipotent stem cell was experimentally demonstrated,[58] the existence of the pluripotent stem cell can be deduced from studies on the clonality of hemopoietic stem cells in patients with chronic myelocytic leukemia[59] and polycythemia vera.[60]

Various hemopoietic populations, with the exception of some of the mature elements, are present in the same tissues (hemopoietic tissues). In an adult mouse most of the hemopoietic stem cells are found in bone marrow, with decreasing numbers in the spleen and peripheral blood, respectively. In man, under normal conditions, bone marrow is a primary source of hemopoietic stem cells. With regard to the hemopoietic cells ontogeny, they appear first in the yolk sac and after migration into the embryo are detected initially in the liver and later in the spleen and bone marrow. As has been mentioned previously, hemopoietic stem cells and their progenitors are comparatively rare within hemopoietic cell populations. It has been calculated that 1 cell in 1000 mouse marrow cells is a multipotential stem cell and 1 cell in 300 to 400 marrow cells is a granulocytic progenitor cell.[53]

Lymphocytes originate also from hemopoietic stem cells and represent a very heterogeneous population of cells. Depending on the type of the progenitor lymphocyte descends from and on the lymphocyte's tissue migration pathway, these cells may become T cells (migration and differentiation via thymus) or B cells (most probably affected by bone marrow). Both B cells and T cells can be subdivided further into distinct subpopulations on the basis of their functional characteristics (helper T cells, suppressor T cells, cytotoxic T cells, antibody producing B cells, suppressor B cells, etc.). There are other subpopulations of lymphocytes, such as natural killer (NK) cells and killer (K) cells, originating from hemopoietic stem cells, which appear also to be heterogeneous. The exact pathway of these cells and their tissue influences has not yet been determined, even though the importance of intact bone marrow for generation and maintenance of fully functional NK cells is indicated from strontium-89 and bone marrow reconstitution experiments.[61,62] Lymphoid progenitor cells reside in both hemopoietic compartment and in specialized lymphoid organs.

For most optimal hemopoietic and lymphoid reconstitution of heavily irradiated recipients by transplanted bone marrow cells, not only the presence of pluripotential hemopoietic stem cells is essential, but also several other conditions are required. Beside the necessary space for transplanted cells to lodge in (which is provided by destruction of host cells by irradiation), local environment and regulatory humoral factors have to be available. The local environment, for instance, appears to be a very important factor in determining the differentiation pathway of hemopoietic stem cells.[63-65] Since the discussion on the environmental and humoral hemopoietic regulators is out of the scope of this chapter, the interested reader is referred to other articles.[50-53]

The distortions in hemopoietic stem cells or their regulators result in serious hemopathies of both benign and malignant origin, as exampled by disorders such as aplastic anemia, polycythemia vera, myelofibrosis, chronic myelocytic leukemia, acute myelocytic leukemia, etc.

B. Types of Bone Marrow Transplants

Bone marrow transplantation can be subdivided into four groups according to histogenetic relationship between the donor and the recipient: (1) autologous, (2) isogeneic (syngeneic), (3) allogeneic (homologous), and (4) xenogeneic (heterologous). The corresponding bone marrow transplants (also called grafts) are designated autograft, isograft (syngeneic graft), allograft (homograft), and xenograft (heterograft), respectively. Autologous bone marrow transplantation represents the situation in which bone marrow graft is taken from and returned to the same individual; an example of such a situation would be the collection of bone marrow cells from the leukemic patient that had been brought into remission, their storage by freezing, and transplantation of these cells back to the patient in the case of leukemia relapse. Isogeneic (syngeneic) marrow transplantation is the event when the donor and the recipient are genetically identical; an example of isogeneic transplantation is exchange of marrow grafts between identical (monozygotic) twins in humans or in animals between members of the same inbred strain. Allogeneic (homologous) transplantation is the case in which the marrow donor and recipient are genetically dissimilar, even though belonging to the same specie. The last group of bone marrow transplants, which is not presently clinically applicable, is xenogeneic (heterologous) transplantation, i.e., exchange of marrow grafts between members of different species. Outcome of bone marrow transplantation and its terminology is summarized in Table 3.

Table 3
TERMINOLOGY AND OUTCOME OF BONE MARROW GRAFTING

Type of marrow graft	Donor-recipient relationship	Outcome of transplantation (complications)
Autograft	Graft obtained from and returned to the same individual	Take
Isograft (Syngeneic graft)	Graft exchanged between identical twins, or members of inbred strain	Take
Allograft (Homograft)	Graft exchanged between genetically dissimilar individuals of the same specie	Failure (HVGR & GVHR)
Xenograft (Heterograft)	Graft exchanged between members of different species	Failure (HVGR & GVHR)

1. Autologous and Isogeneic Marrow Transplants

The first two types of transplantation, namely the autologous and isogeneic, do not present any difficulties from immunogenetic point of view, since the donor and the recipient are genetically identical. However, there are certain obstacles also to these types of transplants. Autologous bone marrow transplantation, for instance, is not always practical, since not all leukemia patients are brought into remission. Another disadvantage of this procedure is that remission patients, due to the vigorous therapy, may possess far too low number of hemopoietic cells to establish a successful graft. Technical problems, connected with preservation and storage of bone marrow cells, can also present a serious problem. Finally, there is high likelihood that remission marrow contains residual leukemic cells or their precursors.

In the case of isogeneic marrow transplantation, the impediment is represented by the low frequency of monozygotic twins available. Only 1 in 300 patients has available an identical twin. Moreover, a monozygotic twin is not necessarily the most ideal donor. If the hemopathy is genetic in origin, the twin is also prone and perhaps the most likely to contract the disease. This is a very pertinent point in the case of leukemia, because it has been shown that there is a 10 to 20% probability that the monozygotic twin of a sibling with leukemia will develop the disease.[28]

2. Allogeneic and Xenogeneic Marrow Transplants

When allogeneic (or xenogeneic) bone marrow transplantation is approached, the picture becomes more complicated because of the genetic disparity between the donor and the receipient. Allogeneic bone marrow transplantation is more perplexing in general than transplantation of solid tissue allografts. For comparison, whereas only unilateral histocompatibility (i.e., the donor may not express a single antigen which is not present in the recipient) is required for successful take of solid tissue grafts, bilateral compatibility (i.e., all antigens expressed by the donor have to be present in the recipient) is required for the establishment of bone marrow grafts. If these conditions are not met, serious and often fatal complications for the patient may occur after allogeneic marrow transplantation. First, if the donor expresses antigen(s) which the recipient lacks, the recipient's immune system recognizes this "foreign" structure(s) and initiates an immune response which leads to the rejection of marrow transplant. Such reactivity is designated as host-versus-graft reaction (HVGR). The second complication presents itself when the recipient's cells exhibit antigens which are not present in the donor. Under these circumstances the donor bone marrow cells recognize these antigenic differences and mount the reactivity directed against the recipient's tissues; such reactivity, if strong, may result in the recipient's destruction. The latter phenomenon is designated graft-versus-host reaction (GVHR). GVHR could be realized, provided that the immunocompetent cells, with recognition properties or their precursors are present in the graft; thus, GVHR is not to be expected where solid tissue transplants are involved. In contrast, GVHR often endangers bone marrow reconstitution, since bone marrow cell inoculum contains a certain percentage, (although under normal circumstances relatively low), of immunocompetent cells, with the ability to recognize histoincompatible tissues and to exhibit antihost reactivity. In fact, the number of immunocompetent cells present in bone marrow can sometimes be quite large since often at the time of marrow collection contamination with blood, containing high numbers of immunocompetent cells occurs. As a result, strong GVHR may occur soon after bone marrow transplantation. This type of GVHR is called acute GVHR, denoting its prompt effect. Moreover, hemopoietic stem cells present in transplanted bone marrow develop progressively into immunocompetent cells and will also with time recognize host alloantigens and initiate antihost-directed activity. This type of GVHR is designated delayed or chronic, to indicate its late occurrence. Even though chronic GVHR is less harmful than its acute version, it still presents a serious complication for bone marrow reconstitution.[66] The degree of HVGR and GVHR varies significantly with the degree of genetic disparity between the donor and the recipient. In general, the higher the genetic differences, the more vigorous and fatal are both reactions.

Rejection of bone marrow grafts is another barrier to successful bone marrow reconstitution. Rejection of marrow grafts can occur despite the irradiation or drug-suppression of prospective bone marrow recipients. The presence of preformed antibodies, due to the immunization of the recipient through multiple transfusions of blood products, presents one mechanism of rejection. Recently a suggestive higher rate of human bone marrow transplant failures, with increasing number of blood or platelet transfusion, was observed.[67] Additional strong evidence for the concept that a prior immunization is an important factor involved in marrow graft rejection comes from marrow transplantation studies in canine models; these studies have shown a close correlation between the failure of bone marrow grafts and the number of transfusions administered.[68,69] Since the bone marrow donor-recipient pairs are, as a rule, matched for both serologically-defined and lymphocyte-defined antigens at major histocompatibility complex (MHC), HLA in man, other than currently identifiable antigens must be responsible for this type of rejection.

However, it is not likely that preimmunization of the recipient is the only cause of bone marrow graft rejection in man, since the cases where no correlation between marrow graft failure and previous transfusions were detected. Rejection of human marrow grafts in the absence of any previous presensitization and the converse, successful takes in spite of multiple previous transfusions, have been described.[67] It is relevant to mention in this regard the murine bone marrow transplantation studies, since these could be relevant for unexplained failures of human marrow grafts. In mice, bone marrow immunogenetics is strongly contrasted to classical transplantation immunogenetics. The outcome of murine allogeneic and xenogeneic allografts cannot be predicted on the basis of MHC differences.[72] Major histocompatibility complex-incompatible hemopoietic allografts or even hemopoietic xenografts, are often accepted (and not rejected as would be expected according to transplantation laws) by certain mouse recipients. The acceptance of allogeneic or xenogeneic hemopoietic transplants cannot be attributed to the low responsiveness of recipient mice to hemopoietic transplants in general, since the same mice are able to reject hemopoietic allografts or xenografts from other strains of mice or rats.[73-75] The lack of correlation between expression of antigens controlled by classical histocompatibility genes (in mice H-2) and marrow graft take (or lack of take) indicates that H-2 genes do not appear to be involved in the control of bone marrow graft rejection.[73] This statement is strengthened by the observation that the F_1 hybrids are not universal acceptors of parental bone marrow grafts.[70,71] Series of genetic studies which followed these initial observations revealed that two types of genes are involved in murine bone marrow graft rejection. The first class of genes, designated Hemopoietic-histocompatibility genes (abbreviated Hh-genes) is involved in the control of the cell surface determinants, Hh antigens, expressed in contrast to classical H-2 antigens only on hemopoietic tissues and their malignant counterparts, (thus, designated Hh genes).[70-73] The Hh genes are multiple and polymorphic, and most of them are linked to the D-region of H-2 on murine chromosome 17.[73] There is an indication that one (perhaps more) Hh locus may also be linked to the K region of H-2.[74] Although most of the Hh genes are linked to murine MHC, they are distinguishable entities from classical H-2 genes for their noncodominant inheritance (lack of expression in heterozygous F_1 hybrid mice), unique tissue distribution of their products, and the capability to elicit specific host-anti-graft reaction(s) after total body irradiation. The independent segregation of H-2 and Hh genes in certain strains of mice is another example of distinctiveness of these two types of genes. The function of Hh genes is a control over expression of Hh antigens on the cell surface. The Hh antigen's expression appears to depend on homozygosity for Hh gene.[72]

Immune responsiveness to Hh antigens is directed by another class of genes, designated Immune response (IR) genes.[72,75] Even though the presence of the Hh antigen on donor bone marrow cells and the lack of its expression by the recipient is one of the requirements for marrow rejection, there is another condition necessary; the Hh-incompatible recipients must possess the relevant IR gene(s) to be able to recognize and/or react to foreign Hh antigens. When the Hh-incompatible recipient is a genetic nonresponder, to a particular Hh antigen, the transplanted hemopoietic cells will proliferate without impairment, despite the donor-recipient incompatibility. The immune response genes are not linked to murine MHC,[72,74] are multiple, and are inherited as dominant traits.[74]

From an immunological angle, anti-bone marrow graft directed immunity deviates substantially from conventional transplantation immunity.[72] The cells involved in bone marrow graft rejection are relatively radioresistant, thymus independent, mature late in the life (3 weeks after birth), and exhibit prompt rejection (within several hours after graft introduction) without previous immunization. In contrast, cells mediating rejection of other tissue grafts, for example, skin, are impaired by irradiation, are dependent on thymus for their function, are active almost immediately after birth, and require stimulation with antigen and certain time elapse (several days) before rejection is realized.

The bone marrow graft effector cells resemble natural killer cells by their characteristics.[76-78] The similarity between natural killer cells and bone marrow effector cells is illustrated in Table 4. Thus, natural killer cells could be an important component of bone marrow transplantation immunity.

From the studies in mice, it is obvious that bone marrow transplantation reaction deviates severely from the classical immunogenetic laws. Similar differences between solid tissue and bone marrow graft immunogenetics may exist in man and could account for some of the unexplained patterns in clinical bone marrow grafting. Hence, understanding of the mechanism and genetic control of murine marrow transplantation could lead to our better understanding of human bone marrow transplantation and to the improvements in donor selection, development of new typing techniques, and finally, could allow modulation of rejection.

Despite the above mentioned complications associated with HVGR and GVHR, allogeneic bone marrow transplantation is a plausible approach to the cure of various hemopathies, such as leukemia, since via immunosuppressive therapy both HVGR and

Table 4
SIMILARITIES BETWEEN MURINE NATURAL KILLER
CELLS AND BONE MARROW GRAFT EFFECTOR CELLS

Natural occurrence (no sensitization required for function)
Prompt reactivity (within several hours)
Thymus independence
Bone marrow dependence
Late maturation
Partial declination with age
Relative radioresistance
Sensitivity to: strontium-89, cyclophosphamide silica, carrageenan, *Corynebacterium parvum,* glucan, cortisone acetate, tolerance-induction

Table 5
MAJOR CAUSES OF BONE MARROW
GRAFT FAILURES

Nontake	Insufficient preparation of the recipient, (conditioning, number of marrow cells injected)
Rejection	Host's recognition of foreign histocom-patibility antigens expressed on marrow graft (host-versus-graft reaction)
GVHR	Donor's recognition of foreign histocom-patibility antigens expressed on recipi-ent's tissues (graft-versus host reaction)
Infections	Especially viral

GVHR can be mitigated. In contrast, xenogeneic transplantation appears presently to be unrealistic for clinical application. Dicke et al. attempted to use the xenogeneic bone marrow transplantation model in order to protect rhesus monkeys from the effect of lethal irradiation. However, their results were quite discouraging;[79] they observed fatal GVHR combined with failure of hemopoietic repopulation after transplantation of human bone marrow cells.

3. Complications Associated with Bone Marrow Transplantation

There are two major problems surrounding bone marrow transplantation procedures that are relevant for all types of marrow transplants; failure of marrow graft to take and infections of the recipients. The failure of marrow transplants to engraft could be caused by several reasons, one of them being an insufficient preparation of the recipient for bone marrow transplantation. The leukemic patients, for instance, must be given before transplantation total body irradiation (and frequently certain chemotherapy) in an attempt to eradicate the leukemic cells. If the leukemic cells are not eliminated, their continuous proliferation would lead to a relapse of the disease, despite the successful bone marrow reconstitution.

Another important factor for optimal reconstitution is the number of bone marrow cells injected. Since the hemopoietic cells are rather infrequent with regard to other cell populations, high numbers of bone marrow cells have to be injected. It has been established in man that the minimal number of cells necessary for engraftment is in the range of 0.5×10^8 to 1×10^8 cells/kg body weight. In addition, sufficient space and stimuli must be provided in order to achieve optimal growth of bone marrow cells. The latter two conditions are fulfilled by irradiation, which via destruction of host hemopoietic tissues,[65] provides both space and necessary environment composed of radioresistant regulatory cells.[80]

Infections present a critical problem in marrow transplantation, especially in leukemia. It has been estimated that more than 50% of transplanted patients died from intestitial pneumonia or other infections.[81] In the majority of transplanted patients, the pneumonia has been found to be caused by viral agents, e.g., cytomegalovirus or *pneumocystis carinii*. The immunosuppressive effect of conditioning regimen, such as irradiation and possible other types of therapy coupled with the relatively late and often incomplete immune reconstitution, favor the infection. Also complications connected with GVHR are additive in this regard. The major causes of bone marrow graft failures are illustrated in Table 5.

III. RESULTS OF CLINICAL BONE MARROW TRANSPLANTATION IN LEUKEMIA

Bone marrow transplantation in leukemia should accomplish two aims; to allow eradication of leukemic cell population by antileukemic agents and to restore normal hemopoiesis. Its success depends on the effectiveness of antileukemic therapy and type, quality, and number of bone marrow cells injected. Its strategy is to eradicate leukemia with high dose chemotherapy treatments that would otherwise be lethal for the leukemic patient.

A. Isogeneic Transplantation

Acute leukemia is the most frequent type of leukemia in which bone marrow transplantation is applied. In isogeneic transplant recipients (transplants between identical twins) the engraftment is almost a rule since the donor and the recipient have identical genetic makeup. The initial isogeneic marrow transplantation studies involving patients with acute lymphoblastic leukemia were performed by the Seattle group. In these studies supralethal doses of total body irradiation were used as pretransplantation conditioning regimen. Even though all of the transplanted patients achieved hemopoietic recovery, transplantation was not therapeutically successful since leukemia recurred within several weeks.[82] In the subsequent group of patients, cyclophosphamide therapy was added to the total body irradiation regimen in order to eradicate more effectively leukemic cells present in the recipient. In most cases, immunotherapy composed of infusion of donor's lymphocytes and irradiated DMSO-preserved leukemic cells was given for several weeks to leukemic patients. The rationale for the involvement of immunotherapy was to potentiate patient's antileukemia defense.[83] Together, 23 isogeneic transplantations were done by the Seattle bone marrow transplantation team using this regimen. Some of the leukemic patients were followed as long as 10 years after transplantation.[84] The results of these studies showed that more than 70% of transplanted patients attained complete remission and almost 30% of them are leukemia free at the present time, i.e., 6 to 10 years after transplant. These are very promising results, indicating that recurrence of leukemia after isogeneic transplantation may be controlled if chemotherapy combined with radiation and immunotherapy is applied. In spite of these encouraging data, other types of bone marrow transplants must be explored since the patients with identical twins are infrequent.

B. Autologous Transplantation

The summary of the results of autologous bone marrow transplantation performed by several transplantation teams are illustrated in Table 5. As can be seen from the table, in most cases of the autologous bone marrow transplantation situation the takes of bone marrow grafts were achieved,[85-90] although graft failures were also observed.[91,92] Similarly to isogeneic bone marrow transplantation, the recurrence of leukemia presents a serious problem. In fact, under the autologous transplantation circumstances, the patient may be more disposed to leukemia recurrence, since it is highly likely that in addition to the presence of leukemic cells persisting after chemo- and radiation therapies, the bone marrow cell pool, collected in the remission of the disease, contains leukemic cells or their precursors. The leukemic cells in remission marrow are difficult to detect since the presently available techniques for their detection, such as cytogenetic analysis, are highly insensitive; in addition they are useful only in 70% of cases of acute leukemia that have chromosomal abnormalities.[79] It has been calculated that the total number of leukemic cells in the marrow in leukemia remission can be as high as 10^7.[35] Hence, the number of residual leukemic cells collected in remission may be as great as 10^4 to 10^5 cells when one estimates that 1% of entire bone marrow supply is collected for transplantation.[79]

However, there are currently several new techniques explored, aimed at elimination or at least reduction of leukemic cells from normal tissues. Some of these are of physical nature and are based on differential sensitivity of leukemic and normal cells to osmotic shock,[94] freezing and thawing,[95] hyperthermia,[96] or their different densities.[97-99] The density fractionation technique is the most common technique used in clinics and has been described in detail before.[100] Briefly, it is the discontinuous albumin gradient technique, consisting of albumin solutions of different concentrations (25%, 23%, 21%, 17%). The bone marrow cells are suspended in the top (17%) albumin layer. After centrifugation, five fractions are obtained that differ with regard to the cell distribution based on their densities. Leukemic cells of AML patients were demonstrated to be in the lighter fractions, whereas at least 50% of hemopoietic (colony forming) cells are in the middle and lower fraction.[117] Even though not absolute, this technique allows separation of leukemic cells from human hemopoietic cells. Other techniques aimed in separation of leukemic and normal hemopoietic cells are based on differential sensitivities of these two cell populations to drugs or on the differences in their cell surface characteristics. Thus, it may be possible in the future with combination of these various techniques to eliminate most, if not all of the leukemic cells from autologous bone marrow graft.

In autologous bone marrow transplantation cases another point of solemn concern is the quality of bone marrow cells collected in remission, since these cells were exposed often to megadose chemotherapies and also to storage procedures. Schaefer et al.[101] observed, for instance, significant decrease of hemopoietic progenitors (GM-CFC) in cryopreserved bone marrow after longer storage. It has also been reported that there are differences in self-replicating properties between hemopoietic stem cells in remission marrow and those from normal individuals.[102] These observations must be kept in mind when long-term stored bone marrow cells are employed for engraftment.

C. Allogeneic Transplantation

Total body irradiation alone has been found insufficient to eradicate leukemia also under allogeneic bone marrow transplantation condition. Various drugs, such as cyclophosphamide,[103] piperazinedione,[104] as well as combination chemotherapy, e.g., SCARI (ARA-C, thioguanine, cyclophosphamide, daunorubicin) in one case[35,105] and CRAB (BCNU, cyclophosphamide, ARA-C) in the other[106] was added in order to ameliorate recurrence of leukemia. Addition of cyclophosphamide to the total body irradiation significantly increased the number of surviving leukemia patients. From 196 leukemic patients that received HLA-compatible allogeneic bone marrow grafts, 15% represent the long-term survivors (more than 2 years). Thirty eight percent of the patients experienced relapse and died of leukemia.[35] The rest of the patients died of GVHR, infection, or persistence of leukemia.

When the SCARI combination therapy regimen was added to irradiation prior to allogeneic marrow transplantation, substantial diminution in leukemia recurrence was observed; however, due to its toxicity, such regimen did not improve survival of leukemic patients significantly. The median survival was 196 days and leukemia-free survival of 11 months was accomplished in 27% of the patients. The results of transplanted leukemia patients receiving CRAB chemotherapy protocol and irradiation were not impressive either; 10 patients were treated and 4 of these relapsed with leukemia, 3 died of sepsis, 2 of interstitial pneumonitis, 1 of GVHR, and 1 of liver disease.[106] The median survival was 57 days and none of the transplanted patients survived over 2 years. The results of allogeneic transplantation of Dicke et al.,[104] combining peperazionedione chemotherapy with total body irradiation, showed the median survival time of 90 days and the longest survivor more than 1 year.[104]

Another transplantation group conducted allogeneic transplantation of leukemic patients with chemotherapy alone. High doses of cyclophosphamide were used in these studies (200 to 240 mg/kg body weight, administered in four consecutive day doses of 50 to 60 mg/kg). Even though initial antileukemic effect was observed, recurrence of leukemia was manifested at later time intervals in most of the transplanted patients; patients surviving more than 150 days showed leukemia relapse.[107,108] Graft-vs-host disease and interstitial pneumonitis represented other complications of this transplantation regimen. In some of the patients conditioned only with cyclophosphamide, graft failure was noticed (13% of patients).

In summary, recurrence of leukemia, frequent infections, GVHR, and lack of engraftment are complications connected with human allogeneic marrow transplantation.

Acute GVHR can be seen already within 7 days after marrow transplantation and is caused by the presence of lymphocytes (T cells) contaminating the bone marrow inoculum. Delayed GVHR begins usually within a month post-grafting and is caused by maturation of transplanted hemopoietic cells into immunocompetent lymphocytes. Acute GVHR could be mitigated by marrow fractionation using the already described discontinuous albumin density gradients, since the majority of lymphocytes involved in GVHR is present in different fractions than hemopoietic cells.[104] Dicke has shown[35] that fraction of bone marrow cells obtained after discontinuous albumin gradient separation, containing low numbers of PHA responsive T cells, exhibited less severe GVHR after allogeneic transplantation than unfractionated marrow.[104] Delayed GVHR, of course, cannot be mitigated by density gradient fractionation. Methotrexate[111] and antilymphocyte reagents[112] have been suggested as useful agents in mitigation of GVHR. However, the activity of the latter preparation varies broadly from batch to batch. Furthermore, the usefulness of methotrexate in GVHR has not been firmly established either. It has also been indicated by murine experimental studies that delayed GVHR could be prevented by bacterial decontamination before marrow transplantation.[113,114] These data were confirmed in a primate experimental model.[109] Moreover, in man after complete bacterial decontamination, only 1 patient from 10 was confronted with GVHR after transplantation.[115] Interestingly, relationship has been established between GVHR and leukemia; it has been suggested that an indirect relationship between recurrence of leukemia and GVHR exist; the higher the degree of GVHR, the less chance of recurrence of leukemia. Specifically, it was observed that the leukemic patients undergoing II to IV grade degree of chronic GVHR after allogeneic transplantation experienced 13 times less leukemia recurrence than leukemic recipients that received isogeneic transplant, 11 times less than allogeneic transplant recipients without GVHR, and 7 times less than recipients of allogeneic grafts with GVHR of Grade I degree.[35] The fact that despite the GVHR antileukemic effect, the outcome of allogeneic transplantation is not as good as the syngeneic one, is due mainly to the mortality from GVHR, bone marrow graft rejection, and infections.

As has been indicated before, GVHR is directly related to the genetic disparity be-

Table 6

RESULTS OF BONE MARROW TRANSPLANTATION IN LEUKEMIA

Type of leukemia	Type of treatment	Results	Number of patients	Ref.
AML, ALL	Piperazinedione & TBI	14/28 CR MD (4 + MO) MS (7 + MO)	28	85
ALL	Combination chemo. & TBI	1/3 DR	3	86
CGL-BC	Various chemo. & TBI	5/7 Chron. phase	7	87
AML in remission	Cytoxan & TBI (1000r)	5/5 Full HEM. Recovery	5	88
AML, ALL	Cytoxan & TBI (1000r)	6/6 CR MD (4MO)	6	89
AML	Thioguanine ARA-C cytoxan CCNU	1 CR 2 PR	3	90
CGL-BC	Cytoxan & TBI (1000r)	2 Chron. phase 2 Graft fail. 3 Partial engraftment	7	91, 92
ALL	TVI (470r)	1/3 CR(3 + MO)	3	185

Note: CR — complete remission; MD — Median duration; DR — Delayed recovery; CGL-BL — Chronic granulocytic leukemia, blast crisis; PR — Partial remission; MS — Medial survival; TBI — Total body irradiation.

tween the donor and recipient. Thus, the selection of donor-recipient pairs genetically identical at MHC is also an important factor in controlling GVHR. Even though the identity in MHC lessens the degree of GVHR, it does not always prevent it.[116] It is suggested that except for currently defined MHC loci, other genes both linked and nonlinked to MHC control GVHR.[69] The ideal donor recipient pairs are MHC-identical related individuals. However, because of low frequency of these donors (∼ 25%), allogeneic transplantation is often performed with MHC compatible, unrelated individuals. The available clinical data indicate that GVHR in nonrelated MHC compatible donor-recipient pairs is more vigorous.

IV. CONCLUDING REMARKS

It is obvious that bone marrow transplantation presents a viable therapeutic approach not only to the treatment of leukemia, but also to the other types of hemopathies, immunodeficiencies, and solid malignancies. Since this approach is relatively new, there are many pressing questions which have to be subjected to continuous studies in man and further experimentation in animal models. Some of these are prevention of bone marrow graft rejection and graft-versus-host reaction, improvement in the speed and quality of marrow reconstitution, improvement in typing techniques for donor-recipient selection, and investigation of new immunomodulating agents which would improve the graft-versus-host reaction and rejection of bone marrow grafts (perhaps via induction of suppressor cells) and also augment hemopoiesis. Furthermore, our thorough understanding of the genetic control and mechanism of bone marrow graft rejection could make bone marrow transplantation useful and viable clinical therapy.

ACKNOWLEDGMENTS

I wish to express my thanks to Dr. Karel Dicke for providing the data for Table 6, and to Jackie Salters and Geraldine Harrison for their expert secretarial assistance in the preparation of this manuscript.

REFERENCES

1. Cowdell, R. H., Phizackerley, P. J. R., and Pyke, D. A., Constitutional anaemia (Fanconi's Syndrome) and leukemia in two brothers, *Blood,* 10, 788, 1955.
2. Schroeder, T. M. and Kurth, R., Spontaneous chromosomal breakage and high incidence of leukemia in inherited disease, *Blood,* 37, 96, 1971.
3. Ozsoylu, S. and Hicsonmez, G., Leukemia presenting as aplastic anaemia, *J. Pediatr.,* 81, 187, 1972.
4. Jenkins, D. E. and Hartman, R. C., Paroxysmal nocturnal hemoglobinuria terminating in acute myeloblastic leukemia, *Blood,* 33, 274, 1969.
5. Holden, D. and Lichtman, H., Paroxysmal nocturnal hemoglobinuria with acute leukemia, *Blood,* 33, 283, 1969.
6. Kaufmann, R. W., Schechter, G. P., and McFarland, W., Paroxysmal nocturnal hemoglobinurea terminating in acute granulocytic leukemia, *Blood,* 33, 287, 1969.
7. Bloomfield, C. D. and Brunning, R. D., Acute leukemia as a terminal event in nonleukemic hemapoietic disorders, *Semin. Oncol.,* 3, 297, 1976.
8. Gatti, R. A. and Good, R. A., Occurrence of malignancy in immunodeficiency diseases. A literature review, *Cancer,* 28, 89, 1971.
9. Girdwood, R. H., Blood disorders due to drugs and other agents, *Excerpta Medica,* 1973.
10. Le Noir, C., Sur un cas de purpura attribué e l'intoxication par la benzine, *Soc. Med. Hop.,* 14, 1251, 1897.
11. Forni, A. and Vigliani, E. C., Chemical leukemogenisis in man, *Semin. Haematol.,* 7, 211, 1974.
12. Pierre, R. V., Preleukemic states, *Semin. Hematol.,* 11, 73, 1974.
13. Aksoy, M., Erdem, S., and DinCol, G., Leukemia in shoe workers exposed to benzene, *Blood,* 44, 837, 1974.
14. DeGowin, R., Benzene exposure and aplastic anaemia followed by leukemia 15 years later, *JAMA,* 185, 748, 1963.
15. Vigliani, E. C. and Saita, G., Benzene and leukemia, *N. Engl. J. Med.,* 271, 872, 1964.
16. Lebon, J. and Messerschmitt, J., Myelose aplastique d' origine médicamenteuse myéloblastose aigue terminale reflexions pathogéniques, *Le Sang,* 26, 799, 1955.
17. O'Gorman Hughes, D. W., The varied pattern of aplastic anaemia in childhood, *Aust. Paediatr. J.,* 2, 228, 1966.
18. Cohen, H. J. and Huang, A. T. F., A marker chromosome abnormality: occurrence in chloramphenicol-associated acute leukemia, *Arch. Intern. Med.,* 123, 440, 1973.
19. Awwaad, S., Khalifa, A. S., and Kamel, K., Vacuolization of leukocytes and bone marrow aplasia due to chloramphenicol toxicity, *Clin. Pediatr.,* 14, 449, 1975.
20. Goh, K. O., Chloramphenicol, acute leukemia, and chromosomal vacuolizations, *South. Med. J.,* 64, 815, 1971.
21. Scheuer-Karpin, V. R., Ein toxisches agents in der leukämiegenese, *Z. Inn. Med.,* 13, 416, 1958.
22. Fraumeni, J. F., Bone marrow depression induced by chloramphenicol or phenylbutazone, *JAMA,* 201, 828, 1967.
23. Jensen, M. K. and Roll, K., Phenylbutazone and leukemia, *Acta Med. Scand.,* 178, 505, 1965.
24. Leavesley, G. M., Stenhouse, N. S., Dougan, L., and Woodliff, H. J., Phenylbutazone and leukemia. Is there a realtionship? *Med. J. Aust.,* 2, 963, 1969.
25. Hamer, J. W. and Gunz, F. W., Multiple etiological factors in case of acute leukaemia, *N.Z. Med. J.,* 71, 141, 1970.
26. Bull, O. and Skobba, T. J., Acutt myelogen leukemi, Sekvele Ved. oksyfenbutazone-indusert aplastisk anemi, *Tidsskr. Nor. Laegforen,* 94, 1319, 1974.
27. Cronkite, E. P., Moloney, W., and Bond, V. P., Radiation leukemogenesis: an analysis of the problem, *Am. J. Med.,* 28, 673, 1960.
28. Miller, R. W., Death from childhood leukemia and solid tumors among twins and other sibs in the United States, 1960-1967, *J. Natl. Cancer Inst.,* 46, 203, 1971.
29. Gallo, A. C. C., Yang, S. S., and Ting, R. C., RNA-dependent DNA polymerase of human acute leukemic cells, *Nature (London),* 228, 927, 1970.
30. Dmochowski, L., Recent studies on leukemia and solid tumors in mice and man, *Bibl. Haematol.,* 30, 285, 1968.

31. Bennett, J. M., Catovsky, D., Daniel, M. J., Flandrin, G., Galton, P. A. G., Gralnick, H. R., and Sultan, C., Proposals for the classification of the acute leukemias, *Br. J. Haematol.*, 33, 451, 1976.

32. Gralnick, H. R., Galton, P. A. G., Catovsky, D., Sultan, C., and Bennett, J. M., Classification of acute leukemia, *Ann. Intern. Med.*, 87, 740, 1977.

33. Moore, M. A. S., Williams, N., and Metcalf, D., In vitro colony formation by normal and leukemic human hemopoietic cells; interaction between colony forming and colony stimulation cells, *J. Natl. Cancer Inst.*, 50, 603, 1973.

34. Moore, M. A. S., Spitzer, G., Williams, N., Metcalf, D., and Buckley, J., Agar culture studies in 127 cases of untreated acute leukemia; the prognostic value of reclassificiation of leukemia according to in vitro growth characteristics, *Blood*, 44, 1, 1974.

35. Dicke, K. A., Zander, A. R., Verma, D. S., Spitzer, G., and Vallekoop, L., The treatment of acute leukemia, in *Transplantation Surgery*, Kuntz, S. L., Ed., Marcel Dekker, New York, in press.

36. Jacobson, L. O., Simmons, E. L., Marks, E. K., Robson, M. J., Bethard, W. F., and Gaston, E. O., The role of the spleen in radiation injury and recovery, *J. Lab. Clin. Med.*, 35, 746, 1950.

37. Lorenz, E., Uphoff, D., Reid, T. R., and Shelton, E., Modification of irradiation injury in mice and guinea pigs by bone marrow injections, *J. Natl. Cancer Inst.*, 12, 197, 1951.

38. Ford, C. E., Hamerton, J. L., Barnes, D. W. H., and Loutit, J. F., Cytological identification of radiation chimeras, *Nature (London)*, 177, 452, 1956.

39. Nowell, P. C., Cole, L. J., Habermeyer, J. G., and Roan, P. L., Growth and continued function of rat marrow cells in X-irradiated mice, *Cancer Res.*, 16, 258, 1956.

40. Vos, O., Davids, J. A. G., Weyzen, W. W. H., and van Bekkum, D. W., Evidence for the cellular hypotheses in radiation protection by bone marrow cells, *Acta Physiol. Pharmacol. Neerl.*, 4, 482, 1956.

41. Lindsley, D. T., Odell, T. T., Jr., and Tausche, F. G., Implantation of functional erythropoietin elements following total-body irradiation, *Proc. Soc. Exp. Biol. Med.*, 90, 512, 1955.

42. Mitchison, N. A., The colonization of irradiated tissue by transplanted spleen cells, *Br. J. Exp. Pathol.*, 37, 239, 1956.

43. Till, J. E. and McCulloch, E. A., Direct measurement of the radiation sensitivity of normal mouse bone marrow cells, *Radiat. Res.*, 14, 213, 1961.

44. Brecher, G. and Smith, W. W., Dissociation between spleen colony formation and bone marrow recovery in colchicine-treated irradiated mice, *Radiat. Res.*, 25, 176, 1965.

45. Savage, A. M., Hematopoietic recovery in endotoxin-treated lethally X-irradiated BUB mice, *Radiat. Res.*, 23, 180, 1964.

46. Wu, A. M., Till, J. E., Siminovitch, L., and McCulloch, E. A., A cytological study of the capacity for differentiation of normal hemopoietic colony-forming cells, *J. Cell Physiol.*, 69, 177, 1967.

47. Welshons, W. J., Detection and use of cytological anomalies in the mouse, in *Mammalian Cytogenetics and Related Problems in Radiobiology*, Pavan, C., Chagas, C., and Frota-Pessoa, O., Eds., Pergamon Press, Oxford, 1964, 233.

48. Lewis, J. P. and Trobaugh, F. E., Jr., Haematopoietic stem cells, *Nature (London)*, 204, 589, 1964.

49. Jurášková, V. and Tkadleček, L., Character of primary and secondary colonies of haematopoiesis in the spleen of irradiated mice, *Nature (London)*, 206, 951, 1965.

50. Quesenberry, P. and Levitt, L., Hematopoietic stem cells, *N. Engl. J. Med.*, 301, 755, 1979.

51. Quesenberry, P. and Levitt, L., Hematopoietic stem cells, *N. Engl. J. Med.*, 301, 819, 1979.

52. Quesenberry, P. and Levitt, L., Hematopoietic stem cells, *N. Engl. J. Med.*, 301, 868, 1979.

53. Metcalf, D., An outline of hemopoiesis and current terminology, in *Hemopoietic Colonies. In Vitro Cloning of Normal and Leukemic Cells*, Springer-Verlag, New York, 1953, 5.

54. Maximov, A. A., Relation of blood cells to connective tissues and endothelium, *Physiol. Rev.*, 4, 533, 1924.

55. Metcalf, D. and Moore, M. A. S., Haemopoietic cell, in *Frontiers in Biology*, North Holland, Amsterdam, 1971.

56. Bradley, T. R. and Metcalf, D., The growth of mouse bone marrow cells in vitro, *Aust. J. Exp. Biol. Med. Sci.*, 44, 287, 1966.

57. Axelrad, A. A., McLeod, D. L., Shreeve, M. M., and Heath, D. S., Properties of cells that produce erythrocytic colonies in vitro, in Hemopoiesis In Culture: Second International Workshop, DHEW Publication No. (NIH) 74-205, Robinson, W. A., Government Printing Office, Washington, D.C., 1973, 226.

58. Pike, B. L. and Robinson, W. A., Human bone marrow colony growth in agar gel, *J. Cell Physiol.*, 76, 77, 1970.

59. Whang, J., Frei, E., III, Tjio, J. H., Carbone, P., and Brecker, G., The distribution of the Philadelphia chromosome in patients with chronic myelocytic leukemia, *Blood*, 22, 664, 1963.

60. Adamson, J. W., Fialkow, P. J., Murphy, S., Prchal, J. F., and Steinmann, L., Polycythemia vera: stem cell and probable clonal origin of the disease, *N. Engl. J. Med.*, 295, 913, 1976.

61. Haller, O. and Wigzell, H., Suppression of natural killer cell activity with radioactive strontium. Effector cells are marrow-dependent, *J. Immunol.*, 118, 1503, 1977.

62. Haller, O., Hansson, M., Kiessling, R., and Wigzell, H., Role on nonconventional natural killer cell resistance against syngeneic tumor cells in vitro, *Nature (London)*, 270, 609, 1977.

63. Curry, J. L., Trentin, J. J., and Wolf, N., Hemopoietic spleen colony studies. II. Erythropoiesis, *J. Exp. Med.*, 125, 703, 1967.

64. Schooley, J. C. and Garcia, J. F., Some properties of serum obtained from rabbits immunized with human urinary erythropoietin, *Blood*, 25, 204, 1965.

65. Lange, R. D., McDonald, T. P., and Jordan, T., Antisera to erythropoietin: partial characterization of two different antibodies, *J. Lab. Clin. Med.*, 73, 78, 1969.

66. van Bekkum, D. W., Hostile grafts, in *Advance in Transplantation*, Daussett, J., Hamburger, J., and Mathé, G., Eds., Williams & Wilkins, Baltimore, 1967.

67. Storb, R., Prentice, R. L., and Thomas, E. D., Marrow transplantation in treatment of aplastic anemia. An analysis of factors associated with graft reaction, *N. Engl. J. Med.*, 296, 61, 1977.

68. Storb, R., Epstein, R. B., Rudolph, R. H., and Thomas, E. D., The effect of prior transplantation on marrow grafts between histocompatible canine siblings, *J. Immunol.*, 105, 627, 1970.

69. Storb, R., Rudolph, R. H., Graham, I. C., Theodore, C., and Thomas, E. D., The influence of transfusion from unrelated donors upon marrow grafts between histocompatible canine siblings, *J. Immunol.*, 107, 409, 1971.

70. Lotzová, E. and Cudkowicz, G., Hybrid resistance to parental NZW bone marrow grafts. Association with the D-end of H-2, *Transplantation*, 12, 130, 1971.

71. Lotzová, E. and Cudkowicz, G., Hybrid resistance to parental WB/Re bone marrow grafts, *Transplantation*, 13, 256, 1972.

72. Lotzová, E., Resistance to parental, allogeneic and xenogeneic hemopoietic grafts in irradiated mice, *Exp. Hematol.*, 5, 215, 1977.

73. Lotzová, E., Involvement of hemopoietic-histocompatibility genes in allogeneic bone marrow transplantation in mice, *Tissue Antigens*, 9, 148, 1977.

74. Cudkowicz, G. and Lotzova, E., Hemopoietic cell-defined component of the major histocompatibility complex of mice. Identification of responsive and unresponsive recipients to bone marrow transplants, *Transplant. Proc.*, 5, 1399, 1973.

75. Lotzová, E., Dicke, K. A., Trentin, J. J., and Gallagher, M. T., Genetic control of bone marrow transplantation in irradiated mice: classification of mouse strains according to their responsiveness to bone marrow allografts and xenografts, *Transplant. Proc.*, 9, 289, 1977.

76. Lotzová, E. and Savary, C. A., Possible involvement of natural killer cells in bone marrow graft rejection, *Biomedicine*, 27, 341, 1977.

77. Lotzová, E. and McCredie, K. B., Natural killer cells in mice and man and their possible biological significance, *Cancer Immunol. Immunother.*, 4, 215, 1978.

78. Lotzová, E., Analogy between rejection of hemopoietic transplants and natural killing, in *Natural Cell-Mediated Immunity Against Tumors*, Herberman, R. B., Ed., Academic Press, New York, 1980, 1117.

79. Dicke, K. A., Lotzova, E., Spitzer, G., and McCredie, K. B., Immunobiology of bone marrow transplantation, *Semin. Hematol.*, 15, 263, 1978.

80. van Bekkum, D. W. and de Vries, M. J., *Radiation Chimeras*, Academic Press, New York, 1967, 20.

81. Johnson, F. L., Thomas, E. D., Buckner, C. D., Clift, R. A., Fefer, A., and Storb, R., The current status of bone marrow transplantation in cancer treatment, *Cancer Treatm. Rev.*, 1, 81, 1974.

82. Thomas, E. D., Lochte, H. L., Jr., Cannon, J. H., Sahler, O. D., and Ferrebee, J. W., Supralethal whole body irradiation and isologous marrow transplantation in man, *J. Clin. Invest.*, 38, 1709, 1959.

83. Thomas, E. D., Herman, E. C., Jr., Greenogli, W. B., Hager, E. B., Cannon, J. H., Ferrebee, J. W., and Sahler, O. D., Irradiation and marrow infusion in leukemia, *Arch. Intern. Med.*, 107, 829, 1961.

84. Fefer, A., Einstein, A. B., Thomas, E. D., Buckner, C. D., Clift, R. A., Glucksberg, H., Neiman, P. E., and Storb, R., Bone marrow transplantation for hematolocytic neoplastica in 16 patients with identical twins, *N. Engl. J. Med.*, 290, 1389, 1974.

85. Dicke, K. A., Zander, A. R., Spitzer, G., Vellekoop, L., Verma, D. S., Lafferty, M., and Litam, J., Autologous bone marrow transplantation in adult leukemia in relapse, *Lancet*, 1, 514, 1979.

86. Wells, J. R., Billing, R., Herzog, S. A., Feig, S. A., Gale, R. P., Terasaki, P., and Cline, M. J., Autotransplantation after in vitro immunotherapy of lymphoblastic leukemia, *Exp. Hematol.*, 7, 164, 1979.

87. Goldman, J. M., Autografting cryopreserved buffy coat cells for chronic granulocytic leukemia in transformation, *Exp. Hematol.*, 7, 389, 1979.

88. Fay, J. W., Silberman, H. R., Moore, J. O., Noell, K. T., and Huang, A. T., Autologous marrow transplantation for patients with acute myelogenous leukemia — a preliminary report, *Exp. Hematol.,* 7, 302, 1979.

89. Herzig, G. P., Phillips, G. L., Mill, W., Napombijara, C., Bernard, S., and Wolff, S., Treatment of hematological malignancy with cyclophosphamide, total body irradiation and autologous bone marrow transplantation, *Blood,* 52, 253, 1978.

90. Gorin, N. C., Najman, A., David, R., Stachowiak, J., HirschMarie, F., Muller, J. Y., Petit, J. C., Leblanc, G., Parlier, Y., Jullien, A. M., Cavalier, J., Salmon, Ch., and Duchamel, G., Autogreffe de moelle osseuse apres chimiotherapie lourde Nlle, *Presse. Med.,* 7, 4105, 1978.

91. Buckner, C. D., Clift, R. A., Fefer, A., Neiman, P. E., Storb, R., and Thomas, E. D., Treatment of blastic transformation of chronic granulocytic leukemia by high dose cyclophosphamide, total body irradiation and infusion of cryopreserved autologous marrow, *Exp. Hematol.,* 2, 138, 1974.

92. Buckner, C. D., Stewart, P., Clift, R. A., Atkins, L., and Webster, E. W., Treatment of blastic transformation of chronic granulocytic leukemia by chemotherapy, total body irradiation and infusion of cryopreserved autologous marrow, *Exp. Hematol.,* 6, 96, 1978.

93. McGovern, J. J., Russell, P. S., Atkins, L., and Webster, E. W., Treatment of terminal leukemic relapse by total body irradiation and intravenous infusion of stored autologous bone marrow obtained during remission, *N. Engl. J. Med.,* 260, 675, 1959.

94. Ben-Sasson, S., Shaviv, R., Bentwich, Z., Slavin, A., and Doljanski, F., Osmotic behaviour of normal and leukemic lymphocytes, *Blood,* 46, 891, 1975.

95. Farrant, J., Knight, S. C., O'Brien, J. A., and Morris, G. J., Selection of leukemic cell population by freezing and thawing, *Nature (London),* 245, 322, 1973.

96. Kase, K. and Hahn, B. M., Comparison of some response to hyperthermia by normal human diploid cells and neoplastic cells from the same origin, *Europ. J. Cancer,* 12, 481, 1976.

97. Metcalf, D., The discrimination of leukemic from normal cells, *Biomedicine,* 18, 264, 1973.

98. Moore, M. A. S., Williams, N., and Metcalf, D., Characterization of in vitro colony forming cells in acute and chronic myeloid leukemia, in *The Nature of Leukemia,* Vincent, P. C., Ed., Australian Cancer Society, Sydney, 1972, 135.

99. Dicke, K. A., Stevens, E. E., Spitzer, G., McCredie, K. B., and Bottino, J. C., Autologous bone marrow transplantation in a case of adult acute leukemia, *Transplant. Proc.,* 9, 193, 1977.

100. Dicke, K. A., van Noord, M. J., Maat, B., Schaefer, U. W., and van Bekkum, D. W., Attempts at morphological identification of the hemopoietic stem cell in primates and rodents, in *Hemotopoietic Stem Cells CIBA Foundation Symposium,* Wolstenholme, G. E. W. and O'Connor, M., Eds., Elsevier, Amsterdam, 1973, 47.

101. Schaefer, U. W., Nowrousian, M. R., Ohl, S., Boecker, W. R., Scheulen, M. E., Schilcher, B., and Smith, C. G., Autologous bone marrow transplantation. The influence of prolonged cytotoxic chemotherapy, in *Haematology and Blood Transfusion,* Thierfelder, X., Rodt, H., and Kolb, H. J., Eds., Springer-Verlag, New York, 1980.

102. Schaefer, U. W., Transplantation of fresh allogeneic and cryopreserved autologous bone marrow (BM) in acute leukemia, *Exp. Hematol.,* 5, 101, 1977.

103. Thomas, E. D., Buckner, C. D., Banaji, M., Clift, R. A., Fefer, A., Flournoy, N., Goodell, B. W., and Hickman, R. O., One hundred patients with acute leukemia treated by chemotherapy, total body irradiation and allogeneic marrow transplantation, *Blood,* 49, 511, 1977.

104. Dicke, K. A., Spitzer, G., Peters, L., Stevens, E. E., Hendriks, W., and McCredie, K. B., Approaches to graft-versus-host disease following bone marrow transplantation in monkeys and man, *Transplant. Proc.,* 10, 217, 1978.

105. Weiden, P. L., Fluornoy, N., Thomas, E. D., Prentice, R., Fefer, A., Buckner, C. D., and Storb, R., Antileukemic effect of graft-versus-host disease in human recipients of allogeneic marrow grafts, *N. Engl. J. Med.,* 300, 1068, 1979.

106. O'Leary, M., Ramsay, M. K. C., and Nesbit, M. E., Bone marrow transplantation for hematologic malignancy, in *Graft-Versus-Leukemia in Man and Animal Models,* O'Kunewick, J. P. and Meredith, R., Eds., CRC Press, Boca Raton, Fla., in press.

107. Elbenfein, G. J., Borgaonkar, D. S., Saral, R., Bias, W. B., Burns, W. H., Sensenbrenner, L. L., Tutschka, P. J., Zaczek, B. S., Zander, A. R., and Epstein, R. B., Cytogenetic evidence for recurrence of acute myelogenous leukemia after allogeneic bone marrow transplantation, *Blood,* 52, 627, 1978.

108. Tutschka, P. J., Santos, G. W., and Elfenbein, G. J., Allogeneic bone marrow transplantation as therapy for leukemia — Baltimore experience, in *Graft-Versus-Host-Leukemia in Man and Animal Models,* O'Kunewick, J. P. and Meredith, R., Eds., CRC Press, Boca Raton, Fla., in press.

109. Dicke, K. A., van der Waay, D., and van Bekkum, D. W., The use of stem cell grafts in combined immune deficiencies, *Birth Defects XV,* 1, 389, 1975.

110. Dicke, K. A. and van Bekkum, D. W., Preparation and use of stem cell concentrates for restoration of immune deficiency diseases and bone marrow aplasia, *Rev. Europ. Clin. Biol.,* 17, 645, 1972.

111. Thomas, E. D., Storb, R., Clift, R. A., Fefer, A., Johnson, L., Neiman, P. E., Lerner, K. G., Glucksberg, H., and Buckner, D. C., Bone marrow transplantation, *N. Engl. J. Med.*, 292, 832, 1975.

112. Weiden, P. L., Doney, K., Storb, R., and Thomas, E. D., Anti-human thymocyte globulin (ATG) for prophylaxis and treatment of graft versus host disease in recipients of allogeneic marrow grafts, *Transplant. Proc.*, 10, 213, 1978.

113. van Bekkum, D. W., Roodenburg, J., Heidt, P. J., and van der Waaij, D., Mitigation of delayed secondary disease of allogeneic mouse radiation chimeras by changing the intestinal microflora, *Exp. Hematol.*, 1, 289, 1973.

114. van Bekkum, D. W., Rodenburg, J., Heidt, P. J., and van der Waaij, D., Mitigation of secondary disease of allogeneic mouse radiation chimeras by modification of the intestinal microflora, *J. Natl. Cancer Inst.*, 52, 401, 1974.

115. Vossen, J. M., Guiot, H. F. L., and Dooren, L. J., Suppression of clinical graft versus host disease by control of microflora in children treated with bone marrow transplantation, *Exp. Hematol.*, 7, 11, 1979.

116. Speck, B., Dooren, L. J., and DeKoning, J., Clinical experience with bone marrow transplantation: failure or success, *Transplant. Proc.*, 3, 409, 1971.

117. Dicke, K. A., personal communication, 1980.

Chapter 7

BREAST CANCER: EFFECT OF RADIATION TREATMENT ON IMMUNE STATUS

Donald E. Carlson

Breast cancer is the leading cause of cancer death among females.[1] It is important to keep in mind that the term "breast cancer" is used for a heterogeneous group of cancers of the breast — heterogeneous in terms of the grade of malignancy, site or origin, histological type, and presence or absence of surface markers such as estrogen receptors.[2,3] Although breast cancer may be viewed naively as a localized disease, in fact a clinically evident tumor must be recognized as a systemic entity. The mere fact that some 25% of patients with clinically negative lymph nodes result in treatment failures following surgery suggests a systemic disease extending beyond the defined region of surgical intervention.[4] Within a given group of breast cancer patients with clinically similar diseases, responses are rarely uniform.[5]

This consideration together with additional data to be discussed in some detail below provides evidence for existence of host-mediated mechanisms which may specifically or nonspecifically modulate local and systemic tumor growth and dissemination. To understand these mechanisms and to utilize them to therapeutic advantage it is necessary to deal with a number of questions which may now only be indirectly or partially addressed. These relate to both basic tumor biology and to the immune response. For example, the general level of immune competence appears to decrease with advancing disease,[6] yet there are no highly accurate means for quantifying the total tumor burden, and the immunological events which may limit tumor growth are yet to be described. The nature of the tumor-specific antigens is not well-understood; the question of whether there is a specific antigen common to all tumors of the breast is open.

The principal treatment of breast cancer has been a matter of discussion in the recent past. While advanced cancers continue to be treated primarily by radical surgery, in many cases together with adjuvant radiotherapy or chemotherapy,[4,7] "early" breast cancers may be treated with apparently equal long-term survival by minimal surgery and radiotherapy.[8] While precise dose and fractionation schedules may vary between centers, a typical radiation therapy course will deliver significant doses to axillary, infra-, and supraclavicular nodes, as well as to the internal mammary chain.[9] In fact, a portion of the thymus may be contained in the irradiation field. While the effects of ionizing radiation on populations of cells participating in immune responses are discussed in detail elsewhere in this volume, it may seem initially that any radiation dosage to lymphoid tissues, particularly those near the tumor mass, might tend to diminish antitumor immune responses and render the patient less capable of combating ongoing or potentially recurrent disease. In fact, Sternsward voiced this argument based on peripheral lymphoid counts and mortality data.[10] The validity of the quoted mortality data has been rebutted by Levitt et al.,[11] yet the effect of radiation therapy on lymphocyte counts appears to be real.[12] The central question which remains is the extent to which a patient's true antitumor immune capability can be determined from peripheral lymphocyte activities, and the extent to which this may be affected by radiation therapy.

Several lines of evidence together suggest that there are specific immune responses against breast tumors. Plausible evidence for host resistance obtains from recurrence data in patients following mastectomy, such as reported by Harris et al.[13] They reported an incidence of second primary tumors at 2.8% per year through the sixth postoperative year; the incidence for years 7 to 13 remained constant, then increased at an annual rate of 6.8% for years 13 to 16 inclusive. These frequencies suggest that the immune system may have been stimulated by the first tumor, which acted to suppress the second tumor. That late, aggressive occurrences are seen several years after initial treatment is consistent with this view. Encouraging results in chemotherapeutic regimens including immunopotentiators such as BCG and *C. Parvum* are consistent with immune stimulation.[14,15]

Attempts have been made to characterize tumor specific antigens from breast carcinomas.[16] In a recent study, Mesa-Tejada et al.[17] reported that an antigenic component prepared from sections of human breast carcinoma cross-reacted to a 52,000 dalton group-specific glycoprotein of murine mammary tumor virus (MMTV), using an indirect immunoperoxidase method. These workers found that nearly half of randomly selected breast carcinomas were cross-reactive, and that some 64% of invasive tumors with an intraductal component were positive. In contrast, all normal and benign tissues were negative for the antigen, and carcinomas from sites other than breast were nearly uniformly negative.[17] While these data suggest a viral etiology for certain breast carcinomas, frequencies of cross-reactivity are not sufficiently strong to establish this antigen as a TSTA. In fact, the data of Rauch et al.[18] suggest a close relationship between tumor-specific antigens and HLA determinants. The question of whether tumor antigen(s) represent modified HLA antigens has not been resolved. The implications of the latter are far reaching, both in terms of carcinogenic mechanisms and in possible heterogeneity of antigens relative to attempts at utilizing adjuvant immunotherapy.

Evidence for the presence of circulating tumor antigens in breast cancer patients has been reported by several groups.[19-21] Breast cancer cells appear to shed cell surface glycoproteins both in vitro and in vivo, and these may combine with antibody to form immune complexes.[22] Immune complexes from a breast cancer patient when characterized yielded an IgG component with high affinity for saline extracts of malignant breast tissue, relative to those from normal tissue or benign breast disease.[23] Quite possibly antigen shedding, through binding to circulating immunoglobulin, may constitute a form of blocking that allows initial immunological escape or continued growth of the tumor. Serum blocking factors (SBF) may interfere with in vitro correlates of cell-mediated immunity. Yonemoto et al.[24] reported that SBF levels correlated with tumor burden and clinical stage, and in a later report characterized these factors as Ig antigen complexes.[25] While neither the Ig or antigen fraction alone showed blocking activity, the restored complex blocked in relation to its concentration in LAI cultures.

Direct evidence for cell-mediated responses against autochthonous tumors is difficult to achieve for the human. One very interesting attempt is reported by Kiricuta et al.[26] in which breast cancer fragments were placed in culture together with fragments of axillary lymph nodes. Lymphocytes migrated from the nodal explants to tumor explants and infiltrated the tumor fragments with evidence of cytotoxicity. Migration was greater when axillary lymph nodes showed hyperplasia of the paracortical area and/or sinus histiocytosis. Histologic type and tumor grade were not correlated with migration, but there was a strong negative correlation between migration and presence of metastases in the lymph node explant, and the extent of metastatic spread in vivo. Migration was absent in patients with more than three metastatic nodes.[26] If these results could be generalized to all breast cancer patients, and if tumor cytotoxicity occurred by means of cells migrating from regional lymph nodes, it would seem that radiation therapy might be contraindicated only for patients with very early disease, since nodal involvement suggests subclinical spread in other nodes.

The majority of attempts to monitor immune competence of breast cancer patients have utilized either delayed hypersensitivity reactions by skin testing, or some parameter of peripheral blood cells. The latter include in vitro cytotoxicity tests,[27] blast transformation by mitogens,[28] various rosette-forming tests,[29] migration inhibition assays,[30] leukocyte adherence inhibition tests,[31] and peripheral counts. With some variation, correlates of cell-mediated immunity tend to diminish only with quite advanced disease. One recent report by Goust et al.[32] is interesting in that a subpopulation of active T cells (TEa) appears to be elevated in a majority of Stage I breast cancer patients. This subpopulation is thought to play a role in immune surveillance, and if so, may represent a correlate of increased immune activity in early clinically evident disease.[32]

A number of reports using techniques listed above have established that radiation therapy results in significant peripheral lymphopenia.[10,33-36] Jenkins et al.[33] provide a reasonably complete study of this type. They evaluated total leukocyte, granulocyte, and lymphocyte counts as well as stimulation by mitogens Con A, PWM, and PHA, on breast cancer patients before, during, and after external beam therapy. All parameters decreased during the course of therapy, and there appeared to be no statistical difference in depression between patients who had or had not undergone mastectomy, nor with clinical stage of disease.[33] Using rosette assays, Blomgren et al.[37] presented data suggesting that peripheral B cells were depressed to a greater extent than T cells, although results with mitogens appear less clear-cut relative to a differential B cell depression.[35] Peripheral lymphocyte depression appears to persist for as long as 22 months.[36]

The questions of the anatomic site and volume irradiated relative to peripheral lymphopenia have been addressed. Results of Nordman and Toivanen[36] using a small patient sample might suggest that a smaller treatment volume may produce suppression of shorter duration. Raben et al.,[34] on the other hand, with an equally small sample compared rosette formation of cells from breast cancer patients versus patients irradiated for abdominal cancers and found no significant difference in suppression. They concluded that the thymus need not be in the radiation field for depression of T cells. Chee et al.[38] in a larger study evaluated lymphocyte replicating ability in patients undergoing radiotherapy for cancers at various sites, including those whose treatment included considerable exposure of major blood vessels, bone marrow, and lymphoid tissue. In only one category, osteogenic sarcoma which involved the lower femur and knee and which received 7000 rad, was lymphocyte depression absent. Significantly, the treatment volume did not include red marrow or lymphoid tissue.[38] On the basis of these studies it seems reasonable to attribute lymphopenia to direct radiation exposure of lymphoid cells or their precursors.

Attempts have been made to relate the degree of lymphopenia to prognosis. While trends tend to be mixed, with a rough correlation of these parameters suggested by Baral et al.,[39] and Papatestas et al.,[40] others tend to not predict survival on this basis. Indeed, considering the complexity of both immune responses and of breast cancer, a simple correlation of this type would be unexpected.

A lymphocyte population which mediates antibody-dependent cellular cytotoxicity (ADCC) against nucleated cells has been studied in patients who received radiation therapy for a variety of cancers including breast.[41,42] The active cells, known as "killer" or K cells, are neither T or B cells since they do not form rosettes or bear surface immunoglobulin. Originally termed null cells since they were thought to bear no surface markers, they now are known to possess Fc receptors which interact with specific IgG on the surface of target cells. Target cell lysis does not require complement. K cell activity, using ascitic P-815 murine mastocytoma cells coated with rabbit antimastoma cell antibody, was determined by ^{51}Cr release using mononuclear cells of breast cancer patients before, during, and after 4500 rad delivered in 3 weeks.[42] Suppression was not noted during the first week of therapy, but became severe by the fourth week (the week following the end of therapy), and thereafter K cell activity increased generally throughout the following 22 weeks. Patients with no residual tumor evidenced significantly greater recovery of K cell activity than those with either persistent tumor or distant metastases. K cells are relatively radioresistant with D_0 values of about 3 krad.[43] The delay in numerical decrease after the beginning of radiotherapy may be explained on the basis of killing the more radiosensitive precursor cells. The significance of the decrease in K cell activity is unknown at this time; if K cells are cytotoxic to tumors in vivo, they might be expected to localize at the site of tumor foci. If so, they would be vulnerable to cell killing by radiation and would be expected to appear in fewer numbers in the peripheral circulation if disease were persistent.

While in vitro tests of cell-mediated immunity have provided few insights to tumor-host relationships in the human, and have added little to our overall understanding of radiation effects on host antitumor immunity, they may hold some promise for aiding investigators in understanding some aspects of mechanisms involved. Recent work with animal models has established that immune responses are under strict genetic control and are very closely regulated through interaction of one or more cell populations.[44] The first suggestion of cell regulation in breast cancer patients was by Blomgren et al.,[6] who were evaluating impaired lymphocyte responses to PPD tuberculin in patients using in vitro blastogenesis to PPD. They showed that cultures from breast cancer patients, but not healthy controls, increased in activity when depleted of adherent monocytes. Reactivity to PHA was also increased by monocyte depletion of patients' cells, but not controls. Subsequent work by Juhlin et al.[45] showed that nonspecific inhibitor cells appeared after radiation therapy for breast carcinoma. Using an MLC technique, they demonstrated that cells obtained after radiotherapy could inhibit both stimulator and responder capacities of cryopreserved lymphocytes obtained from patients before therapy, when added to the cultures. The group further demonstrated that while peripheral lymphocyte counts fell to less than 50% of preirradiation values, the number of monocytes was not altered, and there was no relationship between PPD responses and lymphocyte:monocyte ratios.[46] By comparing cutaneous hypersensitivity with in vitro blastogenesis to PPD of the same patients' cells, there appeared to be a strict parallel. These authors argue that while the total number of monocytes is not increased, the percent of activated monocytes within the population is elevated. Data of Ghossein et al.[47] are consistent with this interpretation in that lysozyme levels, associated with this interpretation in that lysozyme levels, associated with increased monocyte proliferation or hyperfunction, are not elevated in patients after radiotherapy. Blomgren et al.[48] subsequently were able to activate monocytes in vitro by lipopolysaccharide (LPS) and to simulate responses of irradiated breast cancer patients by lymphocytes from healthy donors.

The precise significance of these findings at the clinical level is unclear; activated macrophages are thought to play an active role in host response to tumors.[49,50] The significance of impaired T lymphocyte responses to various mitogens following radiation is not known.

A major question relates to whether breast cancer patients who have undergone radiation therapy are immunosuppressed to the point that responses against residual local or disseminated disease are futile. The data presented above shed little light on this matter.

Results with immunopotentiating agents tend to suggest that immune responses against autochthonous tumors may be stimulated somewhat. Interesting, but somewhat inconclusive, results have been obtained with the agent levamisole (LMS).[51,52] Levamisole is an antihelmenthic drug, considered to be an immunomodulator by restoring immune responses in compromised hosts, but appears to not stimulate above normal levels. The agent improves T cell or macrophage-dependent function such as DTH, GVH, and blood clearance of colloidal particles. Levamisole seems not to directly influence B cells. While BCG reportedly stimulates suppressor cells in mice, LMS does not.[53] Nathanson et al.,[54] who showed that LMS increased monocyte chemotaxis in man, imply that LMS may act by enhancing the movement of monocytes out of peripheral blood and into tumor sites. While LMS alone was reported to be without value in the treatment of very advanced cancers,[51] a clinical trial employing radiation alone versus radiation plus LMS suggests that LMS may be of value for breast cancer,[52] despite problems in design of the trial.[55] Although patients were assigned alternately to treatment group, and doses were calculated to central-axis and not to the tumor per se, the results merit attention. The patients were Stage III breast carcinoma and received 7000 rad to chest wall and supraclavicular area and 3000 rad to the posterior axillary field. Patients who received LMS had a mean disease-free interval of 25 months, versus 9 months with radiation alone. The percentage of patients with positive skin tests to DNCB and *Candida albicans* was greater for those who received LMS, and lymphocyte counts were increased at 20 months in patients in the LMS group, while those who received radiation alone showed only a slight increase in lymphocyte counts.[52] The extent to which these trends are duplicated in a rigorously designed and executed trial remains to be seen.

Given that host responses against the tumor may influence the ultimate outcome of radiation therapy, in the absence of definitive means of quantitating antitumor immunity, one approach to obtaining information indirectly has been with clinical trials of pre- and postoperative radiation. In particular, preoperative radiation might be expected to reduce tumor burden and to allow the ongoing host responses an opportunity to rebound. Postoperative radiation, on the other hand, should be no more suppressive to immunologically active cell populations than radiation delivered before surgery.

The Stockholm cancer trial, still in progress, was designed to reveal any differences in clinical indices between patients who received surgery alone, or surgery either preceded or followed by 4500 rad over 5 weeks.[7,56] Recent data covering 159 of 960 patients for whom 5 years has elapsed indicate that preoperative radiation may result in improved survival, reduced incidence of local and regional recurrence, and distant metastases.[57] Trends for patients who received radiation after surgery, or surgery alone, are nearly equivalent at this point. These results are consistent with the notion that preoperative radiation reduced tumor burden, allowed the host antitumor activity to recover during the 6-week interval between radiation and surgery, thereby reducing residual disease.[58] The validity of this implication must await further information.

In summary, there are significant gaps in our knowledge of tumor biology and of immune processes. To understand the implications of radiation effects on host-tumor interactions, it is necessary to first understand the system to be perturbed. Additional information must be obtained about the structure of tumor-specific antigens. This in turn will resolve the issue of whether there is a unique antigen for all breast cancers or even for cancers of a given histological type. Knowledge of antigenic structure and specificity will enable the establishment of strategies aimed at specific immunotherapy. A second area relates to the identity of cytotoxic cells in breast cancer, their frequency, distribution, specificity, and regulation. Knowledge of the activity of particular cell subsets would allow the clinician to monitor immune status and optimize various therapeutic procedures. The understanding of cell regulation will likely allow establishment of therapies to correct regulatory defects. It would not be surprising to find ultimately that the event or agent which produces malignant transformation may be responsible also for a defect in immunologic recognition and/or regulation.

REFERENCES

1. Seidman, H., Silverberg, B. S., and Bodden, A., Probabilities of eventually developing and of dying of cancer, *Ca*, 28, 33, 1978.
2. Fisher, B., Hanlon, J. T., Linta, J., and Fisher, E. R., Natural history of breast cancer: a brief overview, in *Immunotherapy of Cancer: Present Status of Trials in Man,* Terry, W. D. and Windhorst, D., Eds., Raven Press, New York, 1978, 621.
3. Lee, S. H., Cancer cell estrogen receptor of human mammary carcinoma, *Cancer,* 44, 1, 1979.
4. Fisher, B., Slack, N., Katrych, D., and Wolmark, N., Ten year follow-up results of patients with carcinoma of the breast in a co-operative clinical trial evaluating surgical adjuvant chemotherapy, *Surg. Gynecol. Obstet.,* 140, 528, 1975.
5. Fisher, B., Golinger, R. C., Kelly, M., and Ruth, D., Variation of macrophage migration by a factor from regional lymph node cells of breast cancer patients, *Cancer,* 42, 2097, 1978.
6. Blomgren, H., Baral, E., Petrini, B., and Wasserman, J., Impaired lymphocyte responses to PPD tuberculin in advanced breast carcinoma, Increased reactivity after depletion of phagocytic or adherent cells, *Clin. Oncol.,* 2, 379, 1976.
7. Wallgren, A., A controlled study: preoperative versus postoperative irradiation, *Int. J. Radiat. Oncol. Biol. Phys.,* 2, 1167, 1967.
8. Alpert, S., Ghossein, N. A., Stacey, P., Migliorelli, F. A., Efron, G., and Krishnaswamy, V., Primary management of operable breast cancer by minimal surgery and radiotherapy, *Cancer,* 42, 2054, 1978.
9. Fletcher, G. H., *Textbook of Radiotheraphy,* Lea & Febiger, Philadelphia, 1973, chap. 6.
10. Stjernsward, J., Decreased survival correlated to local irradiation in "early" operable breast cancer, *Lancet,* 2, 1285, 1974.
11. Levitt, S. H., McHugh, R. B., and Song, C. W., Radiotherapy in the postoperative treatment of operable cancer of the breast, *Cancer,* 39, 933, 1977.
12. Lundell, G., Effects of radiation therapy on blood-borne leucocytes in patients with mammary carcinoma, *Acta Radiol. (Ther.),* 13, 407, 1974.
13. Harris, R. E., Lynch, H. T., and Guirgis, H. A., Familial breast cancer: risk to the contralateral breast, *J. Natl. Cancer Inst.,* 60, 955, 1978.
14. Morton, D. L. and Goodnight, J. E., Clinical trials of immunotherapy. Present status, *Cancer,* 42, 2224, 1978.
15. Pinsky, C. M., De Jager, R. L., Wittes, R. E., Wong, P. P., Kaufman, R. J., Mike, V., Hansen, J. A., Oettgen, H. F., and Krakoff, I. H., Corynebacterium Parvum as adjuvant to combination chemotherapy in patients with advanced breast cancer: preliminary results of a prospective randomized trial, in *Immunotherapy of Cancer: Present Status of Trials in Man,* Terry, W. D. and Windhorst, D., Eds., Raven Press, New York, 1978, 647.
16. Leung, J. P., Bordin, G. M., Nakamura, R. M., DeHeer, D. H., and Edington, T. S., Frequency of association of mammary tumor glycoprotein antigen and other markers with human breast tumors, *Cancer Res.,* 39, 2057, 1979.
17. Mesa-Tejada, R., Keydar, I., Ramanarayanan, M., Ohno, T., Fenoglio, C., and Spiegelman, S., Immunohistochemical evidence for RNA virus related components in human breast cancer, *Ann. Clin. Lab. Sci.,* 9, 202, 1979.
18. Rauch, J. E., Shuster, J., Thomson, D. M. P., and Gold, P., Isolation of HLA and tumor antigens by means of affinity chromatography employing anti β_2-microglobulin (β_2m) antiserum, *Cancer,* 42, 1601, 1978.
19. Schwartz, M. K., Estrogen receptors and tumor associated antigens in breast cancer, *Ann. Clin. Lab. Sci.,* 9, 258, 1979.
20. Lopez, M. J. and Thomson, D. M. P., Isolation of breast cancer tumor antigen from serum and urine, *Int. J. Cancer,* 20, 834, 1978.
21. Lerner, M. P., Anglin, J. H., and Nordquist, R. E., Cell surface antigens from human breast tumor cells, *J. Natl. Cancer Inst.,* 60, 39, 1978.
22. Nordquist, R. E., Anglin, J. H., and Lerner, M. P., Antigen shedding by human breast cancer cells *in vitro* and *in vivo, Br. J. Cancer,* 37, 776, 1978.
23. Papsidero, L. D., Harvey, S. R., Snyderman, M. C., Nemoto, T., Valenzuela, L., and Chu, T. M., Characterization of immune complexes from the pleural effusion of a breast cancer patient, *Int. J. Cancer,* 21, 675, 1978.
24. Yonemoto, R. H., Fujisawa, T., and Waldman, S. R., Effect of serum blocking factors on leukocyte adherence inhibition in breast cancer patients: specificity and correlation with tumor burden, *Cancer,* 41, 1289, 1978.
25. Tanaka, F., Yonemoto, R. H., and Waldman, S. R., Blocking factors in sera of breast cancer patients, *Cancer,* 43, 838, 1979.

26. Kiricuta, J., Todorutiu, C., Mulea, R., and Risca, R., Axillary lymph-node and breast carcinoma interrelations in organ culture, *Cancer*, 42, 2710, 1978.
27. Deodhar, S. D., Crile, G., Jr., and Esselstyn, C. B., Jr., Study of the tumor cell-lymphocyte interaction in patients with breast cancer, *Cancer*, 29, 1321, 1972.
28. Whittaker, M. G. and Clark, C. G., Depressed lymphocyte function in carcinoma of the breast, *Br. J. Surg.*, 58, 717, 1971.
29. Nemoto, T., Han, T., Minowada, J., Angkur, V., Chamberlain, A., and Dao, T. L., Cell-mediated immune status of breast cancer patients: Evaluation by skin tests, lymphocyte stimulation, and counts of rosette-forming cells, *J. Natl. Cancer Inst.*, 53, 641, 1974.
30. Black, M. M., Zachran, R. E., Shore, B., Dion, A. S., and Leis, H. P., Jr., Cellular immunity to autologous breast cancer and RIII-murine mammary tumor virus preparations, *Cancer Res.*, 38, 2068, 1978.
31. Goldrosen, M. H., Summary and future prospects of leukocyte adherence inhibition, *Cancer Res.*, 39, 660, 1979.
32. Goust, J. M., Roof, B. S., Fudenberg, H. H., and O'Brien, P. H., T-cell markers in breast cancer patients at diagnosis, *Clin. Immunol. Immunopathol.*, 12, 396, 1979.
33. Jenkins, V. K., Olson, M. H., Ellis, H. N., and Cooley, R. N., Effect of therapeutic radiation on peripheral blood lymphocytes in patients with carcinoma of the breast, *Acta Radiol. Ther.*, 14, 385, 1975.
34. Raben, M., Walch, N., Galili, U., and Schlesinger, M., The effect of radiation therapy on lymphocyte subpopulations in cancer patients, *Cancer*, 37, 1417, 1976.
35. Slater, J. M., Ngo, E., and Lau, B. H. S., Effect of therapeutic irradiation on the immune responses, *Am. J. Roentgenol.*, 126, 313, 1976.
36. Nordman, E. and Toivanen, A., Effects of irradiation on the immune function in patients with mammary, pulmonary, or head and neck carcinoma, *Acta Radiol. Ther.*, 17, 3, 1978.
37. Blomgren, H., Glas, U., Melen, B., and Wasserman, J., Blood lymphocytes after radiation therapy of mammary carcinoma, *Acta Radiol. Ther.*, 13, 185, 1974.
38. Chee, C. A., Ilberry, P. T. L., and Rickinson, M. A., Depression of lymphocyte replicating ability in radiotherapy patients, *Br. J. Radiol.*, 47, 37, 1974.
39. Baral, E., Blomgren, H., Petrini, B., Wasserman, J., Ogenstad, J., and Silversward, C., Prognostic relevance of immunologic variables in breast carcinoma, *Acta Radiol. Ther.*, 16, 417, 1977.
40. Papatestas, A. E., Lesnick, G. J., Genkins, G., and Aufses, A. H., The prognostic significance of peripheral lymphocyte counts in patients with breast carcinoma, *Cancer*, 37, 164, 1976.
41. Stratton, M. L., Herz, J., Loeffler, R. A., McClurg, F. L., Reiter, A., Bernstein, P., Danley, D. L., and Benjamini, E., Antibody-dependent cell-mediated cytotoxicity in treated and nontreated cancer patients, *Cancer*, 40, 1045, 1977.
42. McCredie, J. A., MacDonald, H. R., and Wood, S. B., Effect of operation and radiotherapy on antibody-dependent cellular cytotoxicity, *Cancer*, 44, 99, 1979.
43. MacDonald, H. R., Bonnard, G. D., Sordat, B., and Zawodnik, S. A., Antibody-dependent cell-mediated cytotoxicity: heterogeneity of effector cells in human peripheral blood, *Scand. J. Immunol.*, 4, 487, 1975.
44. Broder, S. and Waldmann, T. A., The suppressor-cell network in cancer, *N. Engl. J. Med.*, 299, 1281 and 1335, 1978.
45. Juhlin, I., Blomgren, H., and Wasserman, J., Evidence for the appearance of non-specific inhibitor cells in the blood after radiation therapy for breast carcinoma, *Cancer Lett.*, 3, 311, 1977.
46. Blomgren, H., Wasserman, J., Baral, E., and Petrini, B., Evidence for the appearance of non-specific suppressor cells in the blood after local radiation therapy, *Int. J. Radiat. Oncol. Biol. Phys.*, 4, 249, 1978.
47. Ghossein, N. A., Keiser, H. D., Brooks, T. L., and Samuels, B., Absence of non-organ specific autoimmune reactions in patients treated by curative radiotherapy, *Int. J. Radiat. Oncol. Biol. Phys.*, 5, 535, 1979.
48. Blomgren, H. and Wasserman, J., Activation of monocytes in vitro to produce lymphocyte dysfunctions, *Int. J. Radiat. Oncol. Biol. Phys.*, 5, 221, 1979.
49. Holderman, O. A., Klein, E., and Casale, G. P., Selective cytotoxicity of peritoneal leukocytes for neoplastic cells, *Cell. Immunol.*, 9, 339, 1973.
50. Alexander, P., Eccles, S. A., and Gauci, C. L., The significance of macrophages in human and experimental tumors, *Ann. N. Y. Acad. Sci.*, 276, 124, 1976.
51. Symoens, J. and Rosenthal, M., Levamisole in the modulation of the immune response: the current experimental and clinical state, *J. Reticuloendoth. Soc.*, 21, 175, 1977.
52. Rojas, A. F., Mickiewicz, E., Feierstein, J. N., Glait, H., and Olivari, A. J., Levamisole in advanced human breast cancer, *Lancet*, 1, 211, 1976.

53. Bruley-Rosset, M., Florentin, I., Kiger, N., Davigny, M., and Mathé, G., Effects of Bacillus Cal-mette-Guerin and levamisole on immune responses in young adult and age-immunodepressed mice, *Cancer Treat. Rep.*, 62, 1641, 1978.

54. Nathanson, S. D., Zamfirescu, P. L., Portaro, J. K., deKernion, J. B., and Fahey, J. L., Acute effects of orally administered levamisole on random monocyte chemotoxis in man, *J. Natl. Cancer Inst.*, 61, 301, 1978.

55. Rozencweig, M., Heuson, J. C., Von Hoff, D. D., Mattheiem, W. H., Davis, H. L., and Muggia, F. M., Breast cancer, in *Randomized Trials in Cancer: A Critical Review by Sites*, Staqnet, M. J., Ed., Raven Press, New York, 1978, 231.

56. De Schryver, A., The Stockholm breast cancer trial: preliminary report of a randomized study con-cerning the value of preoperative or postoperative radiotherapy, *Int. J. Radiat. Oncol. Biol. Phys.*, 1, 601, 1976.

57. Wallgren, A., Arner, O., Bergstrom, J., Blomstedt, B., Granburg, P.-O., Karnstrom, L., Raf, L., and Silversward, C., Preoperative radiotherapy in operable breast cancer, *Cancer*, 42, 1120, 1978.

58. Blomgren, H., Lymphopenia and breast metastases, *Int. J. Radiat. Oncol. Biol. Phys.*, 2, 1177, 1977.

Chapter 8

RADIOTHERAPY, IMMUNITY, AND CERVICAL CARCINOMA

David M. Mumford and Nancy McCormick

TABLE OF CONTENTS

I. INTRODUCTION

In the past decade, the question of possible interplays between immunity and cancer has gained enhanced significance. Immunity is now believed to be involved in the host's resistance to many forms of cancer. Both humoral (antibody) and cell-mediated immune mechanisms have been shown to influence the biological progression of a variety of tumor types in experimental animals and in man.

Immune events associated with human cervical carcinoma have been demonstrated.[1] However, the significance of these findings is still somewhat unclear. As a result, active immune investigations are ongoing in an attempt to ascertain the dynamics and importance of immune changes found in cervical cancer patients. In particular, studies are focusing on the possible role of immunity in etiologic events, tumor progression, and in the prediction of prognosis. Moreover, immunotherapeutic efforts, as a form of adjuvant treatment for cervical cancer, are underway. We recently reviewed many of the reported immune-cervical cancer relationships.[1]

However, this latter survey only incidentally considered the effects of radiation therapy on the immune status of cervical carcinoma patients. The present article will attempt to look at the interaction of immunity, cervical cancer, and radiation treatment more extensively. Before so doing, it might be wise to briefly summarize some of the better known immune-cervical cancer associations.

II. BACKGROUND COMMENTS

The foremost finding of immune-related events in cervical carcinoma patients has been the suggested relationship between herpes virus infection and the development of carcinoma of the uterine cervix. Following the early report of Naib in 1966, investigators from many laboratories have concluded that herpes simplex virus — type 2 (HSV-2) infections may predispose to cervical cancer.[2-5] Earlier studies focused on the incidence or prevalence of serum antibodies to herpesvirus in women with various stages of carcinoma-*in-situ* and cervical carcinoma when compared to appropriate control groups. Later, neutralizing and complement fixing antibodies to new HSV-induced antigens in tissue culture cells were also found in a significant percentage of American women with cervical carcinoma.[6]

Other immune reactions which lend support to a putative change in the immunity of cervical cancer patients are (1) spontaneous "cervical cancer cures", (2) histologic evidence of immune reaction at tumor sites and/or in regional lymph nodes, (3) changes in general cell-mediated immune function as measured by skin tests or by a variety of in vitro assays, e.g., the lymphocyte transformation test, macrophage migration inhibition test, etc., (4) changes in CEA levels during the course of disease or after treatment, and (5) detection of antibody to cervical cancer tumor-associated or tumor-specific antigens.[1] These lines of evidence tend to substantiate that immunity may play some role in host defense against cervical cancer. If immunity does play a part in the patient's response to cervical cancer, it is a factor which should be more intensively studied because cervical cancer is a significant human malignancy.

According to the American Cancer Society's estimates, approximately 20,000 cases of invasive cervical carcinoma occurred in 1978, and 40,000 new cases of *in situ* cervical cancer were found.[7] Persistence or recurrence of this tumor was a probable cause of death for some 7400 women. Many of these patients had received irradiation as a prime form of therapy. Despite the treatment failures, irradiation continues to be a successful component of cancer management. Nonetheless, additional information, such as the interaction between immunity and irradiation, is needed to increase treatment efficiency.

Radiation therapy for cervical cancer began shortly after the turn of the century.[8] Intracavitary radiation was first used although subsequently found to have frequent complications. In 1924 supplemental external X-ray to the lateral pelvic wall was introduced.[9] After World War II, surgery became a viable alternative therapy for patients with early cervical carcinoma.[10,11] This surgical progress was possible because of vast improvements in anesthesia and supportive care — especially the availability of antibiotics. However, refinements of radiotherapy techniques and the development of new ionizing modalities kept radiotherapy technology in the forefront for treatment of frankly invasive cervical carcinoma. Depending on the stage of the disease, the patient's status, the availability of facilities, and the skill and experience of the physician, surgery or radiation (or occasionally the combination of the two) have been successfully utilized. Combined external and internal radiation is most frequently used when radiotherapy of cervical cancer is elected. Important to the planning of any management program for cervical cancer is the relationship of the disease stage to the probability of neoplastic involvement of pelvic and para aortic lymph nodes.[9] When efforts are made to include para aortic lymph nodes in the radiation field, tumor destruction may be increased, but so too is the complication rate. In this situation, the wider radiation fields, must not only be balanced against increased irradiation complications, but also against other more recently recognized factors such as the possible immune role of the regional lymph nodes and systemic immunity in combating tumor spread. Only recently has the significance of regional lymph nodes in combating tumor spread and facilitating tumor rejection been recognized. These findings have come especially from reports on breast carcinoma, but also include cervical cancer as well. Undoubtedly an interaction often exists between cervical carcinoma, the regional lymph nodes, and the local and systemic processes of host immunity to tumor.

Unfortunately, there may also be host or tumor factors which decrease host resistance. These may suppress the body's normal immune response to a variety of general antigens or to the fairly specific tumor-associated ones. It has been demonstrated that in some human tumors, as well as in animal tumor models, "blocking antibodies" may arise which inhibit the effective action of the immune system against the tumor. Moreover, suppressive substances may be produced by a tumor or perhaps other body cells (liver?) which inhibit immune reactivity at local tumor sites or affect the general immune system. Circulating serum inhibitory factors are often demonstrated by incubating a normal person's lymphocytes in vitro with serum, serum fractions, or tumor extracts from a cancer patient. Inhibition of immune responsiveness of normal lymphocytes to defined antigens or mitogens in the face of the possible suppressive substances is tested. The test antigens may be common nontumor or specific tumor antigens. Local or circulating suppressive substances have been described in patients who have not received irradiation, but they sometimes occur in patients receiving irradiation.

III. RADIATION EFFECTS ON IMMUNITY

Radiation energy is known to alter immune reactivity in a variety of ways. This has been discussed in Chapters 1 and 2 of this book. A good review of the available experimental evidence for irradiation effects on immune reactivity has recently been published.[12] A few brief comments will be made on this relationship, with emphasis on their application to cervical cancer. While immunity undoubtedly may cause tumor destruction or inhibition of tumor progression in some instances, it, in turn, is often susceptible to the tumor killing properties of radiotherapy. Accordingly, prudence dictates that treatment plans for cervical cancer should utilize irradiation for maximal tumor kill while considering ways to minimize adverse irradiation effects on the immune system. Tumor killing radiation programs which leave host immune defenses with a high reactive capacity should be sought. Or, if immunosuppression is unavoidable, radiotherapy should be used in a manner in which immune reactivity can recuperate as rapidly as possible. Having said this, one should also emphasize another point. The current dogma of cancer immunology teaches that host resistance to tumor mass is probably most effective when the tumor dose per site is low — probably less than 10^6 to 10^8 cells and preferably less than 100,000 tumor cells.[13] Advocates of the role of immunology and immunotherapy therefore should temper their enthusiasm and recognize the priorities of first assuring adequate tumor kill before devising elaborate immunotherapeutic regimens to mop up residual tumor cells.

Before describing some of the effects of radiotherapy on immunity — which usually results in the deterioration but occasionally the improvement of immune function — several more cautions should be stated. These concern patient and tumor characteristics as well as the appropriateness of some of the immune tests used to monitor immune changes in human patients. The comments include the circumstances under which the assays should be used as well as limitations in interpretation(s). Variables which may affect immune function, or our understanding of the immune events postradiotherapy include: the patient's immune status before treatment; the size and nature of the tumor especially its antigenicity; the type and timing of the immune test(s); the dose of radiotherapy used; the response of the tumor to irradiation in terms of tumor kill; the area of tumor treated and of nontumor tissue exposed: and the age, as well as the general medical status of the patient.

Even without considering the direct effect of radiation on immune cells, the response of the tumor to irradiation may determine not only the remaining tumor mass but the immune response to that mass. Too much tumor residual mass may overwhelm the immune system. Too little may produce a suboptimal tumor antigen dose. There seems to be an ideal dose schedule and mode of presentation for any antigen (including tumor antigens) in order for maximal immune reactivity to occur. This ideal may vary from patient to patient, or within the same patient at different periods of time.

Alteration or absence of tumor antigen may also occasionally pose a problem. In some cases it has been reported that specific tumor reactivity may be lacking due to the complete absence of tumor antigen or its alteration into an ineffective immunizing form.[14] This can conceivably occur even though there is an ideal residual tumor mass. The action of blocking antibodies, enzymatic degradation action, or other digestive or coating processes may be responsible for tumor antigen alteration. Of course, more commonly, factors arise prior to, during, or after irradiation because of its direct radiotherapy effects which cause alteration — usually depression — of local or systemic tumor immunity. These inhibitory events usually involve direct action of irradiation on the patient's lymphocytes or other cells involved in the immune sequence.

The selection of the proper immune assay, its technical considerations and its timing, is crucial in attempts to serially assess immune responsiveness of cancer patients. For instance, the time of immune testing is important — pretreatment? during therapy? or post-therapy? Immediate, intermediate, or evaluations at distant intervals may each provide differing evaluations of the patient's "presumed" immune reactivity state. Interpretations ascribed to findings at any one time may (or may not) be valid at another. When depression occurs with radiotherapy, the most common cause is an immediate immune depression due to damage to circulating lymphocytes. This immune depression, revealed by immune profiling, can only be reversed once (and if) lymphocyte renewal occurs. In other instances depression may reflect immunosuppression due to tumor, serum, or blocking factors.

Another caveat concerns the limitation of any one immune assay used to measure "true" immune function. Tests vary in sensitivity, scope, reproducibility, and specificity. Moreover, at a given moment, only certain of the patient's immune functions (humoral or cell-mediated) may be altered or depressed. Consequently, depending on the test(s) that is used, a depressed, normal, or augmented immune state present might (or might not) be revealed. In such situations, batteries of tests are more apt to show significant changes than is a single assay. Finally, it should be noted that there may be differences between results from assays thought to measure the same immune function. This is particularly true when comparing certain in vivo and in vitro tests. For example, evaluations of in vivo skin tests compared to in vitro cell-mediated immune tests may not correlate as measures of delayed type hypersensitivity. Several investigators, including ourselves, have found this to be particularly true when following cervical carcinoma patients after radiotherapy.

A summary of the above comments should be made. One has to be judicious in the selection of immune assays employed. The timing reproducibility and individual interpretation given results from immune testing must be done in a somewhat cautionary manner. Unfortunately, at our current level of knowledge, no one test is an infallable indicator of immune status. Furthermore our increasing awareness indicates that the immune system is a complex syncytium of ever changing events. This realization emphasizes that any one assay at any one time in any one patient can only measure a small portion of the total reactivity of that individual.

IV. RADIATION EFFECTS ON LYMPHOCYTES

After the somewhat generalized overview above, what special comments can be made about immune assessments of patients receiving radiation therapy — especially for cervical carcinoma?

Radiotherapy to the pelvic area results in a large number of lymphocytes being damaged or destroyed. This may occur because (1) the area and dose of radiation used in carcinoma of the pelvic area is larger than is often used for treatment of carcinoma of other organs (e.g., the dosage of radiotherapy may be as high as 5000 to 6000 rads for whole pelvis external radiation in advanced cervical carcinoma patients; (2) lymphocytes and other immune associated cells in regional lymph nodes, as well as recirculating in the lymph ducts which later flow into the thoracic duct, may be at risk. Irradiation to tumor and regional areas may damage immune competent or immune progenitor cells in situ or in transit. Hence this irradiation effect may markedly diminish the functional capabilities of immune competent cells, their life span, or their reproductive potential even if immediate destruction does not occur; (3) the volume of bone marrow in the pelvic area is estimated to be 40% of the body's total.[15] Consequently, a major part of the generating hematopoietic area is at risk in widespread irradiation for cervical cancer; (4) there are major blood vessels in the pelvic area with significant circulating populations of immune competent cells; (5) there may be exposure of gut-associated lymphoid tissue to irradiation damage;[16] and (6) irradiation may cause a specific stress factor which in itself may be immunosuppressive.[17]

We now know that there are multiple subpopulations of lymphocytes. So when speaking of radiation effects on lymphocytes, the situation may be quite complex and depend on the cell type involved. Functional studies of lymphocyte surface markers reveal that T and B cells are the major subpopulations of lymphocytes. T (thymic-dependent) lymph cells are primarily involved in cell-mediated immunity, and B (bursal cells from the bone marrow in humans) are precursors of antibody producing cells. The most commonly employed techniques distinguishing these two categories depend on the ability of the T cells to rosette with sheep erythrocytes. Therefore T cells are also called E rosetting cells. B lymphocytes require a more complex erythrocyte-antibody-complement (EAC) system to rosette. Other types of lymphocytes have recently been described including K (killer), null, suppressor, and helper cells. Studies of the effect of irradiation on some of these lymphocyte subpopulations have been reported, but in most cases they have not. In addition, the significance of the findings even when reported are often still uncertain.

A. Radiotherapy and Lymphocyte Numbers

It is well established that following radiotherapy for many human cancers, there is a reduction in total numbers of lymphocytes which may last for months or even years. This reduction is also thought to be true for patients with gynecological malignancies. [16,18-22] Yamagata followed the lymphocyte counts of a group of patients with cervical carcinoma, before, during, and after radiotherapy. During radiotherapy, the total lymphocyte counts were reduced to 20 to 50% of values found before treatment.[19] These patients averaged 500 mm³ lymphocytes during radiation therapy. Shortly after treatment, lymphocyte counts tended to increase but none approached normal values until at least 3 months post-therapy. In most (70%) patients, however, mild or moderate lymphopenia persisted for at least 2 years. However, 5 years post-therapy almost all surviving patients had normal lymphocyte counts. Other investigators have reported that patients with carcinoma of the cervix have a significant fall in absolute numbers of lymphocytes after radiotherapy[21,22] which can persist for more than 5 years.[21] Halili reported that patients treated by radiotherapy for various gynecological malignancies took 3 to 15 years post-treatment to regain normal lymphocyte counts.[23] One speculation to account for the differences in reports may be depended on the fact that the degree of lymphopenia after radiation therapy may be related not only to the dose of radiation but also to the time of immune profiling. For example, with pelvic radiation doses up to 1000 rad there was a 40% reduction of lymphocyte count when tested at an intermediate interval, while the report of 3000 to 5000 rads resulting in only a 23% reduction of lymphocytes was because immune assessment was done immediately after therapy.[24]

DiSaia correlated the length of survival of certain advanced stage cervical cancer patients with their preradiotherapy lymphocyte counts.[25] This study indicated that the initial lymphocyte count was strongly correlated with the length of patient survival.

Total lymphocyte counts less than 1000 mm³ at the beginning of radiotherapy had a considerably worse prognosis than those in patients with a greater initial count. Indeed, all patients who were alive at 23 months had pretherapy counts greater than 1000 mm³. Although there is no compelling evidence to indicate that prognosis is altered by the immediate decrease in lymphocytes after radiotherapy,[26] the determination of lymphocyte counts *before* therapy may give a good indication of the patient's response as measured by length of survival after radiotherapy. The implication of this observation for the role of immunity in cervical cancer provides interesting but far from clear speculation.

B. The Effect of Radiotherapy on Lymphocyte Subpopulations

A few studies have been done with cervical carcinoma patients to determine radiation effects on lymphocytes subpopulations. In one study of patients with localized mammary or pelvic malignancies of various types, the effects of radiotherapy on lymphocytes subpopulations were studied.[20] T and B cell determinations were performed prior to, immediately after therapy, and 4 to 6 weeks post-treatment. Levels of total E rosetting cells (T cells) and erythrocyte-antibody-complement (EAC) rosetting cells (B cells) before treatment was not significantly different from the normal controls. Immediately following treatment, the percent T cells decreased significantly while EAC rosettes were unaffected. By 4 to 6 weeks after therapy, the percentage of T cells continued to decrease although the percentage of B cells remained unchanged.

T cell changes were further studied since it is known that there are even subpopulations within the T cell classification which have different testing or functional characteristics. T cells were differentiated by their ability to form high or low affinity rosettes. The relative proportion of T cells forming high affinity E rosettes (HA-E) was not reduced after therapy. The authors concluded that radiation predominatly affected the subpopulation of T cells which do not form high affinity E rosettes. This probably means that the T cell subpopulation responsible for high affinity E rosettes is relatively radio resistant.

In the same report patients were also subdivided into two groups; (1) those who received radiation to the thymus and mediasternal blood vessels area (mammary cancer) and (2) those who received radiation to pelvic blood vessels (pelvic malignancies). Immediately after radiotherapy the level of T cells was significantly lower in patients who received pelvic radiation, but not in those who received mediasternal and thymic irradiation. However, by 4 to 6 weeks post-therapy both groups of patients showed a significant depression of E rosettes. The author concluded that irradiation to the thymus was not necessary for the reduction in T cells, and that irradiation to pelvic vessels caused a greater effect than to the mediasternal vessels.[20] However, other factors such as the total amount of hemopoietic material exposed in the pelvic area vs. the thorax, the total lymph node mass exposed etc., was not considered, so one would have to ponder the validity of the conclusions that the primary irradiation effect on lymphocytes in the pelvis was due to a reduction in the level of T lymphocytes in major vessels of that area. In another study, cervical carcinoma patients with localized tumors (stages 1 and 2) had decreased T cell (detected by E-rosetting) and B cell (detected by IF) percentages following irradiation therapy.[22] Levels did not return to normal until 12 months post-therapy. However, at the 1-year period, the absolute lymphocyte count was still depressed.

In contrast to the reports of Raben and Hancock, Rand[20-22] found untreated advanced stage cervical carcinoma patients had T cell percentages which were significantly lower than control subjects. E rosetting cell levels returned to normal in 6 weeks after radiotherapy and remained so thereafter. However, absolute T cell numbers were not significantly different in the untreated patients prior to therapy, but did drop significantly after treatment. B lymphocytes possessing surface membrane immunoglobulin (Sm-Ig-B), stainable by IF, were reduced by radiation for up to 5 years. The absolute number of EAC rosette-forming B cells, nonetheless increased when the counts were expressed as a percentage of the total lymphocyte count. In the same study, null cells (cells with neither surface markers of T or B cells) were also reduced after radiotherapy. The authors suggest that null cells may represent a pool of uncommitted reserve lymphocytes. Therefore part of the radiation induced lymphopenia may in part be due to a reduction in absolute numbers of null cells.[21] In patients with various pelvic malignancies (cervical, ovarian, and endometrial carcinoma), a rapid decrease in circulating T and B lymphocytes following radiotherapy, as measured by rosette testing, was found.[16] Byfield also reported that the magnitude of the decrease in T and B lymphocytes during radiotherapy was related to the dose of irradiation employed.[24]

As can be seen, although different methods for the assessment of T and B cell function were used in the studies cited above, certain generalizations can probably be made. Radiotherapy may depress the percentage of T cells (as measured by E rosetting) in cervical carcinoma patients.[20,22] The length of time for cells to return to normal levels varies from within 6 weeks[21] to 12 months.[22] B cell levels, as measured by EAC testing were not significantly decreased by radiotherapy.[20,21] However, B cell levels, determined by IF staining (Sm-Ig-B), were decreased significantly following treatment.[21,22] The proportion of B cells detected by the latter method, only return to normal after 1 year[22] or up to 5 years.[21] The discrepancy between levels reported for EAC rosette forming B cells and Sm-Ig-bearing B cells may represent variations of the respective tests in detecting subtypes of B lymphocytes which bear only one surface marker. Other explanations include reactions with "activated" T cells forming EAC rosettes or a failure to exclude all monocytes.

C. In Vitro Tests of Lymphocyte Function

A short-term (3 to 7 days) tissue culture method is commonly employed to measure in vitro cell-mediated responses of lymphocytes. This assay has been variously called the lymphocyte transformation test (index) lymphocyte proliferation index, lymphocyte stimulation test, etc. The in vitro test measures the ability of lymphocytes to respond to nonspecific substances such as mitogens from plant lecithins or to specific antigens to which the individual is known (or presumed) to be sensitive. The usual mitogens utilized are phytohemagglutinin (PHA), concanavalin A (ConA), and pokeweed mitogen (PWM). The former is thought to be more reactive to T cell function and the latter, to B cell function. "Specific" antigens used have included PPD, "strep" antigens, mumps, *Candida albicans,* etc.

Varied responses after radiotherapy in patients with gynecologic malignancies have been described for lymphocyte stimulation assessment. Most investigators have noted a depression in responsiveness to mitogens (particulary PHA) immediately after pelvic radiotherapy.[18,19,22] In some reports, the response to mitogens remains low through the 3 to 12 months follow-up period.[18,22] By contrast, during this time in vivo skin testing, as a measure of cell-mediated immunity, in one report remained normal.[22] Stratton reported immediate impairment of PHA responsiveness after radiotherapy in a variety of cancer patients including some with gynecological malignancies.[16] He noted that some recovery may occur as early as 3 weeks post-therapy, but chronic depression of lymphocyte function may persist for years. Yamagata in a long-term study confirmed the lingering effect of irradiation on lymphocytes.[19] Depressed lymphocyte stimulation function occurred in some cervical carcinoma patients for years after radiotherapy. Even in these patients, however, there was a gradual shift towards a higher reactivity with time (2 to 10 years) until by 10 years post-therapy, none of the patients tested had depressed response to mitogens. In this study lymphocyte reactivity recovered more slowly than did the total peripheral lymphocyte count. Fifty percent of the patients had normal lymphocyte counts 5 years after radiotherapy. It should be noted that all patients with recurrent cervical carcinoma had depressed lymphocyte reactivity although total peripheral lymphocyte counts were variable. Patients with unexpectedly good results showed both a higher total lymphocyte count and better functional lymphocyte reactivity than did those with poorer response. In preliminary findings from our own series of 35 cervical cancer patients studied with lymphocyte transformation assays, the effects of radiotherapy on lymphocyte reactivity were studied by dividing the patients into three groups (Figure 1). Group 1 had no recurrence of disease at the 12-month follow-up; group 2 had a recurrence of disease, either local or with distant mestastasis by 12 months; and group 3 had carcinoma *in situ* (CIS) but received no radiotherapy and served as "disease controls".[27] Depression of lymphocyte response to all three mitogens (PHA, ConA, PWM) usually occurred 1 month post-therapy. There was a recovery of lymphocyte response in all groups of patients with the exception of the recurrent disease group. Statistical analysis of data by student's T test for changes in lymphocyte reactivity indicated that (1) the pretreatment response to all mitogens in the recurrent cancer group was not statistically different from the other two groups, however, (2) in the recurrent cancer group, there was a statistically significant decreased responsiveness to all mitogens within 1 month post-therapy. Moreover, responses to PHA and PWM, but not to ConA, continued to be significantly decreased at the 8 months follow-up.

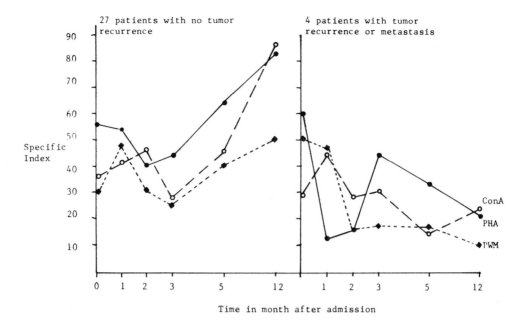

FIGURE 1. The means of the in vitro lymphocyte transformation responses of cervical cancer patients.

Although most investigators have found that the ability of lymphocytes to synthesize DNA on stimulation by mitogens in vitro is quite radiosensitive and becomes depressed, there are some reports of increased mitogen responsiveness in patients following radiotherapy. For example, McCredie found a 50% increase in lymphocyte DNA synthesis after PHA stimulation in patients irradiated for cervical carcinoma.[15] This increase persisted for 60 months following therapy even though during this time total peripheral lymphocyte counts decreased by as much as one third. In our current study, we did find some examples of patients (particularly with minimal disease) in which increased postirradiation lymphocyte stimulation also occur.

The lymphocyte stimulation index has been used in other ways to determine immune responsiveness. It is known that certain serum factors inhibit the proliferation of normal lymphocytes. Thus, studies have been conducted in which a patient's serum is added to the tissue culture media when testing the lymphocytes of normal individuals stimulated by mitogens or antigens. Yamagata showed that serum inhibition occurred in some cervical cancer patient's serum when tested against normal lymphocytes challenged by mitogens.[19] Interestingly, some individuals with preirradiation treatment serum inhibition were found to diminish or loose this inhibitory effect during radiotherapy. In patients with poor prognosis usually there was no loss, change, or increase in inhibition strength during therapy. Patients without later recurrent disease showed no serum inhibition effects after cessation of radiotherapy — often in spite of weak responses by their own lymphocytes to mitogens. The authors concluded that studying the depressive effect of a patient's serum might give important information about dosage and therapeutic effects of irradiation. It was suggested that such testing might also distinguish between patients who are likely to have an early disease recurrence. If serum inhibition is present, the patient is likely to develop recurrent cancer, while a low lymphocyte count and weak lymphocyte reactivity may merely reflect a persistent radiation effect.[19] Hancock also noted the disappearance of a serum inhibitory factor in four cervical carcinoma patients after radiotherapy.[22]

Another cell-mediated in vitro immune assay measures the ability of a patient's leukocytes to migrate in the presence of antigen(s) that are known to inhibit the migration if the individual is sensitive to the antigen(s). Menczer used the leukocyte migration inhibition test to evaluate specific cell-mediated immune responses to a soluble tumor extract from endometrial adenocarcinoma patients.[28] It was found that if the patient's tumor was localized and confined to the uterine cavity, the test was positive in all patients before any treatment or radiotherapy. In one patient, however, who had received preoperative radiotherapy, the test was negative. In other patients 6 to 9 months after therapy which included radiotherapy, the leukocyte migration inhibition test was negative. The authors suggested that this negative response might be due to the lack of antigenic stimulation rather than a change in host immune reactivity.

V. RADIATION EFFECTS ON OTHER CELLS

A. Phagocytic Cells and Macrophages

Cells of the mononuclear phagocyte series are found widely distributed throughout the body, in tissues, blood, and in lymphoid organs. They are known to form an important part of the host's defense mechanism including, presumably, tumor resistance. The circulating phagocytic mononuclear cells are known as monocytes and those in tissues are described as macrophages. There may be transient periods of such cells' lives in which the phagocytic cell circulates and then takes up residence in a specific tissue. The macrophage is important in immune reactivity because it has the capacity of binding and engulfing particular materials (including antigens) and can, under certain circumstances, also take up soluble molecules of antigens as well. The macrophage is capable of various secretory functions including the production of enzymes, certain complement proteins, interferon, and factors which are known to modulate the function of surrounding cells — particularly of the immune system. Some investigators claim that under special conditions, macrophages can secrete certain cytotoxins which kill tumor cells. Thus macrophages have come to be considered as important cells in some cell-mediated immune responses which result in tumor destruction as well as in the inflammatory processes which are often important to tumor destruction.[26]

Ghossein analyzed the differential counts of peripheral blood specimens of gynecological patients with various localized tumors after radical radiotherapy. There was no significant drop in the number of monocytes in spite of the marked decrease in lymphocytes as well as total leukocytes.[26] Rotman reported a significant increase in absolute monocyte numbers in 29 patients with tumors of the pelvic area (including cervical carcinoma) and of the thorax after radiotherapy. Monocytes in these patients rose from 299 to 411 mm³ about 3 weeks after therapy.[29] Monocytosis has been associated with various clinical conditions such as (1) various malignancies, perhaps in response to tumor associated antigens,[26] (2) after injection of epinephrine,[29] or (3) after injection of antigen. Rotman commenting on these known responses has suggested that the increase in monocytes after radiotherapy may be due to protein release from irradiated tissues which then act as antigens.[29]

The polymorphonuclear leukocyte is usually the most common circulating white blood cell and generally represents about 50 to 60% of the total white blood cell population of blood. These neutrophils are important in inflammation mediated by pyrogenic bacteria, in reactions involving antigen-antibody-complexes and in acute noninfectious inflammations. Thus alteration in neutrophilic activity might be important in host defense against tumors.

Significant drops in neutrophils have occurred after radiation in both pelvic and thoracic tumor patients.[29] This decrease in polymorphonuclear cells averaged from 3060 mm³ to 2383 mm³, was not nearly as marked as the decrease in lymphocytes in the same study. The decrease in neutrophils was slightly more marked in patients receiving pelvic irradiation than those with thoracic exposure.[29] Hancock reported that the absolute number of neutrophils may remain depressed after radiotherapy for 3 to 12 months.[22]

Irradiation to large areas of the body can reduce the number of neutrophils by damaging precursor cells in the bone marrow.[26] However, the mature neutrophil itself appears to be quite radioresistant. Relatively few studies have been done on the effect of irradiation on neutrophil function in contrast to numbers, but Hancock reports that neutrophil activity, as measured by the nitro blue tetrazolium (NBT) phagocytic test, was unchanged after radiotherapy even though the numbers of neutrophils were depressed.[22]

B. Eosinophils

The eosinophil is commonly associated with the cellular component involved in the immediate allergic reaction and is normally found in the blood of humans in small percentages (less than 5%). There are reports of eosinophilia after radiotherapy, particularly when the irradiated region is abdominal or pelvic.[29] The mean increase in eosinophilia is apparently greater following pelvic irradiation than in other areas.[29] This irradiation — induced eosinophilia — is sometimes as high as 30 to 40% of the total white blood count. In one study, 45% of the gynecological cancer patients had a fivefold or greater increase in eosinophils immediately after radiotherapy.[30]

Eosinophilia is associated with favorable prognosis in some reports. There are indications that the ability to produce an eosinophilia depends upon the integrity of the cell-mediated and humoral immune mechanisms.[31,32] Ghossein has suggested that irradiation damage can cause an alteration of cells in such a way that they appear foreign to the host. In turn, these antigens may stimulate an immune response which may induce release of eosinophils. He also suggested that eosinophils phagocytize antigen-antibody complexes and thereby may be an important ingredient in inflammatory reactions which modify delayed type hypersensitivity.[33] Muggia suggests that radiation damage to mucous cells may attract eosinophils and stimulate their activity.[34]

VI. EFFECT OF RADIOTHERAPY ON IN VIVO CELL-MEDIATED IMMUNITY

The primary in vivo assessment of delayed type hypersensitivity reactivity is measured with various types of skin tests. A de novo antigen such as DNCB (dinitrochlorobenzene) is one to which most people have not been exposed. Thus, sensitization to it can be used as an indication of the patients current ability to induce immune reactivity to a new antigen. Assessment of "recall antigens" (antigens to which the individual may have been exposed in the past) have also been employed. However, these tests measure an established immune responsiveness, not necessarily the ability to respond to a new antigen which requires a somewhat different immune sequence. There are a number of reports attempting to correlate the patients' ability to respond to skin tests and prognosis of the tumor type involved. Most of these citations have been studies through relatively short or intermediate follow-up periods and have, unfortunately, focused on tumors other than cervical carcinoma.[35-39] When examined, in contrast to the decrease reactivity reported for some in vitro tests of cell-mediated immunity, skin reactivity to recall antigens in gynecologic tumor patients (during and following radiotherapy) have been normal.[22,23,40] Even though T and B cell numbers dropped immediately after radiation therapy, the skin test responses remained normal in cervical carcinoma patients.[22,40] Cheek found radiation therapy did not effect cervical cancer patients mumps skin tests as has been reported for patients whose thymus has been irradiated.[40]

Responsiveness to de novo antigens has been thought to be a better prognostic indicator for some tumor types than recall antigens.[35,38] In Halili's study of the long-term effect of radiotherapy on the primary immune response of gynecological patients 3 to 15 years after treatment, the skin test patterns were similar to that of normals.[23] Of the 52 cancer patients, 87% responded in a positive manner — a proportion similar to that expected in the normal population. Patients who were disease free had a DNCB reactivity of 73% 3 to 5 years post-therapy, while those free of disease at 5 years had a reactivity rate of 96%. The state of DNCB reactivity before treatment may be an important indicator according to some authorities. Haza reported that patients with the ability to respond positively to DNCB sensitization prior to radiotherapy had a significant better chance of survival after 1 year.[41] Nalick also reported that gynecological patients with normal delayed type hypersensitivity reactions to standard recall skin test antigens as well as to the de novo antigen DNFB (dinitroflurobenzene) had a better prognosis than did those with impaired reactivity.[42] In our preliminary studies, primary sensitization to DNCB occurred in approximately 50% in all groups of patients and did not appear indicative of prognosis. Also the majority of cervical carcinoma patients in our study do not appear to be highly reactive to recall antigens before irradiation therapy and anergic or weakly positive reactions were not infrequent after treatment.[27] Patients who had a favorable response and no recurrence of tumor 12 months post-therapy had fewer anergic reactions than did the group of patients who developed either local or distal recurrences. We found some augmented responses to some recall antigen skin tests after treatment in certain stages of cervical cancer. This latter type of enhanced reactivity has been described by other investigators for other human tumors following radiotherapy.[43,44] Enhanced responses to DNCB after treatment has also been found in other tumor types in some studies.[45]

VII. EFFECT OF RADIOTHERAPY ON ANTIBODY PRODUCTION

A. Serum Immunoglobulins

Various changes in the serum immunoglobulin levels in untreated cervical carcinoma patients have been reported. Plesnicar found statistically significant higher levels of serum IgG in patients with Stage I disease when compared to Stage IV patients.[46] In advanced disease, IgM levels were below that of controls, but did not differ from those with early stage disease. Vaudevan found that untreated cervical carcinoma patients had raised levels of IgM and IgA.[47] After radiotherapy these levels returned to normal. In contrast, Hancock found no significant changes in any of the immunoglobulin levels in cervical carcinoma patients when compared to pretreatment levels.[22] Halili followed patients with various gynecological malignancies for 3 to 15 years after radiotherapy and reported all serum immunoglubulin levels were within the normal range.[23]

The differences in the two reports are somewhat unsettling, but may be due to differing sampling times, assay techniques, etc. Although there may be some alteration of various serum Ig classes before radiotherapy, there is no good indication that levels are abnormal after treatment, particularly long-term. It should be noted that there are many variables that may alter immunoglobulin levels, (stress, diet, age, concomitant disease, etc.). Wide variations within the normal range exist and careful controls are needed. One of the most fruitful approaches may be to use each patient as her own control and look for serial changes over time. Even here, interpretation of changes must be guarded.

B. Antitumor Antibodies

Cancer cells may have antigens on their surfaces which are normal, fetal or tumor-induced. Different antigens may react with the host's immune system to produce so called tumor-specific auto-antibodies which can be detected by various techniques, especially cytotoxic and immunofluorescent methods.

Christensen et al. studied complement-dependent cytotoxic antibodies to surface antigens on herpes simplex virus type 2 (HSV-2) infected cells and to cervical carcinoma cell lines derived from women with various stages of cervical carcinoma.[48] Patients were divided into three groups, (1) severely ill, (2) survivors with advanced disease, and (3) survivors with less advanced disease. The severely ill group of patients had the strongest cytolytic activity to the cervical cell lines. The opposite was noted for cytolysis of the HSV-2 infected cells. Patients with less advanced cancer had significantly higher cytolytic activity than those who were severely ill or had advanced cancer. During therapy the cytolytic reactivity to the cervical carcinoma cell lines decreased while a rise in cytolytic activity to HSV-2 infected cells was observed. Long-term survivors have a high cytolytic activity to HSV-2 but not to cervical carcinoma cell lines. The stronger cytolysis of the cervical cell lines from patients with a growing neoplasm may be due to continuous antigen stimulation which induces antibody against a component on the tumor cells. The low anti HSV-2 reactivity in patients with progressing cervical lesions could be due to their impaired antibody production to this type of antigen, to the absorption of circulating antibody on the tumor cells, or to some other phenomenon. Einhorn did a similar, but not identical, study of cervical carcinoma patients.[49] His results were inconclusive. Patients with antibodies to the HeLa cell line (derived from a cervical cancer patient) tended to do better than those patients without antibodies. He also noted an increased number of patients reacting to HeLa cell lines after radiotherapy, but the changes were not statistically significant. All seven patients who had antibodies to the HeLa cells before radiation therapy had no evidence of tumor during the follow-up period. However, 5/22 (20%) of the patients with antibodies to HeLa cell after treatment, and 17/54 (31%), without antibodies on any occasion, developed a recurrence. In an earlier study, after irradiation of the uterus, there was a significant increase in serum antibodies to eipthelial cells of the portico and cervical glands cells as detected by IF in gynecological tumor patients.[50] This irradiation effect was not thought to be due to manipulation of the uterus during the application of the radium.

VIII. EFFECT OF RADIOTHERAPY ON OTHER IMMUNE FEATURES

A few comments might be made about the effect of radiation on some other immunologically associated events in gynecologic malignancies. One substance that has been studied is the change in levels of carcinoembryonic antigen (CEA) in cervical carcinoma patients. This antigen was originally described by Gold in patients with cancer of the colon, but is now known to be present in a variety of neoplastic conditions including cervical carcinoma.[51] It is also demonstrable in low levels in the sera of many normal persons.[51] The elevation of titers of CEA in cervical carcinoma patients may be quite high. Plasma CEA levels above 2.5 ng per ml have been found in 40 to 80% of patients with invasive squamous carcinoma of the cervix.[52-54] Elevation of CEA levels in cervical carcinoma may correlate with the extent of the disease. One study of stage I cervical carcinoma patients reported elevated CEA levels in approximately 40% of the cases.[54] In four patients (stage IV) the incidence was 80%.

Longitudinal changes of CEA levels in cervical carcinoma patients following radiotherapy have been reported with differing results. In Donaldson's study, the initial incidence of raised CEA levels in 75 patients with various stages of cervical carcinoma was 65%.[54] Thirty-two of the patients were also followed during radiotherapy, and CEA levels rose above the preirradiation levels in 81% of the women. In a recent study by Kjostad approximately 80% of the women with squamous carcinoma of the cervix were described as either reacting to radiological or surgical treatment with a significant fall in plasma levels of CEA.[55]

Donaldson's studies described three distinct patterns of CEA changes following radiotherapy. Some patient's levels declined to normal and were associated with a disease-free state. This lowering occurred 12 to 16 weeks after therapy. Some patient's levels declined to almost, but not quite, normal levels and were associated with heavy cigarette smoking, or in one case, persistent disease; and in three patients, the decline to normal levels was followed by a subsequent rise to abnormal levels.[54] This latter was associated with recurrence of tumor. An earlier report by Disaia did not find these patterns.[56] The reasons for the difference between the results of Donaldson and Disaia are not understood. The time required for the CEA levels in treated patients to return to normal in Donaldson's studies were also different from that expected from previous reported changes of CEA levels postsurgery. Following surgery, normal CEA antigen levels were often found as soon as 6 weeks postoperation.[53] What may be noteworthy, however, is that five to seven patients with recurrent disease in Donaldson's study had an increase in CEA levels which preceded the clinical recognition of tumor recurrence by at least 1 to 4 months. Thus determinations of CEA, while certainly not specific for cervical cancer, may be useful in following a patient's progress during and after irradiation therapy.

IX. EFFECT OF RADIOTHERAPY ON REGIONAL LYMPH NODES

Histological and morphologic evaluation of cervical carcinoma tissues and regional lymph nodes have often suggested that certain immune cell types can be correlated with clinical prognosis. Gusberg showed that the more profuse the mononuclear infiltration of the stroma around the cervical tumor, the more favorable the response to radiotherapy.[57] Surprisingly, lymphocyte infiltration of the tumor itself did not correlate with the favorable response so that the location of the infiltrate was more important than was the type of cell involved in the response. Graham reported that the presence of large numbers of mast cells and histiocytes in the stroma around invasive cervical carcinoma sites gives significantly greater survival rates following radiotherapy than similar tumors without such cells.[58] Patients with tumor positive lymph nodes sometimes had a higher cure rate with radiotherapy than those treated with alone. The phenomenon of concomitant immunity may partially explain this paradox. In this situation, primary tumor may inhibit the growth of the secondary foci of the same tumor in some incompletely understood manner. Studies in animal models have shown that the surgical removal of certain tumors is associated with a rapid loss of tumor-specific cellular immunity, the development of enhancing tumor antibodies, and the appearance of metastatic deposits that were thought to be derived from previously dormant tumors in the blood or lymph organs of the host animal.[59,60] Concomitant immunity, although an experimental animal phenomenon, has not yet been conclusively observed in man.

The destruction of tumors by irradiation, in contrast to surgical removal, may result in a prolonged increase in tumor-specific immunity which prevents growth of secondary foci.[60] This heightened immunity may be the result of local and systemic release of large amounts of tumor material following local irradiation. Indeed, increased tumor-specific humoral and cell-mediated responses following local radiation have been observed in man.[50,61]

X. SUMMARY

There seems little doubt that immune events are associated with human cervical can-

Table 1
REPORTED IMMUNOLOGICAL CHANGES POSTRADIOTHERAPY IN GYNECOLOGICAL TUMOR PATIENTS[a]

Test	After radiotherapy	Ref.
T and B cells		
T cells (E rosettes)	Decrease	16, 20, 22
T cells (HA-E rosettes)	No change	20
B Cells (EAC rosettes)	No change	20, 21
B cells (detectable by IF)	Decrease	21, 22
Lymphocyte transformation indices		
To mitogens (PHA, ConA, PWM)	Decrease	18, 19, 22
Serum inhibition factor (against normal control lymphs)	In some cases diminished or lost	19, 22
Leukocyte migration inhibition		
(to tumor antigen)	Neg in some cases	19, 22
Skin tests		
In vivo DTH to recall antigens	Normal response	22, 23, 40
Peripheral blood cell count		
Lymphocyte	Reduced	16, 18-22
Monocytes	Sig increase	29
PMM	Sig decrease	22, 29
Eosinophils	Increase	29, 30
Serum immunoglobulin		
	No change or a return to normal	22, 47
Complement dependent cytotoxic antibody		
+ HSV-2 infec cells	Cytolytic activity increased	48
+ Cervical cancer cells	Cytolytic activity decreased	48
Carcinoembryonic antigen (CEA)		
	Variable, may increase or decrease	54, 55

[a] Patients usually compared to normal controls or themselves over time.

cer or that immunity can be altered by irradiation treatment (Table 1). We are only beginning to get a glimmering of the significance of these interactions for patients treated with radiotherapy for cervical carcinoma. More extensive studies are sorely needed to document the interplay between immunity and irradiation in these patients so current treatment regimes can be devised which yield maximal therapeutic benefits. If the future holds immunotherapy as an important adjuvant therapy for cervical carcinoma, additional understanding will be even more vital for its effective application.

REFERENCES

1. Mumford, D. M., Kaufman, R. H., and McCormick, N., Immunity, herpes simplex virus and cervical carcinoma, *Surg. Clin. N. Am.*, 58, 39, 1978.
2. Naib, Z. M., Nahmias, A. J., and Josey, W. E., Cytology and histopathology of cervical herpes simplex infection, *Cancer*, 19, 1026, 1966.
3. Nahmias, A. J., Josey, W. E., Naib, Z. M., Antibodies to herpes virus hominis types I and II women with cervical cancer, *Am. J. Epidemiol.*, 89, 547, 1969.
4. Catalano, L. W., Jr. and Johnson, L. D., Herpes virus antibody and carcinoma in situ of the cervix, *JAMA*, 217, 447, 1971.
5. Rawls, W., Gardner, H. L., Flanders, R. W., Lowry, S. P., Kaufman, R. H., and Melnick, J. L., Genital herpes in two social groups, *Am. J. Obstet. Gynecol.*, 110, 682, 1971.
6. Aurelian, L., Schuman, M. B., Marcus, R. L., and Davis, M. J., Antibody to HSV-2 induced tumor specific antigens in serums from patients with cervical cancer, *Science*, 181, 161, 1973.
7. *American Cancer Society* Fact and Figures, 1978.
8. Cleaves, M., Radium: with preliminary note on radium rays in the treatment of cancer, *Adv. Ther.*, 21, 667, 1903.
9. Brady, L. W., Radiotherapy treatment of cervical cancer, in *Gynecologic Oncology*, McGowan, L., Ed., Appleton-Century-Crofts, New York, 1978, 217.
10. Meigs, J. V. and Liu, W., Surgical and pathologic classification for cancer of the cervix, *Surg. Gynecol. Obstet.*, 100, 55, 1955.
11. Brunschwig, A., The surgical treatment of cancer of the cervix state I and II, *Am. J. Roentgenol. Radium. Ther. Nucl. Med.*, 102, 147, 1968.
12. Anderson, R. E. and Warner, N. L., Ionizing radiation and the immune response, *Adv. Immunol.*, 24, 215, 1976.
13. Braunschwig, A., Southam, C. M., and Levin, A. G., Host resistance to cancer, clinical experiments by homotransplants, autotransplants and admixture of autologous leucocytes, *Ann. Surg.*, 162, 416, 1965.
14. Southam, C. M., Cancer-specific antigens in man, in *Immunological Diseases*, 2nd ed., Samter, M., Ed., Little, Brown & Co., Boston, 1971, chapter 42.
15. McCredie, J. A., Inch, W. R., and Sutherland, R. M., Effect of postoperative radiotherapy on peripheral blood lymphocytes in patients with carcinoma of the breast, *Cancer*, 29, 349, 1972.
16. Stratton, J. A., Byfield, P. E., Byfield, J. E., Small, R. C., Benfield, J., and Pilch, Y., A comparison of the acute effects of radiation therapy including or excluding the thymus, on lymphocyte subpopulations of cancer patients, *J. Clin. Invest.*, 56, 88, 1975.
17. Binhammer, R. T. and Croker, J. R., Effect of X-irradiation on the pituitary adrenal axis of the rat, *Radiat. Res.*, 18, 429, 1963.
18. Jenkins, V. K., Olson, M. H., Ellis, H. N., and Dillard, A., *In vitro* lymphocyte response of patients with uterine cancer as related to clinical stage and radiotherapy, *Gynecol. Oncol.*, 3, 191, 1975.
19. Yamagata, S. and Green, G. H., Radiation-induced immune changes in patients with cancer of the cervix, *Br. J. Obstet. Gynaecol.*, 83, 400, 1976.
20. Raben, M., Walach, N., Galili, U., and Schlenger, M., The effect of radiation therapy on lymphocyte subpopulations in cancer patients, *Cancer*, 37, 1417, 1976.
21. Rand, R. J., Jenkins, D. M., and Bulmer, R., T- and B-lymphocyte subpopulations following radiotherapy for invasive squamous call carcinoma of the uterine cervix, *Clin. Exp. Immunol.*, 33, 159, 1978.
22. Hancock, B. W., Bruce, L., Heath, J., Sugden, P., Ward, A. M., and Chir, B., The effects of radiotherapy on immunity in patients with localized carcinoma of the cervix uteri, *Cancer*, 43, 118, 1979.
23. Halili, M., Bosworth, J., Romney, S., Moukhtar, M., and Ghossin, N. A., The long term effect of radiotherapy on the immune status of patients cured of a gynecologic malignancy, *Cancer*, 37, 2875, 1976.
24. Byfield, P. E., Stratton, J. A., and Small, R., Lymphocyte response after radiotherapy, *Lancet*, 1, 309, 1974.
25. DiSaia, P. J., Morrow, C. P., Hill, A., and Mittelstaedt, L., Immune competence and survival in patients with advanced cervical cancer: peripheral lymphocyte counts, *Radiat. Oncol.*, 4, 449, 1978.
26. Ghossein, N. A. and Bosworth, J. L., Immunocompetence in radiation therapy patients, in *The Handbook of Cancer Immunology*, Vol. 4, Water, H., Ed., Garland STPM Press, New York, 1978, 161.
27. Munford, D. M., unpublished data, 1978.
28. Menczer, J., Dor, J., Soffer, Y., and Serr, D. M., Cell-mediated immunity in patients with endometrial adenocarcinoma, *Gynecol. Oncol.*, 6, 223, 1978.

29. Rotman, M., Ansley, H., Rogow, L., and Stowe, S., Monocytosis: a new observation during radiotherapy, *Int. J. Radiat. Oncol. Biol. Phys.,* 2, 117, 1977.

30. Ghossein, N. A., Bosworth, J. L., Stacey, P., Muggia, F. M., and Krishnaswarmu, V., Radiation — related eosinophilia, *Radiology,* 117, 413, 1975.

31. Ponzio, N. M. and Speirs, R. S., Lymphoid cell dependence of eosinophil response to antigen. III. Comparison of the rate of appearance of two types of memory cells in various lymphoid tissue at different times after priming, *J. Immunol.,* 110, 1363, 1973.

32. Speirs, R. S., Speirs, E. E., and Ponzio, N. M., Eosinophils in humoral and cell mediated responses, in *Developments in Lymphoid Cell Biology,* Gottleib, A., Ed., CRC Press, Boca Raton, Fla., 1974, chap. 11.

33. Ghossein, N. A., Bosworth, J. L., and Bases, R. E., The effect of radial radiotherapy on delayed hypersensitivity and the inflammatory response, *Cancer,* 35, 1616, 1975.

34. Muggia, F. M., Ghossein, N. A., and Wohl, H., Eosinophilia following radiation therapy, *Oncology,* 27, 118, 1973.

35. Eilber, F. P. and Morton, D. L., Impaired immunologic reactivity and recurrence following cancer surgery, *Cancer,* 25, 362, 1970.

36. Maisel, R. H. and Ogara, J. H., Abnormal dinetrochlorobenzine skin sensitization — a prognostic sign of survival in head and neck squamous cell carcinoma, *Laryngoscope,* 84, 2012, 1974.

37. Gutterman, J. U., Mavligit, G., Gottlieb, J. A., Burges, M. A., McBride, C. E., Einhorn, L., Freireich, E. J., and Hersh, E. M., Chemoimmunotherapy of disseminated malignant melanoma with dimethyltriozenocarboramide and Bacillus Calmette-Guerier, *N. Surg. J. Med.,* 291, 592, 1974.

38. Lee, Y. N., Sparkes, F. D., Eilber, F. R., and Morton, D. L., Delayed cutaneous hypersensitivity and peripheral lymphocyte counts in patients with advanced cancer, *Cancer,* 35, 748, 1975.

39. Cunningham, T. J., Dant, D., Wolfgang, P. E., Mellyn, M., Madiolek, S., Sponzo, R. W., and Horton, J., A correlation of DNCB induced delayed cutaneous hypersensitivity reactions and the course of disease in patients with recurrent breast cancer, *Cancer,* 37, 1696, 1976.

40. Cheek, J. H., Damker, J. I., Brady, L. W., and O'Niell, E. A., Effect of radiation therapy on mumps-delayed type hypersensitivity reaction in lymphoma and carcinoma patients, *Cancer,* 32, 580, 1973.

41. Hazra, T. A., Parks, L. C., Inahsigh, A., and Peoples, W., Delayed hypersensitivity to DNCB and survival following radiation therapy in patients with solid malignant tumors, *Radiology,* 115, 429, 1975.

42. Nalick, R. H., DiSaia, P. J., Rea, T., and Morrow, C. P., Immunocompetence and prognosis in patients with gynecologic cancer, *Gynecol. Oncol.,* 2, 81, 1974.

43. Cosimi, A. B., Brunstetter, F. H., Kemmerer, W. T., and Miller, B. N., Cellular immune competence of breast cancer patients receiving radiotherapy, *Arch. Surg.,* 107, 531, 1973.

44. Slater, M., Ngo, E., and Law, B. H. S., Effect of therapeutic irradiation of the immune responses, *Am. J. Roentgenol.,* 126, 313, 1976.

45. Gross, L., Manfredi, O. L., and Protos, A., Effects of cobalt-60 irradiation upon cell-mediated immunity, *Radiology,* 106, 653, 1973.

46. Plesnicar, S., Immunoglobulins in carcinoma of the uterine cervix, *Acta Radiol.,* 11, 37, 1972.

47. Vasudevan, D. M., Balakrishnan, K., and Talwar, G. P., Immunoglobulin in carcinoma of the cervix, *Indian J. Med. Res.,* 59, 1635, 1971.

48. Christenson, B. and Espmark, A., Long term followup studies on herpes simplex antibodies in the course of cervical cancer. II. Antibodies to surface antigen of Herpes simplex virus, *Int. J. Cancer,* 17, 318, 1976.

49. Einhorn, N. and Jonsson, J., Antibodies to a HeLa cell line in carcinoma of the cervix uteri, *Acta Radiol. (Ther.),* 11, 83, 1972.

50. Einhorn, N., Jonsson, J., and Fagraeus, A., Immunological reactions after irradiation of the uterus, *Radiat. Res.,* 40, 456, 1969.

51. Gold, P. and Freedman, S. O., Demonstration of tumor specific antigens in human colonic carcinoma by immunological tolerance and absorption technique, *J. Exp. Med.,* 121, 439, 1962.

52. DiSaia, P. J., Haverback, J., Dyce, B. J., and Morrow, M., Carcinoembryonic antigens in patients with squamous cell carcinoma of the cervix uteri and vulva, *Surg. Gynecol. Obstet.,* 138, 542, 1974.

53. Barrelett, V. and Mach, J. P., Variations of the carcinoembryonic antigen level in the plasma of patients with gynecologic disorders during therapy, *Am. J. Obstet. Gynecol.,* 121, 164, 1975.

54. Donaldson, E., Van Nagell, J. R., Jr., Wood, E. G., Pletsch, Q., and Goldenberg, D. M., Carcinoembryonic antigen in patients treated with radiation therapy for invasive squamous cell carcinoma of the uterine cervix, *Am. J. Roentgenol.,* 127, 829, 1976.

55. Kjorstad, K. E. and Orjaseter, H., Carcinoembryonic antigen levels in patients with squamous cell carcinoma of the cervix, *Obstet. Gynecol.,* 5, 536, 1978.

56. DiSaia, P. J., Morrow, C. P., Haverback, B. J., and Dyce, B. J., Carcinoembryonic antigen in cervical and vulvar cancer patients-serum levels and disease progress, *Obstet. Gynecol.,* 47, 95, 1976.

57. Gusberg, J. B., Yannopoular, K., and Cohen, C. J., Virulence indices and lymph nodes in cancer of the cervix, *Am. J. Roentgenol.*, 111, 273, 1971.

58. Graham, R. and Graham, J., Mast cells and cancer of the cervix, *Surg. Gynecol. Obstet.*, 123, 2, 1966.

59. Gershon, R. K., Carter, R. L., and Kondo, K., Immunologic defenses against metastasis: impairment by excision of an all transplanted lymphoma, *Science*, 159, 646, 1968.

60. Crile, G. and Deadbar, S. D., Role of preoperative irradiation in prolonging concomitant immunity and preventing metastasis in mice, *Cancer*, 27, 629, 1971.

61. Einhorn, N., Klein, G., and Clifford, P., Increase in antibody titer against the EBV-assoc. membrane antigen complex in Burkitt's lymphoma and nasopharyngeal carcinoma after local irradiation, *Cancer*, 26, 1013, 1970.

Chapter 9

RADIATION EFFECT ON IMMUNITY IN CANCER OF THE GENITOURINARY TRACT

Donthamsetti S. Rao and Stefano S. Stefani

TABLE OF CONTENTS

I. KIDNEY

Biological (spontaneous) regression occurs with higher frequency in granular or clear cell carcinoma of the kidney than in any other malignancy.[1] In addition, the prolonged survival even with metastasis and the delayed appearance of local recurrences and metastases, sometimes even after 25 years in apparently cured patients, all suggest that immunologic and/or hormonal factors play a major role in the evolution of renal cell tumors.[1]

A. Pretherapy

The response to recall antigens is depressed in patients with renal cell tumors,[2-4] being more so in patients with advanced than in those with localized disease.[2,3] But in another study, Elhilali et al.[4] failed to observe a significant correlation between extent of the tumor and response to recall antigens. Similar to recall antigens the ability of patients with carcinoma of the kidney to develop cell-mediated immune response to topical application of dinitrochlorobenzene (DNCB) is also depressed.[4] No significant differences in response have been noted between the localized and metastatic group by Elhilali et al. while Morales et al.[3] and Brosman et al.[2] have found a relationship between reactivity and tumor extent. Thus, Brosman et al.[2] obtained positive responses to DNCB in all six patients with localized disease (no invasion of the Gerota's capsule) but in only 7 of 15 patients with distant metastases. Patients with urologic cancer, including kidney malignancies, have normal absolute peripheral lymphocyte count.[5,6] But Morales et al.,[3] studying solely patients with renal cancer over a period of 16 weeks, found that lymphocyte values became significantly lower in a group of 10 patients with metastatic disease than in 8 patients with localized tumors. It must be noted, however, that the metastatic group received BCG immunotherapy during the same period; this could explain the sudden and sharp drop in the absolute count. There is a decreased number of T lymphocytes in patients with renal carcinoma,[7] more pronounced in those with metastatic than in the group with localized disease.[3] The absolute T lymphocyte count further declines with the progression of the disease and deterioration of the patient's condition.[3] There is also a statistically significant depression of the lymphocyte reactivity to PHA stimulation.[3,8] Occasionally there are wide fluctuations in the results of this test in the same patient, to such an extent that some investigators feel it does not play any role in monitoring the evolution of neoplastic process or its response to therapy.[3]

Monocytic chemotactic response is depressed in renal cancer, being greater in patients with metastatic than with localized disease, according to Brosman et al.[2] These investigators claim this test is a reliable and useful measure of monocyte function and correlates well with the clinical course of the disease.

The microcytotoxicity test of Takasugi and Klein, as modified by Hellström et al.,[9] has been used in renal carcinoma patients to assess their cell-mediated immunity. Cole et al.[10] failed to demonstrate cell-mediated immunity in three out of four patients free of disease while it was present in all four patients with clinically active disease. Using the same test, Montie et al.[11] found a higher mean percent cell inhibition in post-nephrectomy patients than in normal controls and prenephrectomy cancer patients, the difference being statistically significant between the pre- and postnephrectomy groups.

B. Post-Therapy

There are few reports dealing with the effect of radiation on immunity in patients with renal cell carcinoma, the number of patients being very small in most of the studies. The results of these investigations vary widely, going from no changes in immune status following radiation[3] to prolonged depression up to 2 years after radiation therapy.[6]

Radiation treatment seems to influence the response to primary and recall antigens. Elhilali et al.,[4] in 38 patients with urologic cancers who received radiation therapy as an adjunct to surgery or as the sole therapy, obtained 40% positive response to recall antigens pretherapy and 27% post-therapy (1 to 12 months); the difference is not statistically significant. In a selected group (but the size of the sample is not given and each patient was tested only pre- or post-therapy) the same authors observed a 64% positive in the recall antigen response in the group tested pre-therapy and a 24% positive in the post-therapy group (p <0.005). Similarly, in this selected group, 62% of the DNCB responses were positive pretherapy as compared to 4% post-therapy (p <0.005). Surprisingly, no appreciable differences were noted, however, as a function of the tumor dose (1600 to 2000 vs. to 7500 rad), whether the patients were tested with DNCB or recall antigens.[4] Similarly, there were no differences before or after radiotherapy in the metastatic disease group. Another study in which DNCB testing was done serially before, 3 and 9 months after the first irradiation, there was no change in skin reactivity in 45 patients, 6 of whom had urinary bladder cancer, suggesting that cancericidal doses of C060 do not impair the cell-mediated immunocompetence.[12]

There are indications that the peripheral total lymphocyte count and the percentage and absolute T lymphocyte count decrease in kidney cancer patients following irradiation. Thus, Catalona et al.[6] compared four patients who received a cumulative tumor dose ranging from 2000 to 9000 rad (three treated for bone metastases and one for the primary kidney tumor) with two nontreated patients. However, we are not given the time lapsed between the irradiation and the testing and we do not know whether the control patients were in the same stage of disease as the treated group. They observed a mean total lymphocyte count of 990 (vs. 1975 for the control, nonirradiated patients) a percent T lymphocyte of 38.3 (vs. 61.0) and an absolute T lymphocyte count of 412 (vs. 1.497). Radiotherapy did not produce any significant alterations in the T lymphocytes according to Morales et al.[3] but it was exclusively used for control of bone pain in only four patients with advanced disease.

There is suggestion that there is some impairment in cell-mediated immunity following irradiation as tested by the microcytotoxicity assay,[10] but this observation is based on only two patients, not enough to allow any conclusion. In summary, there is impairment of cell-mediated immunity in patients with renal cell carcinoma. This depression correlates with the extent of the disease. More controlled studies are necessary to come to any meaningful conclusion regarding the effect of radiation on immunity in patients with renal cell carcinoma.

II. BLADDER

Cancer of the urinary bladder has an unpredictable evolution, in some patients recurring quite early after therapy, in others, with apparently similar characteristics, being completely controlled.[13] Lymphocytic and plasma cell infiltration has been observed more frequently in cancers than in benign or inflammatory bladder conditions and is more prominent in lower grades and stages of bladder cancer than in more aggressive, more advanced conditions.[14] Moreover, in the same patients, the regional lymph nodes show changes indicative of immunologic reactivity; these changes correlate well with prognosis.[15] These observations suggest that immunity influences the course of the disease.

A. Pretherapy

The response to skin stimulation with recall antigens has been found to be significantly depressed in bladder cancer patients by several investigators.[4,16-18] There is some disagreement, however, on the value of these tests as to whether they correlate with the stage of the cancer or its response to treatment. Williams et al.,[17] assessing cutaneous delayed hypersensitivity to three antigens (candida, streptokinase/streptodornase, and PPD), found some correlation only for the response to PPD. In this case, the PPD-negative group had a higher percentage of patients with more advanced tumors than the PPD-positive. By contrast, Brosman et al.[19] found a correlation with the stage of disease only in the response to streptokinase and streptodornase. Finally, Olsson et al.[16] initially reported more depressed skin responses to antigens in the group with active bladder tumor than in the groups with recurrent tumors or free of disease. But a 2-year follow-up did not corroborate their theory of energy in the presence of active tumor.[20] However, they did note the absence of tumor recurrences among those patients who demonstrated delayed hypersensitivity to intracutaneous testing with Keyhold-limpet hemacyanin.

Delayed hypersensitivity response to DNCB is definitely impaired in patients with cancer of the bladder;[18,19,21,22] the difference between one group of 91 such patients and another of 35 healthy controls was statistically significant at the $P <.001$ level.[19] There is also a good correlation between the response rate to DNCB and stage of disease, being higher in earlier cases.[17-19,22] No good correlation exists, however, between locally invasive and metastatic disease.[19] There are conflicting results regarding the prognostic value of this test. For instance, Catalona et al.[22] found, in a group of 19 patients with transitional carcinoma and negative test to DNCB, that 13 had recurrent disease, 11 of whom were dead within 1 year, while all patients in the DNCB-positive group were alive and only 5 (25%) had tumor recurrence. Similarly, Williams et al.[17] in a group of 54 patients observed that those who reacted to DNCB prior to therapy were free of tumor for more than 1 year; among 8 patients who failed to respond to the test, 7 died within 3 months. Less convincing is the observation of DeCenzo et al.:[23] 46 patients with bladder cancer were tested with 2-4 dinitrofluorobenzene (DNFB), a compound chemically similar to DNCB. Only 6 of the 31 patients in the DNFB-positive group were found to have progression of the disease as compared to 7 out of 17 whom were in the DNFB-negative group; however, 12 patients, lost to follow-up, 8 of whom were in the DNFB-positive group, were not counted as failures. Finally, Brosman et al.,[19] reporting on the largest group of bladder cancer patients studied for their response to DNCB, found no correlation between response and prognosis. Truly, they observed that the tumor-free interval was longer in DNCB-positive patients for any stage of disease (superficial or invasive) at 1 year. However, at 2 years, tumor recurrence and survival were the same in both DNCB groups.

Total peripheral lymphocyte count is depressed in bladder cancer.[24] Amin et al.,[24] in a group of 61 patients, found 41% to have lymphopenia (less than 1000 lymphocytes per cu.mm) before the start of radiotherapy, as compared to 6% in a group of healthy subjects, as reported by Zacharski and Luxman.[25] Although presenting unconvincing data to support it, Amin and Lich[24] state that in their study lymphopenia was associated with poorer survival and was common during the end stage of the disease. Catalona et al.[6] observed normal lymphocyte counts in a smaller group of patients with bladder cancer prior to therapy. The rosette assay has been used by Elhilali et al.[26] to study a group of 103 patients with urologic cancer, including 56 bladder cancer patients. They observed a significant decrease in the percentage of T-RFC and a significant increase in the percentage of B-RFC, when compared to results obtained in age-matched control. The group of patients with metastatic disease showed the lowest mean percentage of T-RFC. Similarly, Catalona et al.,[27] comparing the T-RFC values of 21 patients with bladder carcinoma with those of 83 healthy controls, found in the cancer group a significant decrease, although relatively mild, in the mean percentage and mean absolute T lymphocyte count. The drop in the mean absolute T-RFC was more pronounced in the group of patients with advanced (P3 and P4) bladder carcinoma.

Response of peripheral blood lymphocytes to PHA stimulation is reduced in bladder carcinoma patients.[8,26,28,29] Conflicting are, however, the reports dealing with the value of PHA response as a function of the clinical status of disease. Elhilali et al.[26] after dividing their cancer patients into three groups: with metastatic cancer; with localized disease, tumor persistent; and with localized disease, clinically cured; found significant only the difference between the last group with localized disease, clinically cured (PHA index: 68) and the age-matched control (PHA index: 152). Similarly, McLaughlin et al.[8] found no improvement in lymphocyte reactivity after radical operation for localized bladder cancer. Also the depressed lymphocyte reactivity was generally uniform and did not correlate with the clinical stage of the disease. This observation is contrary to that of Catalona et al.[28] who noted normal reactivity in early bladder cancer and impaired reactivity in advanced disease.

Attempts to detect the specific immunity of patients to their tumors — including those of the genitourinary tract — have involved a variety of tests including lymphocyte migration inhibition, lymphocyte adherence inhibition, and lymphocyte mediated microcytotoxicity. While in the past it was postulated that these assays were successful in detecting specific human tumor immunity, more recent evidence has led to the conclusion that, to date, there is no method that reliably detects human tumor-specific immunity in the cancer patient.[31] For this reason, and because it is beyond the scope of this publication, we will not present here a summary of the various investigations in this field of immunity. The changes in tissue blood group antigens, A, B, and H, using the specific red cell adherence (SRCA) have been studied in patients with bladder cancer by several authors.[32-35] Lange et al.,[34] in a group of 75 patients with low stage transitional cell carcinoma, concluded that (1) approximately 90% of patients who retained their antigens do not develop invasive disease, whereas 70% of the patients without these antigens do develop invasive disease over a 5 year or more period, (2) the presence or absence of SRCA reactivity does not correlate exactly with histological grading and therefore suggests that SRCA tests may help along with histological grading in predicting future clinical course, and (3) the analysis of serial biopsies on the same patient appear to increase the predictability.

B. Post-Therapy

In Table 1, we have summarized the experience of other investigators dealing with effect of radiotherapy on immunological profile with bladder cancer. The response to recall antigens is depressed following radiation therapy according to Elhilali et al.[4] They compared 38 patients with genitourinary cancer who received radiation therapy as an adjunct to surgery, or as the sole therapy, with 43 cancer patients who did not receive radiation therapy. It must be noted that the breakdown among cancers of bladder, kidney, and prostate is not given. These patients were skin tested with four microbial recall antigens, 1 to 12 months after completion of radiation therapy and recorded as positive responders if reacting to two or more antigens. There was a diminished response in the irradiated group with localized cancer (27% positive responders vs. 40% in the localized, nonirradiated group), but this difference is not statistically significant. No appreciable difference was noted between the two metastatic disease groups as well as between the group of patients who received 1600 to 2000 rad and that which was treated with doses greater than 2000 rad.[4] This work, the only one we could find in the literature dealing with the effect of radiation on recall antigens, is, in our opinion, unsatisfactory: (1) there is no breakdown among the genitourinary cancers, the authors, failing to recognize that treatment techniques and doses of irradiation are quite different between cancer of the kidney and cancers in the pelvis, (2) the pretherapy values are not given nor are used to assess the post-therapy response, and (3) it is impossible to determine whether the radiation effect, if any, is more pronounced at any specific time during the first follow-up year. One cannot exclude the possibility that patient selection and not radiation is responsible for the small difference in percent of positive responders in the two localized groups. The reports on the effect of radiation on DNCB reactivity are controversial.

Elhilali et al.[4] comparing the same 38 radiation-treated patients with genitourinary cancers discussed above, with a group of 43 patients radiation-untreated, noted not discernible differences between the two groups: 26% positive vs. 29% in the localized group and 32% vs. 30% in the metastatic one. Contrary to expectation, there were only 23% positive responders in the less than 2000 rad group and 33% in the 2000 to 7500 rad group. It is possible, although it is not stated in the paper, that a larger number of patients with more advanced disease who were treated palliatively were included in the less than 2000 rad group. Schellhamer et al.[8] came to the same conclusion in studying patients scheduled to receive preoperative radiation. They observed less response to DNCB in the group of patients with deep tumor invasion that in that with early invastion (P <0.05). This "identifies the higher stage of the disease as the cause for depression of DNCB reactivity rather than the treatment administered."[18] This position is also shared by Catalona et al.[35] Gross et al.[12] studied the effect of radiation on DNCB reactivity in various tumors including bladder cancer and concluded that in 85% of these patients therapeutic doses of C060 irradiation did not adversely affect the cell-mediated immune response. The further deterioration of delayed hypersensitivity response in the remaining 15% of patients is attributed to the effect of natural biological tumor burden rather than to radiation.[12]

Lymphocytes are the most radiosensitive of blood cells. Therefore, in any cancer treatment by radiation, one should expect a certain degree of lymphopenia. Localized irradiation for carcinoma of the breast, as an example, has been shown to reduce absolute lymphocyte counts by more than a third.[37,38] Radiation-induced lymphopenia in cancer of the bladder is not an exception: the number of lymphocytes in the peripheral blood was reduced to less than 50% within 3 weeks after completion of irradiation.[37] Similar postradiotherapy decrease in lymphocytes has been reported by Catalona et al.[6] in a group of patients with urological cancer.

Since the peripheral blood lymphocyte population represents a mixutre of immunologic cells (T, B, Active T, null cells), attempts have been made to investigate whether the lymphopenia induced by local irradiation is due to a reduction of T or B or both cells. The results, unfortunately, are conflicting. Catalona et al.[6] found that radiation produced a reduction in the percentage and absolute T lymphocyte count in 8 bladder cancer patients when compared with 14 nonirradiated patients with a cancer in the same organ. Unfortunately, missing in their report is the interval between irradiation and testing, which could have provided a better understanding of the radiation effect as a function of time. According to Blomgren et al.[37] already within 3 weeks after radiation completion there is a slight, although not significant, increase in the percentage of T lymphocytes, while for Elhilali et al.[26] it takes more than 1 year after radiation to see a drop in the percentage of this lymphocyte subpopulation. In contrast to these observations, Rafla et al.[29] reported no changes shortly after the end of therapy. It should be noted that neither Blomgren et al.[37] nor Elhilali et al.[26] or Rafla et al.[29] dealt in their study with a patient population consisting solely of cancer of the bladder.

The percentage B lymphocyte decreases significantly (from 46.4 to 24.3) within 3 weeks postradiation[37] and rebounds to significantly higher levels more than 1 year later.[26]

Radiation reduces the response to PHA, according to Elhilali et al.[26] and Catalona

Table 1

EFFECT OF RADIATION THERAPY ON IMMUNITY IN BLADDER CANCER

Group tested	No. Pts tested	R. Therapy dose in rad/time	Time immunity tested	Total lymphocytes	Total T-cell	Total B-cell	PHA (mean %)	SRCA/ MLR*	Ref.
Pts with invasive bladder Ca only	16 8	1400—6400/?	No R.T. 2 Mos—34 yrs after R.T.					1/16[f] 8/8 +[f]	Alroy, J. et al, 1978
Pts with bladder Ca only	61	0 ?/?	Before R.T. ?After R.T.	1000/mm³ 41% 82%					Amin, M. et al, 1974
10 GU Ca Pts (includes 7 bladder)	10	3600—8400 4—8 wks	Before R.T. 4—10 Wks after R.T.	1802[d] 788[d]	36.3% 42.3%	46.4%[a] 24.3%[a]	85.1 72.8		Blomgren, H. et al, 1974
Pts with bladder Ca only	8	6400/8 wks	Before R.T. <2 wks after R.T.	1470[d] 570[d]				45,580[c,g] 14,680[c,g]	Blomgren, H. et al, 1977
103 GU Ca Pts (includes 56 bladder)	74 25 14 24	1600—7000?	No R.T. <3 Mos after R.T. 6—12 Mos after R.T. >12 Mos after R.T.		63.1%[b] 63.7% 62.1% 52.4%[b]	21.0%[b] 25.0% 21.9% 21.8%[b]	134.4 60.5 38.7 71.8		Elhilali, M. M. et al, 1976
Pts with bladder Ca only	14	800—5500/?	No R.T. 0—60 Mos after R.T.	1987[d] 823[d]	1201[d] 439[d]				Catalona, P. et al, 1974
41 Pelvic tumors (includes 15 bladder)	36 18	0 ?/?	Before R.T. ~6 wks after R.T.		No change		19%[e] 29%[e]		Rafla, S. et al, 1978

[a] $p < 0.05$
[b] $p < .01$
[c] $p < 0.005$
[d] $p < 0.001$
[e] Peak reactivity
[f] Specific red cell adherence
[g] Mixed lymphocytic reaction

et al.[28] The mean PHA index decreases already during radiotherapy, reaches the lowest point between 6 months to 1 year, and recovers slightly 1 year after irradiation.[26] Catalona et al.[28] made a similar observation. Blomgren et al.[37] observed no change in the PHA response immediately after radiation, while, interestingly, Rafla et al.[9] found an improvement in PHA response post-therapy, in a group of 41 patients with pelvic tumors including 15 with bladder cancer.

Both the responder and stimulator capacities of the peripheral lymphoid cells in the mixed lymphocyte culture are impaired within 14 days after completion of a curative course of external radiotherapy for advanced bladder cancer (T_3 and T_4 — UICC classification).[30] This impairment does not correlate with the extent of radiation-induced lymphopenia.[30]

Similar to surgery, local radiotherapy in tumor doses of 3500 to 8400 R either destroys or diminishes lymphocyte cytotoxicity.[39] This loss, in the absence of tumor recurrence, occurs over a period of about 1 year after radiotherapy.[40] Based on the study of a total of 54 patients with cancer of the urinary bladder, O'Toole et al.[39] suggest that lymphocyte cytotoxicity activity toward bladder-tumor cells reflects the presence of a growing tumor or of a tumor-derived material. Also, that lymphocyte cytotoxicity found within the first year after irradiation may not be long-lasting if the tumor is effectively controlled.

Radiotherapy may also alter the result of the specific red cell adherence test. A retrospective study by Alroy et al.[35] revealed that all patients with invasive carcinoma who had a strongly positive SRCA test had received, some many years before, radiotherapy to the bladder region. None of the patients with negative or weakly positive SRCA tests had been radiated. Thus, they postulated that radiation induces differentiation in tumors, possibly through an enhancement of Golgi apparatus function.

Radiotherapy seems to have little influence on the immunoglobulin levels. Slater et al.[41] performed quantitative assays on IgG, IgA, and IgM on patients with bladder cancer before, during, two weeks, two months and six months after radiotherapy. No significant changes in mean values were observed. In summary, the results of the studies on the effect of radiation on immunity in bladder cancer have been controversial. The immunodepression appears correlated more to the tumor extent rather than the treatment administered. Further studies are recommended for more definite conclusion.

III. PROSTATE

A. Pretherapy

There is considerable controversy regarding the status of immune competence in patients with carcinoma of the prostate. This could partly be attributed to the nonuniform selection of the controls as well as differences in the methodology of testing. The response to recall antigens does not seem to be depressed in prostatic cancer patients.[17,42] Thus, Stefani et al.[42] in a more recent study reported on a group of 65 such patients and found that the percentage of positive responders to the recall antigens was not lower than the control group consisting of patients with benign prostatic hypertrophy.

These observations are contradicting previous reports which found a difference in response between cancer patients and controls.[43,44] The difference may be explained by the selection of the controls; in the first two studies, the controls were age-matched patients with benign prostatic hypertrophy, in the other studies, the control groups included healthy and sometimes not age-matched persons. In contrast, there appears to be full agreement about the observation that there is little difference in responsiveness between the group with early (or localized) and that with late (or metastatic) disease.[17,42,43] Impaired immunocompetence to DNCB stimulation is frequent among patients with prostatic carcinoma and the degree seems to correlate with the stage of the disease. Stefani et al.[42] showed that the sensitivity decreases in patients with metastases (63 vs. 19%) but that it is the same as that in control patients with benign prostatic hypertrophy (51 vs. 63%). These results agree with the findings of some[43,45] but not with all investigators[4,8,17,18,36] who found no demonstrable correlation between DNCB reactivity and stage of the disease. These differences could be due to nonuniform selection of the controls, the use of different staging classification and procedures as well as the method of skin testing.

Several investigators[8,42,46-48] studies the responsiveness of peripheral lymphocytes to phytohemagglutinin in patients with prostatic carcinoma. The majority of them indicated that there is a decreased response and no correlation between the response and the stage of the disease. In contrast, Stefani et al.[42] failed to demonstrate decreased response between the control group (using patients with benign prostatic hypertrophy) and the cancer patients independently of the stage of their disease. Previously reported series[8,47] used healthy controls which, again, may account for the difference. The absolute count of peripheral lymphocytes seems to be normal in patients with prostatic malignancy. However, Stefani et al.[42] found a substantially significant difference between early and advanced cases.

While Thomas et al.[44] did not observe any statistically significant difference in rosette-forming cell levels between controls and patients, Catalona et al.[27] have reported lower T cell percentage and total T cell counts in cases with metastatic prostatic carcinoma. Here again, the patients were compared to healthy subjects who were 10 years younger. Ablin[49] studied the relationship between the level of the three major serum immunoglobulins (IgG, IgA, IgM), the third component of complement (C') C'3 and the clinical stage of the disease. He observed a statistically significant difference in the levels of serum immunoglobulins in patients with prostatic carcinoma compared to those with benign prostatic hypertrophy and healthy adults, but not among the cancer patients as a function of the stage of their disease.

B. Post-Therapy

We have summarized in Table 2, the experience of other investigators dealing with effect of radiotherapy on immunological profile with prostatic cancer. Radiation seems to depress the response to recall antigens especially during the course of radiation. Slater et al.[41] demonstrated in a group of 18 patients with pelvic malignancies (including four prostatic and one bladder carcinoma) a significant decrease in response rate during the course of radiation therapy (from 67% positive to at least one antigen before therapy to 50% during therapy). There was a complete recovery (72%) two months post-therapy and again a drop (60%) at the end of 6 months. The post-therapy drop (1 to 12 months) in percent positive responders was not substantiated in the study by Elhilali et al.[4] which dealt with 38 patients with genitourinary cancer who received radiation therapy as an adjunct to surgery or as the sole therapy. The effect of radiation on DNCB skin reactivity is unclear. Elhilali et al.[4] in the same group of patients noted no significant change following radiation while Ghossein et al.[5] demonstrated an improvement in DNCB reactivity following curative radiation therapy (4000 to 7000 rad) in a group of 144 cancer patients which included 29 with genitourinary tumors. Short-term survival (average follow-up: 18 months) seemed better in those patients who became DNCB positive following radiotherapy. The same group of investigators[51] claim that the DNCB test is a good indicator of tumor response to radiation and prognosis. In a group of 112 patients—including 30 with genitourinary malignancies—tested prior to radiation therapy, 84% of the strong DNCB reactors had an excellent tumor response, while only 48% of the negative reactors had an equiv-

Table 2
EFFECT OF RADIATION THERAPY ON IMMUNITY IN PROSTATIC CANCER

Groups tested	No. Ca. prostate	R. Therapy dose in rad/time	Time immunity tested	Recall antigens % positive	DNCB % positive	Total lymphoc. count	Total T cell	Total B cell	PHA	Mixed lymphoc. reaction	Ref.
10 GU Ca pts: (includes bladder)	3	5400 rad in 6 wks	Before RT			1802[a]	36.3%[a]	46.4%[d]	85.1%		Blomgren, H. et al, 1974
			<3 Wks post RT			788[c]	42.3%[a]	24.3%[d]	72.8%[d]		
	5	5400 rad in 6 wks	Before RT			1880[a]				33,250	Blomgren, H. et al, 1977; Catalona, P. et al, 1974
			≤2 Wks post RT			900[a]				14,430	
	16	0	≤12 MOS post RT			1975[c]	1244[c]				
		3000—11000	≤12 MOS post RT			813[c]	345[c]				
GU Ca Pts (includes bladder & kidney)	74	0					63.1%[c]	21.0%[c]	134±30 SE		Elhilali, M. et al, 1976
	25	1600—7000	≤3 Mos post RT				63.7%	25.0%	61±17 SE		
	24		>12 Mos post RT				52.4%[c]	21.8%[c]	72±49 SE		
Includes bladder & renal Ca	43	0 vs		LOC:40 MET: 43	LOC:29 MET:30						Elhilali, M. et al, 1978
	38	1600—7500	1—2 Mos Post RT	LOC:27 MET:37	LOC:26 MET:32						
	23	1600—2000		27	23						
		vs		33	33						
	9	2000—7500									
144 Pts includes 29 GU Ca	?	4000—7000 4—7 wks	Before RT		59	1807[d]			7299[d]		Ghossein, N., et al 1975
			End of RT		—	834			4199		
			3—6 Mos Post RT		70	1046[d]			4583[d]		
32 Healthy controls vs 90 Ca pts	33	0 7000—7500	1—208 Mos post RT			<36 Mos ↓14/15 Pts >36 Mos ↓3/9 Pts			63×10[3e] 34×10[3e]	31×10[3e] 9×10[3e]	Hoppe, R. T. et al, 1977

18 Pelvic Ca pts	4	4000—7000	Before RT	67	1.691 = 100%	100%	Slater, J. M. et al, 1976
			During RT	50	−55%	−45%	
			End of RT	56	−62%	−25%	
			2 Mos post RT	72	−85%	−45%	
			6 Mos post RT	60	−80%	−122%	

[a] <0.5
[b] <0.1
[c] <0.01
[d] <0.05
[e] <0.001

alent response. In addition, among the positive DNCB responders 70% were alive at 6 months and the group had a median survival of 18 months versus 38% and 10 months, respectively, for the nonreactors.

The absolute peripheral lymphocyte count is depressed during and following irradiation.[6,37,41,50] Slater et al.[41] noted a sharp drop on the absolute lymphocyte count (to about 50% of the pretherapy value) during therapy in the group of patients receiving irradiation to the pelvis. Two weeks post-therapy and up to 6 months the count still remained low, although there was some indication of recovery. Depressed absolute lymphocyte counts persist up to 12 months, according to Catalona et al.[6] and up to 3 years postradiation, according to Hoppe et al.[50] Only after 3 years, there were good signs of recovery: 6 of 9 patients had normal counts.[50] Catalona et al.[6] comparing 6 irradiated patients with 16 nonirradiated patients with prostatic cancer, noted a significant reduction in the percentage of T lymphocyte count (42.3% vs. 59.4%) and in the absolute T lymphocyte count (345/mm³ vs. 1244/mm³) indicating a selective loss of T cells in the lymphocyte population. The depression was more severe among patients with prostatic carcinoma than with other urological malignancies, perhaps because of the propensity of these tumors to metastasize to the bone marrow.[6] Another explanation could be the higher doses usually delivered to prostatic cancers, but in this small group of six, half were treated palliatively for bony metastasis only. Based on all 18 urologic cancer patients examined, Catalona et al.[6] found a reduction in the percent and absolute T lymphocyte count up to 12 months after irradiation. Two of the three patients examined 24 months or more after therapy, had normal T cell levels. In contrast, Hoppe et al.[50] found in nearly all patients tested within 3 years of radiotherapy a T lymphopenia (less than 1100/mm³) and a B lymphopenia (less than 180/mm³) which accompanied the depressed absolute lymphocyte count. But, in the majority of these patients the percentages of T and B cells were within normal range, indicating, in our opinion, how misleading any report based on percentages only can be.

Blomgren et al.[37] in 15 patients with prostatic or urinary bladder carcinoma found a drop in the percent of B lymphocytes and an increase in the percent of T lymphocytes at the end of therapy. The lymphocyte response to PHA stimulation is depressed during and at the end of radiation therapy; there is a drop in response ranging between 25 and 85% of the pretherapy values.[5,37,41] This depression persists for 3 to 6 months according to Ghossein et al.[5] while Slater et al.[41] observe a rebound to more than 20% above pretreatment baseline at 6 months post-therapy. Hoppe et al.[50] state that the PHA response is impaired for extended periods to time (up to 3 years?) after completion of irradiation, but the authors do not present their data as a function of time to make their observation clearer. The effect of radiation on the in vitro lymphocyte transformation to concanavalin A and pokeweed mitogen and PPD stimulation is somewhat similar to that observed for PHA.[37,41]

The reactivity of peripheral lymphocytes in mixed lymphocyte culture (MLC) was found to be depressed at completion of therapy in five patients with poorly differentiated carcinoma of the prostate tested by Blomgren et al.[30] There was a decrease of both the *responder* (response against the lymphocytes of a healthy control) and *stimulator capacities* (capacity to stimulate the lymphocytes of the same control person) to approximately 40% of the original values. The impaired ability of the lymphocytes to respond in the MLC persists up to 52 months, according to Hoppe et al.[50] 70% (31 of 44) of the patients showed MLC responses which were below the lowest limit of normal donors. No significant changes in the mean values of IgG, IgA, or IgM were detected postradiotherapy by Slater et al.[41] However, they observed a significant increase in the IgG levels in 47% (8 out of 17) of patients who developed metastasis or died of their disease during the first year postradiation. But whether this increase is radiation-related or the expression of some changes occurring in terminally ill cancer patients remains to be demonstrated.

In summary, the literature on the effect of radiation on immunity in cancer of the prostate is scanty. Moreover, in most reports, the prostate is grouped with other malignancies, usually in the pelvis, and the number of patients in several studies is too small to allow meaningful conclusions.

IV. TESTIS

Testicular tumors have long been considered to be under some kind of immunologic control because of the observation of spontaneous regression of metastasis[52] and of the frequently observed mononuclear infiltrate in seminomas.[53,54] The degree of infiltration correlates with prognosis, according to Thachray[53] but not according to Johnson et al.[54] Several aspects of the immune response in patients with testicular tumors have recently been investigated, although not in a significant number of studies.

A. Pre- and Post-Therapy

Delayed hypersensitivity response to recall antigens does not seem to be depressed in nonseminomatous testicular tumors, regardless of the stage of disease or whether patients had or had not received systemic chemotherapy one or more months prior to skin testing.[18] Schellhamer et al.[18] tested this same group of 50 patients for their capacity to respond to DNCB stimulation and found no depression in the group of patients with negative retroperitoneal nodes on lymph node dissection. However, the response was impaired in the group of patients with more advanced disease and in the group receiving chemotherapy. We could not find any report dealing with the effect of radiation on the response to primary or recall antigens stimulation.

There is no lymphopenia in seminoma testis, according to Heier et al.,[55] who tested 17 such patients pretherapy. These patients then received radiation treatment with a total tumor dose of 4000 rad in 4 weeks to the right or left iliacal and to all para-aortic lymphnodes. Included in this study were also 30 previously treated (up to 10 years before) patients: 16 who had received a similar treatment, and 14 in whom the mediastinum and left supraclavicular area had been treated as well. During the course of therapy the average lymphocyte count fell from about $2200/mm^3$ to less than $500/mm^3$. Although there was a gradual increase as a function of time post-therapy, lymphopenia persisted up to 3 years after irradiation. The total lymphocyte number was again normal in patients studied 5 and 10 years after treatment.[55] Heier et al.[55] also evaluated, in the same group of patients described above, the effect of radiation on the T and B lymphocytes. The mean percentage of T lymphocytes stayed at normal levels at all intervals studied, while the percentage of B lymphocytes remained higher than the pretherapy values throughout, except at 10 years. Based on this observation, the authors conclude that in the peripheral blood the B lymphocytes recover more rapidly than the T lymphocytes. The blastogenic response of lymphocytes to PHA and mixed lymphocytes stimulation was significantly depressed in a group of 80 disease-free patients with a history of cancer of the prostate, breast, cervix, and testis who were tested one to 208 months after completion of irradiation.[50] We do not know, however, whether there is any difference according to tumor site. In summary, data regarding the effect of radiation on immunity in testicular carcinoma are scanty. Further studies are necessary to come to any meaningful conclusion.

REFERENCES

1. Bloom, H. J. G., Hormone-induced and spontaneous regression of metastatic renal cancer, *Cancer,* 32, 1066, 1973.
2. Brosman, S., Hausman, M., and Shacks, S. J., Studies on the immune status of patients with renal adenocarcinoma, *J. Urol.,* 114, 375, 1975.
3. Morales, A. and Eidinger, D., Immune reactivity in renal cancer: a sequential study, *J. Urol.,* 115, 510, 1976.
4. Elhilali, M. M., Brosman, S. A., Vescera, C., Paul, J. G., and Fahey, J. L., The effects of treatment on delayed cutaneous hypersensitivity responses (DNCB, croton oil, and recall antigen) in patients with genitourinary cancer, *Cancer,* 41, 1765, 1978.
5. Ghossein, N. A., Bosworth, J. L., and Bases, R. E., The effect of radical radiotherapy on delayed hypersensitivity and the inflammatory response, *Cancer,* 35, 1616, 1975.
6. Catalona, W. J., Potvin, C., and Chretien, P. B., Effect of radiation therapy for urologic cancer on circulating thymus-derived lymphocytes, *J. Urol.,* 112, 261, 1974.
7. Carmignani, G., Belgrano, E., Puppo, P., and Cornaglia, P., T and B lymphocyte levels in renal cancer patients: influence of preoperative transcatheter embolization and radical nephrectomy, *J. Urol.,* 118, 941, 1977.
8. McLaughlin, A. P., III and Brooks, J. A., A plasma factor inhibiting lymphocytic reactivity in urologic cancer patients, *J. Urol.,* 112, 366, 1974.
9. Hellström, I., Hellstrom, K. E., Sjögren, H. O., and Watuer, G. A., Demonstration of cell-mediated immunity to human neoplasms of various histological types, *Int. J. Cancer,* 7, 1, 1971.
10. Cole, A. T., Avis, I., Fried, F. A., and Avis, F., Cell-mediated immunity in renal cell carcinoma-preliminary report, *J. Urol.,* 115, 234, 1976.
11. Montie, J. E., Straffon, R. A., Deodhar, S. D., and Barna, B., In vitro assessment of cell-mediated immunity in patients with renal cell carcinoma, *J. Urol.,* 115, 239, 1976.
12. Gross, L., Manfredi, O. L., and Protos, A. A., Effect of cobalt-60 irradiation upon cell-mediated immunity, *Radiology,* 105, 653, 1973.
13. Nichols, J. A. and Marshall, V. F., The treatment of bladder carcinoma by local excision and fulguration, *Cancer,* 9, 559, 1956.
14. Sarma, K. P., Proliferative and lymphoid reactions in bladder cancer, *Invest. Urol.,* 10, 199, 1973.
15. Herr, H. W., Bean, M. A., and Whitmore, W. F., Jr., Prognostic significance of regional lymphnode histology in cancer of the bladder, *J. Urol.,* 115, 264, 1976.
16. Olson, C. A., Rao, C. N., Menzoian, J. O., and Byrd, W. E., Immunologic unreactivity in bladder cancer patients, *J. Urol.,* 107, 607, 1972.
17. Williams, G. and Castro, J. E., The diagnostic and prognostic significance of delayed hypersensitivity skin testing in patients with urological cancer, *J. Urol.,* 47, 97, 1975.
18. Schellhammer, P. F., Bracken, R. B., Bean, M. A., Pinsky, C. M., and Whitmore, W. F., Jr., Immune evaluation with skin testing. A study of testicular, prostatic and bladder neoplasms, *Cancer,* 38, 149, 1976.
19. Brosman, S., Elhilali, M., Vescera, C., and Fahey, J., Immune response in bladder cancer patients, *J. Urol.,* 121, 162, 1979.
20. Olson, C. A., Chute, R., and Rao, C. N., Immunologic reduction of bladder cancer recurrence rate, *J. Urol.,* 111, 173, 1974.
21. Merrin, C. and Han, T., Immune responses in bladder cancer, *J. Urol.,* 111, 170, 1974.
22. Catalona, W. J., Smolev, J. K., and Harty, J. I., Prognostic value of host immunocompetence in urologic cancer patients, *J. Urol.,* 114, 922, 1975.
23. Decenzo, J. M., Allison, R., and Leadbetter, G. W., Jr., Skin testing in genitourinary carcinoma: 2-year follow-up, *J. Urol.,* 114, 271, 1975.
24. Amin, M. and Lich, R., Jr., Lymphocytes and bladder-cancer, *J. Urol.,* 111, 165, 1974.
25. Zacharski, L. R. and Linman, J. W., (cited by Amin, M. and Lich, R., Jr.), Lymphocytes and bladder-cancer, *J. Urol.,* 111, 165, 1974.
26. Elhilali, M. M., Britton, S., Brosman, S., and Fahey, J. L., Critical evaluation of lymphocyte functions in urological cancer patients, *Cancer Res.,* 36, 132, 1976.
27. Catalona, W. J., Potvin, C., and Chretieu, P. B., T Lymphocytes in bladder and prostatic cancer patients, *J. Urol.,* 112, 378, 1974.
28. Catalona, W. J., Tarpley, J. L., Chretien, P. B., and Castle, J. R., Lymphocyte stimulation in urologic cancer patients, *J. Urol.,* 112, 373, 1974.
29. Rafla, S., Yang, S. J., and Meleka, F., Changes in cell-mediated immunity in patients undergoing radiotherapy, *Cancer,* 41, 1076, 1978.
30. Blomgren, H., Wasserman, J., Edsmyr, F., Baral, E., and Petrini, B., Reduction of responders and stimulator capacities of peripheral lymphoid cells in the mixed lymphocyte culture following external radiotherapy, *Int. J. Rad. Oncol. Biol. Phys.,* 2, 297, 1977.

31. Lange, P. H., Genitourinary tumors and immunology, *Proc. Inst. Med. Chicago,* 32, 58, 1978.
32. Kay, H. E. M. and Wallace, D. M., H and B antigens of tumors arising from urinary epithelium, *J. Natl. Cancer Inst.,* 26, 1349, 1961.
33. Decenzo, J. M., Howard, P., and Irish, C. E., Antigens with deletion and prognosis of patients with stage A transitional cell bladder carcinoma, *J. Urol.,* 114, 874, 1975.
34. Lange, P. H., Limas, C., and Fraley, E. E., Tissue blood group antigens and prognosis in low stage transitional cell carcinoma of the bladder, *J. Urol.,* 119, 52, 1978.
35. Alroy, J., Teramura, K., Miller, A. W., III, Pauli, B. N., Gottesman, J. E., Flanagen, M., Davidsohn, I., and Weinstein, R. S., Iso antigens A, B and H in urinary bladder carcinomas following radiotherapy, *Cancer,* 41, 1739, 1978.
36. Catalona, W. J., Chretien, P. B., and Trahan, E. E., Abnormalities of cell-mediated immunocompetence in genitourinary cancer, *J. Urol.,* 111, 229, 1974.
37. Blomgren, H., Wasserman, J., and Lihbrand, B., Blood lymphocytes after radiation therapy of carcinoma of prostate and urinary bladder, *Acta Radiol. Ther. Phys. Biol.,* 13, 357, 1974.
38. McCredie, J. A., Luch, W. R., and Sutherland, R. M., Effect of postoperative radiotherapy on peripheral blood lymphocytes in patients with carcinoma of the breast, *Cancer,* 29, 349, 1972.
39. O'Toole, C., Perlmann, P., Unsgaard, B., Moberger, G., and Edsmyr, F., Cellular immunity to human urinary bladder carcinoma. I. Correlation to clinical stage and radiotherapy, *Int. J. Cancer,* 10, 77, 1972.
40. O'Toole, C., Unsgaard, B., Almgard, L. E., and Johansson, B., The cellular immune response to carcinoma of the urinary bladder: correlation to clinical stage and treatment, *Br. J. Cancer,* 28(Suppl. 1), 266, 1973.
41. Slater, J. M., Ngo, E., and Lau, B. H. S., Effect of therapeutic irradiation on the immune responses, *Am. J. Roentgenol.,* 126, 313, 1976.
42. Stefani, S. S., Menon, M., Canning, J. R., and Clark, S. S., Cell-mediated immune competence in patients with prostatic carcinoma, *J. Urol.,* 120, 431, 1978.
43. Brosman, S., Hausman, M., Shacks, S., Immunologic alterations in patients with prostatic carcinoma, *J. Urol.,* 113, 841, 1975.
44. Thomas, J. W., Jerkins, G., Cox, G., and Lieberman, P., Defective cell-mediated immunity in carcinoma of the prostate, *Invest. Urol.,* 14, 72, 1976.
45. Huus, J. C., Kursh, E. D., Poor, P., and Persky, L., Delayed cutaneous hypersensitivity in patients with prostatic adenocarcinoma, *J. Urol.,* 114, 86, 1975.
46. Robinson, M. R., Nakhla, L. S., and Whitaker, R. H., A new concept in the management of carcinoma of the prostate, *Br. J. Urol.,* 43, 728, 1971.
47. Catalona, W. J., Sample, W. F., and Chretien, P. B., Lymphocyte reactivity in cancer patients — correlation with tumor histology and clinical stage, *Cancer,* 31, 65, 1973.
48. Woodward, W. T., Lymphocyte transformation in carcinoma of the prostate, *Urol. Observ.,* 1, 2, 1973.
49. Ablin, R. J., Serum proteins in prostatic cancer. III. Relationship of levels of immunoglobulins and complement to clinical stage of disease, *Urology,* 7, 39, 1976.
50. Hoppe, R. T., Fuks, Z. Y., Strober, S., and Kaplan, H. S., The long term effects of radiation on T and B lymphocytes in the peripheral blood after regional irradiation, *Cancer,* 40, 2071, 1977.
51. Bosworth, J. L., Ghossein, N. A., and Brooks, T. L., Delayed hypersensitivity in patients treated by curative radiotherapy. Its relation to tumor response and short-term survival, *Cancer,* 36, 353, 1975.
52. Kakizoe, T. and Ogawa, A., Spontaneous regression of pulmonary metastases from testicular tumor — a case report, *Cancer,* 34, 761, 1974.
53. Thachray, A. C., Seminoma. The pathology of testicular tumors, *Br. J. Urol.,* 36, 12, 1964.
54. Johnson, D. E., Gomez, J. J., and Ayola, A. G., Histologic factors affecting prognosis of the pure seminoma of the testis, *South. Med. J.,* 69, 1173, 1976.
55. Heier, H. E., Christensen, I., Froland, S. S., and Engeset, A., Early and late effects of irradiation for seminoma testis on the number of blood lymphocytes and their B and T subpopulations, *Lymphology,* 8, 69, 1975.

Chapter 10

CLINICAL USE OF CARCINOEMBRYONIC ANTIGEN IN THE MANAGEMENT OF PATIENTS WITH CANCER

Paul H. Sugarbaker

TABLE OF CONTENTS

I. INTRODUCTION

Through persistent basic science and clinical research efforts, the CEA blood test has developed into a useful but indeed complex monitor of progression or regression of a wide variety of malignancies. Since the first reports of Gold and Freedman[1] over a decade ago, basic scientists and clinicians have had to work together to develop a role for CEA in taking care of the sick. In few other research settings has the biochemist, immunologist, and oncologist thought together for so long and so hard. Now, after initial over enthusiasm, followed by abandonment by those who were short sighted, emerges a new clinical tool selectively valuable for aiding in diagnosis of primary and recurrent cancer, in assessing prognosis, and in monitoring therapy. Also not only the direct clinical value, but also the value of information gained from the study of CEA as a model of circulating tumor antigens, adds further importance to the study of CEA.

II. CHARACTERIZATION OF THE CEA MOLECULE

Gold and Freedman original studies were interpreted as suggesting that the CEA antigen was produced only by colon cancer cells and was of uniform molecular structure.[1] Further studies by their group in Montreal and numerous other workers has shown CEA production by multiple different tissues; also, the substances that have CEA activity consist of a family of related glycoprotein molecules. The heterogeneity of CEA's molecular structure rests in its carbohydrate portion which may vary from 50 to 75% of its composition.[2,3] The terminal carbohydrate structure is also quite variable, particularly with respect to sialic acid.[2-4] Also several different forms are separable by differences in net change, by ion exchange chromatography, or isoelectric focusing.[3-5]

As opposed to the variable carbohydrate structure, the protein structure of the molecule seems quite uniform. Terry et al.[3] showed a constant sequence of the 24 N-terminal amino acids in several different CEA preparations.

The antigenic determinants of CEA were originally throught to be determined by the carbohydrate portion of the molecule. However, Vrba and co-workers[6] at the Massachusetts General Hospital were unable to competitively inhibit CEA immunoreactivity with a wide variety of simple carbohydrates or carbohydrate chains. Arnon et al.[7] synthesized the amino terminal peptide of CEA and showed it to have CEA immunoreactivity. These data strongly suggest that the internal protein structure of the molecule contains at least part of the antigenic determinants critical for immunoreactivity.

Only occasionally is CEA seen by immunofluorescent or immunoperoxidase studies to be within cancer cells. It accumulates at the cell surface as a glycocalyx.[8] CEA at this extracellular site enters the extracellular space then diffuses into lymphatics and blood capillaries to reach the systemic circulation.

The biologic function of the CEA molecule remains a mystery. Its inconstant presence in a whole host of epithelial tumors plus the fact that its production may cease and the malignant process continue makes its production unlikely as an essential step in the malignant process. It is likely that CEA, like other embryonic antigens and ectopic hormones, is an epigenetic process not essential to the neoplastic event.[9] The degree to which the neoplastic cell machinery reverts to CEA production over and above that produced by normal tissues may be a random and therefore inconsistent event.

III. CEA PRODUCTION AND METABOLISM

It is now well-established that CEA is present in many normal as well as malignant tissues; also that alterations in normal tissue can result in elevated plasma CEA. CEA is present in feces of normal individuals,[10,11] in normal colonic tissue,[12] in normal liver[13] and in bile.[14] The common denominator for increased production of CEA and the resultant plasma elevation is not the presence of a malignancy but a breakdown in the anatomic barrier between an epithelial surface and its underlying tissues. More than likely, the structure that must be disrupted to give CEA elevations is the epithelial basement membrane. This structure is disrupted and would leak CEA molecules into the circulation in inflammatory bowel disease, pancreatitis, gastritis, and the bronchitis that accompanies heavy smoking. As presented later, these are promient causes of nontumor CEA elevations. A tumor also disrupts this basement membrane; after invasion the tumor must release products it produces in normal or increased amounts into the interstitial fluids and hence into lymphatics and blood. Many colonic tumors have no more CEA in their tissue than does normal colonic epithelium.[12,13,15] However normal colonic epithelium excretes CEA into the gut; an invasive adenocarcinoma of the colon lacks this capability. Tumors, and especially large tumors, result in elevated levels of normal substances in the blood, because tumors grow without an excretory system.

Disruptions in the epithelial basement membrane accounts for increased CEA absorption; the other pathophysiologic cause of for CEA elevation is decreased metabolism by the liver. There is strong evidence that CEA degradation and/or excretion takes place almost exclusively in the liver. Schuster et al.[16] injected intravenously into rabbits and dogs small doses of radiolabeled CEA prepared from human tissue. About half the injected material localized in the liver within 5 min. This was followed by a slower rate of continued hepatic uptake. Primus et al.[17] reported that 80 to 90% of intracardiac injected radiolabeled CEA localized in the liver within 5 min. Thomas and Helms[18] found that the half life of intravenously injected CEA in rats was less than 5 min and it localized almost exclusively in the liver. Six to ten percent of the immunologically active injected CEA was detected in the bile within 2 hr. Holyoke et al.[19] and Molnar et al.[14] demonstrated the presence of CEA-like activity in human bile. Go et al.[20] in their duodenal perfusion experiments reported a doubling of CEA concentration in duodenal juice following cholecystokinin-stimulated gall bladder emptying.

Even more direct evidence for a prominent role in CEA metabolism for the liver comes from the clinical studies of Lurie et al.[21] As shown in Figure 1, patients with elevated CEA levels and biliary tract obstruction from stones were studied pre- and postoperatively. CEA levels returned to normal in 7; two patients had unsuccessful operations with retained common duct stones, cholangitis, and liver abscesses and no decline in CEA. A third patient was last to follow-up. Recent studies by Lowenstein et al.[22] show that cirrhotic livers excrete less CEA into the duodenal juice even when plasma CEA levels are elevated. From these studies it becomes clear that decreased excretion of CEA from biliary obstruction or cirrhosis can result in elevated plasma CEA levels.

IV. NONTUMOR CEA ELEVATIONS

The discussion so far has reviewed the nature of the CEA molecule, the pathophysiologic processes responsible for CEA production — both tumor and nontumor — and also, the principle role of the liver in CEA metabolism. However, long before the metabolism of CEA production and excretion were known, Zameheck and his collaborators had established through clinical studies that CEA elevations were resultant from many nontumor disease processes. Working from their clinical base at the Boston City Hospital they noted that alcoholic patients often had CEA levels greater than 2.5 ng/mℓ but less than 10 ng/mℓ. Forty-five percent of 88 patients with alcoholic liver

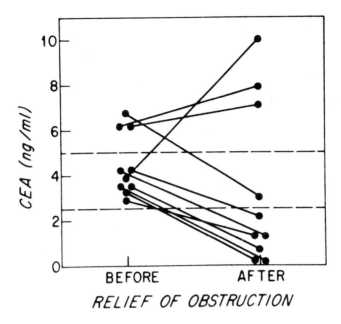

FIGURE 1.   Circulating CEA levels in ten patients before and after relief of biliary tract obstruction. Of the three patients with increased postoperative levels, two had retained common duct stones, cholangitis, and liver abscesses, and the third was lost for follow-up. (From Lurie et al., *JAMA*, 233, 326, 1975. With permission).

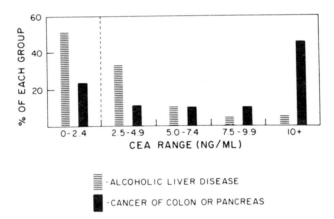

FIGURE 2.   Serum carcinoembryonic antigen (CEA) levels in patients with alcoholic liver disease or cancer. Serum CEA levels of 88 patients with alcoholic liver disease (hatched bars) are compared with serum CEA levels of 86 patients with histologically confirmed carcinoma of the colon or pancreas. The number of patients in each range of CEA levels is expressed as a percentage of the total group. Levels of CEA above 2.5 ng/m*l* of patient serum are positive. (From Moore et al., *Gastroenterology*, 63, 88, 1972. With permission).

disease had positive CEA tests whereas none of 14 patients with nonalcoholic liver disease had positive CEA assays.[23] Further studies showed that CEA could be extracted from the liver of patients with alcoholic liver disease and in lesser amounts from normal liver (see Figure 2). Khoo et al.[13] subsequently determined that the CEA content of normal and cirrhotic livers are not significantly different. Of course, an important task for the oncologist is distinguishing tumor CEA from nontumor CEA elevation. The first successful efforts to do this on a laboratory basis were recently reported from the Boston City Hospital group by Lowenstein et al.[22] Duodenal juice was collected through a double lumen gastroduodenal (Dreiling) tube and CEA outputs determined for 100 min. Normal patients had duodenal CEA outputs of less than 150 ng/min. Six of seven patients with CEA-associated cancers had duodenal outputs of greater than 150 ng/min. The one exception had a plasma CEA level of only 0.6 ng/mℓ. Another patient with a primary carcinoma of the colon had increased duodenal CEA output despite normal plasma levels. Seven of nine patients with benign liver disease or extrahepatic biliary obstruction had normal duodenal CEA outputs. Lowenstein et al.[22] suggest that determinations of duodenal juice CEA may assist the oncologist in two ways: (1) it may detect increased CEA production even prior to the occurrence of elevated circulating levels. This may provide a more sensitive CEA assay system than currently available using plasma sampling, and (2) determinations of duodenal juice CEA may assist in distinguishing between increased plasma CEA due to increased production (by cancer or inflammatory diseases) and that due to impaired metabolism/excretion due to liver disease. Often CEA elevations from alcoholic cirrhosis can be differentiated from elevations due to malignancy by an alcoholic history, hepatomegaly, spider angioma, and a generally lower level of CEA elevation. However, not infrequently none of the obvious signs of alcoholism are present and yet CEA elevations from decreased excretion result. Duodenal juice CEA determinations may become an important clinical tool to help distinguish between cirrhotic and malignant causes of CEA elevation. Zameheck's group also noted that pancreatitis was associated with CEA elevations.[25] Elevations were more frequent in patients with underlying liver disease but liver disease alone did not account for the elevations.

Sharma et al.[26] assayed CEA content from the pancreatic duct obtained at the time of endoscopic retrograde cholangio pancreatography. Mean pancreatic juice CEA in controls, pancreatitis, and pancreatic carcinoma were 8.1 ng/mℓ, 18.6 ng/mℓ, and 309 ng/mℓ, respectively. None of the 32 patients with both pancreatic juice CEA less than 30 ng/mℓ and plasma CEA less than 2.5 ng/mℓ had pancreatic cancer. Sharma suggested that combined measurement of CEA activity in plasma and pancreatic juice may help in diagnosing pancreatic cancer and ruling out pancreatitis.

Gitnick and Molnar[27] have recently examined the transmission of CEA elevations by blood products. In a fascinating study, recipients of CEA positive units of blood were prospectively followed along with recipients of CEA negative blood units matched for race, age, sex, and transfusion volume. Among 50 recipients of CEA positive blood, 23 developed hepatitis while of the 50 recipients of CEA negative blood only 8 developed hepatitis (p <.0005). Among all recipients of CEA positive blood who developed hepatitis and who previously lacked CEA, CEA elevations developed before or at the same time as the first SGPT elevation, peaked with the SGPT, and gradually fell off after the SGPT and returned to normal. Eight recipients of CEA positive blood became CEA positive and failed to develop any laboratory or clinical evidence of hepatitis but carried elevated CEA for the 10 months of follow-up. The authors also noted that plasma of 5 of 19 (26%) hepatitis B patients and 18 or 29 (62%) non A non B hepatitis patients were CEA positive. Gitnick and Molnar conclude: (1) CEA is often an early indicator of developing hepatitis, (2) hepatitis B antigen negative, CEA positive blood units often transmit hepatitis or a chronic CEA carrier state, and (3) sera of patients with non A non B hepatitis are frequently CEA positive (62%).

CEA present in normal colonic mucosa may gain access to the plasma if the basement membrane beneath colonic epithelium is disrupted. By this mechanism patients with inflammatory bowel disease frequently show modest CEA elevations in their plasma. Lo Gerfo et al.[28] reported CEA elevations in 10 of 31 ulcerative colitis patients. Wight and Gazet,[29] Moore et al.,[30] and Rule et al.[31] established that not only one third of ulcerative colitis patients, but also about one third of granulomatous colitis patients will have elevated plasma CEA levels. In an important study, Dilawari et al.[32] determined that the actual CEA values did not correlate with the age of the patient, the activity of the disease, the extent of bowel involvement, or the length of history. Furthermore, in seven colitic patients with severe dysplastic changes in the rectal mucosa, only a single CEA elevation occurred. These dysplastic changes are associated with an unusually high incidence of adenocarcinoma complicating colitis.[33-35] Also in seven patients with established carcinoma in colitis only one had an elevated circulating CEA.

Because only single CEA assays were performed on most patients in the work of Dilawari and co-workers, Gardner et al.[36] followed 57 ulcerative colitis patients with serial CEA levels. In this study, disease severity correlated significantly with peak CEA titers (p <.005). With only one exception, CEA levels elevated during increased disease activity returned to normal with remission. In the Gardner et al.[36] study the extent of colitis did not quite statistically significantly correlate with CEA levels.

Stevens and MacKay[37] determined that heavy cigarette smoking is frequently associated with CEA elevations. In a population study of nearly 1000 Australians age 60 years and older, 13.6% of heavy cigarette smokers who had no detectable cancer had a CEA of 5 ng/ml or greater. Only 1.8% of nonsmokers had CEA elevations. Alexander et al.[38] at the National Institutes of Health further determined that mean CEA in smokers (2.7 ng/ml) was significantly higher than in nonsmokers (1.9 ng/ml) (P <.001). Seventy-six of the 154 smokers who entered the study stopped smoking. Within 3 months, elevated CEA levels declined to within the range of nonsmokers. Alexander and co-workers rightfully suggest that smoking history must be considered in clinical evaluation of elevated CEA levels.

Alexander and co-workers also showed that CEA levels were directly related to age. This fact, little appreciated to date, means that values for the upper limit of normal for CEA should vary for the patient population studied. For example, for a group of premenopausal women with breast cancer, the upper limit of normal for CEA should perhaps be 1.5 ng/ml; on the other hand, for a colorectal cancer population where most patients are 55 years and over, an upper limit of normal should perhaps be 4.0 ng/ml.

Numerous other gastrointestinal inflammatory diseases may show CEA elevations. The author has seen a frequent association of gastritis following partial gastrectomy with elevated CEA levels. The inflamed mucosa of the residual stomach[39] likely allows CEA reabsorption from the bile or from gastric mucus.

Doos et al.[40] reported that 15% of patients with colonic polyps have CEA levels greater than 2.5 ng/ml. These elevated levels do not always decrease when polyps are removed colonoscopically. Alm and Wahren[41] showed that the mildly elevated CEA levels seen in familial polyposis patients may not decline appreciably following colectomy. Also, Guirgis et al.[42] showed that individuals at high genetic risk for development of cancer in cancer family syndromes had higher CEA than relatives at low genetic risk. The relevance of CEA elevations to a precancerous state is yet to be determined, but is of great interest.

The multiple nontumor causes for elevated CEA may cause clinicians considerable difficulty as he/she seeks to utilize the CEA test in patient management decisions. The following suggestions can be made to assist in differentiating tumor from nontumor CEA elevations. The skill with which the clinician makes this differential may in postoperative colorectal cancer patients determine the number of successful second look surgical procedures versus the number of negative exploratory laparotomies that fail to benefit patients. First, the magnitude of the elevation is important; CEA elevations in the 2.5 ng/ml to 10 ng/ml range may be from tumor or nontumor. However, nontumor CEA elevations greater than 10 ng/ml are very unlikely without jaundice and other obvious signs of biliary tract obstruction. Therefore, the patients with moderate CEA elevations (2.5 to 10 ng/ml range) are those likely to create clinical dilemmas. In these patients the clinician must make a search for possible nontumor causes of CEA elevations. Hepatic cirrhosis and hepatitis, heavy smoking, and gastrointestinal inflammatory states are the most common causes of these nontumor elevations. Most commonly, as emphasized by Gardner et al.[36] these conditions are usually in their active state when associated with plasma CEA elevations. If present in a state of complete remission it is not safe to assume they are responsible for an elevated CEA. These clinical entities can be identified by a careful medical history and routine laboratory and radiologic tests. Liver function tests including tests for hepatitis antigens are needed. Sugarbaker et al.[43] suggested that liver biopsy as a routine in all patients undergoing surgery for colorectal cancer should be performed to assist in interpreting postoperative serial CEA assays.

Third, to differentiate tumor from nontumor CEA elevation several sequential CEA assays as opposed to individual determinations may be required. If the titer is progressively rising cancer is the most likely cause; if the serial titers are erratic with both elevated and normal values nontumor causes are more common. Finally in a select few patients if sufficient laboratory expertise is available, duodenal juice CEA[22] and pancreatic juice CEA[26] may be of value.

V. CEA IN THE DIAGNOSIS OF PRIMARY AND RECURRENT CANCER

McNeil and Adelstein[44] in their classic work on interpretation of laboratory tests show how a "laboratory test is only as good as the patient population in whom it is employed." This explains how CEA can be of little or no value in mass screening for cancer, but of great value screening for recurrence in a high risk population such as postoperative colorectal cancer patients. Studies by the National Cancer Institute of Canada,[45] Hansen et al.,[46] and Chu et al.[47] on large populations of asymptomatic individuals showed that few malignancies were detected at great cost. The expense of this type of screening comes not only in performing the large number of CEA assays, but in clinically evaluating the numerous "false positive" tests. False positive tests are expensive in terms of physician time, negative radiologic workups, and patient anxiety. Data obtained from screening populations can be summarized as *too little information too late*. Dykes and King[48] in a collective review found 40% of patients with Dukes A tumors, 65% of Dukes B tumors, and 75% of Dukes C tumors had elevated pretreatment CEA titers. Unfortunately, the patients with bulky primary tumors in whom a low cure rate was expected generally had CEA levels greater than 2.5 ng/ml. Laurence et al.[49] estimated that screening a population for elevated CEA blood levels would detect only 45% of carcinomas of colon, rectum, and stomach. Concannon et al.[50] indicated that CEA may fail to detect 34% of malignant lesions in a population. A good screening procedure should rule out the presence of the disease in question with reasonable accuracy and yield a minimal number of "falsely" elevated results. The isolated CEA test does not fulfill the criteria needed for a good mass screening test for colorectal or other malignancy.

Ona and co-workers[51] at the Mallory Gastrointestinal Laboratory have shown, however, that CEA may be of great value when used in a population of patients suspect of having pancreatic cancer. They report 23 (85%) of 27 patients with pancreatic cancer had elevated CEA assays. The CEA assay was more frequently positive in patients

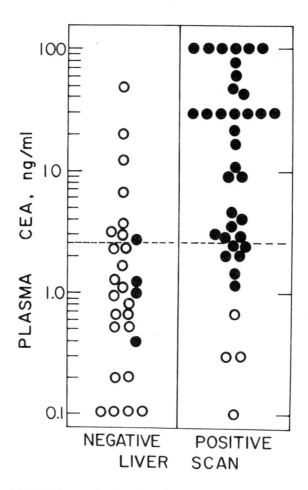

FIGURE 3. Application of the liver scan and CEA assay to detection of hepatic metastases (0 = patients with liver metastases; 0 = patients without liver metastases). CEA values greater than 100 ng/mℓ and values reported as "greater than 20" are drawn as if equal to these numbers for graphical convenience. (From Sugarbaker, Beard and Drum, *Am. J. Surg.,* 133, 531, 1977. With permission).

with cancer of the pancreas than were any other diagnostic test used, including upper gastrointestinal series, hypotonic duodenography, celiac arteriography, and percutaneous transhepatic cholangiography. Also CEA detected liver metastasis with CEA levels of greater than 10 ng/mℓ in more patients than did the liver scan.

All physicians learn to interpret one test in terms of all other clinical and laboratory data that is available. Experience in accurately assimilating relevant clinical information and discarding irrelevant data constitutes what is commonly called "clinical judgment." In "composite testing" the physician selects two clinical and/or laboratory tests that are interpreted as one more accurate test. The composite test may be interpreted in a variety of ways. McCarthy and Hoffer used barium enema and CEA as a composite to detect colon cancer. In 43 of 48 (90%) of colon cancers the barium enema detected the lesion; however, in three of the five false negative examinations CEA was greater than 3 ng/mℓ. If a positive composite test was defined as a positive barium enema and/or positive CEA (greater than 3 ng/mℓ) the percentage of cases detected rose to 95%.

Sugarbaker, Beard, and Drum[53] combined the liver scan and CEA as a composite in patients with suspect hepatic recurrence of breast cancer. In this study the composite test was positive if both tests were positive, negative if both tests were negative, and equivocal (further studies indicated) if the results disagreed. The number of false positive scans was marked reduced by the composite. False positive ratio for the liver scan was 14% and for the CEA assay 25%; however, there were no false positive composite tests (Figure 3). Similar studies have been reported by McCartney and Hoffer.[54]

An interesting new use for anti-CEA antibody has recently been developed by Goldberg et al.[55] at the University of Kentucky. This group took anti-CEA antibody made in goats, coupled it to radioactive iodine and after injecting this into cancer patients performed total body photoscans. Tumor location could be demonstrated at 48 hr after injection in almost all patients studied. Circulating antigen levels up to 350 ng/ml did not prevent successful tumor imaging.

Perhaps the most important and until recently most controversial use of CEA is as an indicator of early recurrent colorectal cancer and guide to selected second look surgery. Early studies by Mach et al.,[56] MacKay et al.,[57] Herrera et al.,[58] Martin et al.,[59] and a prospective study by Sugarbaker et al.[43] suggested that progressively rising serial CEA assays were in many patients the first signal of recurrent cancer. Data presented at the Sixth Meeting of the International Research Group for Carcinoembryonic Proteins held in Marburg/Lahn, West Germany in September of 1978 left no doubt as to the value of postoperative serial CEA assays. Numerous potentially successful second look procedures have been carried out and long-term survivals are expected. Ratcliff et al.[60] from Glasgow, Scotland reported elevated CEA levels preceded clinical evidence of disease in 32 of 35 patients with recurrence. Lead time for CEA was 2 to 29 months with a median of 4 months. Monthly or possibly two monthly postoperative CEA assays must be considered a routine part of every colorectal management plan.

The studies of Sugarbaker et al.,[43] however, emphasized the importance of physical examination as well as serial CEA assays in follow-up. Other tests such as liver scan, barium enema, chest X-ray, and IVP should be considered adjunctive and done on a yearly basis.

The high percentage of early elevations of CEA in patients with hepatic metastases plus the development of resection techniques to remove liver metastases but preserve liver parenchyma[62] suggests that salvage of patients with early hepatic metastatic disease is often possible. Successful resection of metastatic colorectal cancer in the liver similar to the resection of osteosarcoma in the lungs may be possible.[63,64]

Rittgers et al.[65] interjected a timely precautionary note regarding transient CEA elevations occasionally seen following resection of colorectal cancer. Nine of twenty-five patients showed transient elevations without cancer recurrence upon follow-up and close clinical investigation. Trends in serial CEA titers rather than isolated CEA values must be used along with all other clinical and laboratory data available in making the decision to perform second look surgery.

VI. CEA IN ASSESSING PROGNOSIS IN PATIENTS WITH KNOWN MALIGNANCY: USE OF PRETREATMENT CEA ASSAY

Perhaps the most crucial clinical assessment of a patient with cancer is the initial one made immediately after the diagnosis is established and prior to any definitive therapy. This initial workup is a staging process in which adequate judgments must be made often with less than adequate clinical information. The physician, or more often, the oncology team, must plan treatments that properly balance the trauma required in treatment that may afford prolonged survival with the likelihood that a treat-

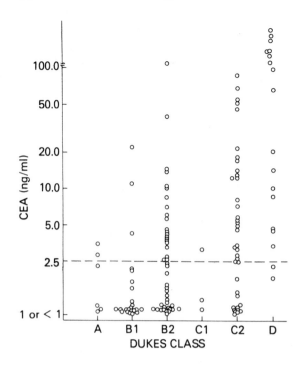

FIGURE 4.   Preoperative CEA levels and Dukes classification of colorectal cancer patients, Peter Bent Brigham Hospital, Boston, Mass.

ment will succeed. Nothing is more discouraging to patient and practitioner than treatments that not only markedly reduce quality of life but also do not prolong survival. For example, a surgical procedure such as an abdomino-perineal resection for rectal cancer should be avoided if at all possible in patients with disseminated disease. In this clinical setting, this procedure would cause much postoperative pain and suffering, put the patient's life at risk, diminish quality of life by necessitating a colostomy and by causing impotence, and do little if anything to add to prolonged survival. Local control of disease within the pelvis is nearly always possible by radiation therapy directed at the perineum and pelvis plus fulguration of the primary tumor.[66]

Laurence et al.[49] suggested that CEA tests done at the time of initial patient evaluation were of prognostic value. This was determined retrospectively by correlating preoperative CEA levels with Dukes Classification in patients with colorectal cancer. The patients with low CEA values often had Dukes A tumors while the patients with high CEA more frequently had Dukes C tumors (see Figure 4). Booth and co-workers[67] provided clinical evidence that patients with undetectable or normal CEA levels have a favorable prognosis whereas the prognosis is poorer in patients with raised preoperative levels. Wanebo and co-workers at the Memorial-Sloan Kettering Cancer Center showed conclusively that recurrence rates were higher in patients with Dukes B and Dukes C lesions who had preoperative levels higher than 5 ng/mℓ. Also as the preoperative CEA level increased, the mean time to recurrence decreased as a linear inverse correlation. As shown in Figure 5, in patients with Dukes' C lesions, the median time to recurrence was 13 months if preoperative levels were higher than 5 ng/mℓ, and 28 months if they were lower. Wanebo et al.[61] concluded that preoperative carcinoembryonic antigen levels in patients with resectable colorectal cancer provided an additional criterion for allocating these patients to groups at high or low risk for recurrence.

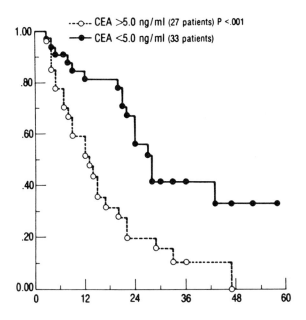

FIGURE 5. Preoperative carcinoembryonic antigen (CEA) levels and postresection recurrence of Dukes' C cancer (the interval since operation, in months, is shown on abscissa, and the proportion free of disease on the ordinate). There was a significant difference in the recurrence rates after resection of Dukes' C cancer, according to the preoperative level. The median time to recurrence was 13 months in the patients with levels >5 ng/mℓ versus 28 months in those with levels <5 ng/mℓ (P <0.001). The proportion free of disease at 30 months was 15% in those with levels >5 ng/mℓ versus 41% of those with levels <5 ng/mℓ. (From Wanebo et al. *N. Engl. J. Med.,* 299, 448, 1978. With permission).

Although preoperative CEA blood tests are prognostic indicators, nevertheless some patients with very large Dukes C, Dukes D, or even metastatic tumors may have normal CEA assays. This is likely due to decreased production or decreased release of CEA by the tumor. Poorly differentiated tumors, even though often of large mass, often are associated with normal circulating CEA values.[12,43,49,68]

Shamberg et al.[69] showed definitively that preoperative plasma CEA levels were statistically significantly related to the degree of tumor differentiation. The consistency of this observation is not always appreciated clinically for primary tumor size also correlates with circulating CEA levels; and, poorly differentiated tumors with lesser CEA production tend to be of larger size and to invade more deeply. Consequently in poorly differentiated tumors the variables of tumor differentiation and tumor size conflict and tend, therefore, to nullify each other.

CEA has been identified as a prognosticator in several other tumors besides colorectal cancer. Kalser et al.[70] found that pancreatic cancer patients with locally unresectable or metastatic carcinoma had a significantly longer survival if CEA was normal at the time of diagnosis. Wang and co-workers[71] showed a relationship between plasma CEA and prognosis in women with breast cancer. Patients after mastectomy with CEA levels above 2.5 ng/mℓ had a significantly (P <0.001) faster recurrence rate than similar patients with CEA levels below this level. At two years after mastectomy the disease had recurred in 65% of the patients with CEA greater than 2.5 ng/mℓ compared to 20% of those with CEA less than 2.5 ng/mℓ. Premastectomy levels of CEA did not

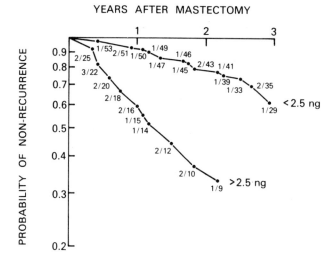

FIGURE 6.   Relationship between postmastectomy CEA levels and recurrence rate of breast cancer. The recurrence rates of women with early breast cancer with <2.5 ng/mℓ CEA are compared with the rate for similar women having >2.5 ng/mℓ CEA (both measured after mastectomy). The numerator of the fractions refer to the number of patients whose disease has recurred while the denominator refers to the number of patients free of the disease. The recurrence rates for the two groups are significantly different (P <0.001). (From Wang et al., *Eur. J. Cancer*, 11, 615, 1975. With permission).

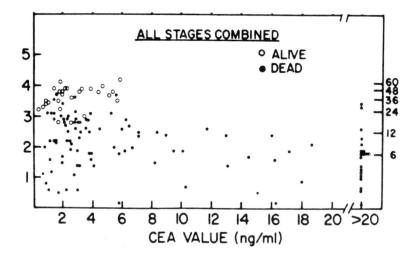

FIGURE 7.   Scattergram of the distribution of preoperative CEA values plotted against the natural log of survival for 130 patients with epidermoid and adenocarcinoma. (From Concannon et al., *Cancer*, 42, 1477, 1978. With permission).

correlate with recurrence rates (see Figure 6). Haagensen et al.[72] and Meyers et al.[73] both also showed a poor prognosis in patients with elevated postmastectomy CEA levels. Haagensen et al.[72] also showed an increased incidence of tumor recurrence with preoperative CEA levels greater than 3 ng/mℓ. Tormey and Waalkes[74] noted that patients with metastatic breast cancer with CEA greater than 5 ng/mℓ prior to treatment had lower response rates and a shorter time to treatment failure that did patients with CEA equal to or less than 5 ng/mℓ.

Dent and co-workers[75] reported from Hamilton, Ontario on the prognostic significance of pretreatment CEA values in patients with bronchogenic carcinoma. The use of the CEA assay for diagnostic purposes was somewhat limited for heavy smokers frequently have elevated CEA levels in the absence of cancer. In groups of nonsmokers, smokers, patients with limited bronchogenic cancer, patients with inoperable cancer, and patients with metastatic cancer there were different and progressively higher mean CEA values.

However, there was much overlap between groups making clinical use of pretreatment CEA levels more difficult. Concannon et al.[76] made the interesting observation that all epidermoid and adenocarcinoma patients in a series of 147 who had pretreatment CEA levels greater than 6 ng/ml died in less than 3 years (see Figure 7). Dent et al.[75] suggested that there may be a CEA level (probably 6 ng/ml) that could with other clinical data be used as a "criteria for inoperability."

Apfel and Peters[77] have presented experimental data to suggest that circulating glycoproteins may suppress immunogenicity and allow tumors to grow out despite host immune surveillance mechanisms. Increasing plasma CEA levels may not only signal an increase in tumor volume but a lesser host resistance to tumor growth. In an interesting study, Lurie et al.[78] correlated circulating CEA level, tumor antigen induced inhibition of mononuclear cell migration (IMM) and skin reactivity to a battery of recall antigens. Disseminated colon cancer was associated with elevated CEA (9/9 patients), absent IMM (7/9), and suppressed skin test reactivity (6/9). Potential surgical cure was associated with normal CEA (4/7), absent IMM (7/7), and increased skin reactivity (6/7). The role circulation CEA or other tumor substances may play in immune suppression in this study was not investigated. However, Aray et al.[79] have shown by in vitro studies that a dose dependent suppression of lymphocyte proliferation is caused by CEA. This suppression was not due to nonspecific cytotoxic activity and both T and B cells were affected by suppression.

VII. SERIAL CEA IN MONITORING CANCER THERAPY

We established earlier in this chapter that progressively rising CEA titers above 10 ng/ml signaled recurrent colorectal or breast cancer. It was shown that high preoperative CEA levels in colorectal, pancreatic, bronchogenic, and breast cancer were associated with a poor response to conventional therapy and/or short disease-free intervals. Serial CEA titers during a period of intensive therapy may also be used as a monitor of the effectiveness of a treatment regimen. After surgical excision of a colorectal cancer, elevated preoperative CEA levels usually fall into the normal range of 2.5 ng/ml or less. Dhar et al.,[80] LoGerfo et al.,[81] Livingstone et al.,[82] Mach et al.,[56] Sorokin et al.,[83] and Oh and MacLean[84] all noted that failure of postoperative CEA values to fall into the normal range was associated with a poor prognosis. In the careful study from the Royal Victoria Hospital, Montreal conducted by Oh and MacLean[84] colorectal cancer patients were divided into three groups according to their preoperative and postoperative CEA levels. Thirty-six patients (Group 1) had preoperative and postoperative CEA values less than 2.5 ng/ml. Eleven patients (Group 2) had a preoperative CEA greater than 2.5 ng/ml but a postoperative value of less than 2.5 ng/ml. Also eleven patients (Group 3) had a preoperative CEA greater than 2.5 ng/ml but the postoperative value failed to decline below 2.5 ng/ml. In Group 1, 14% of patients had recurred, in Group 2 18% of patients had recurred, while in Group 3, 73% of patient had recurred even though mean follow-up was slightly less in Group 3 (see Figure 8).

The studies cited have shown postoperative CEA assays to give a good measure of the adequacy of surgery; in addition pathologic study of the resected specimen provides

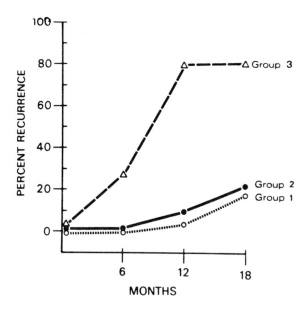

FIGURE 8.   Recurrence rates of colonic cancer after curative surgery (group 1 preoperative and postoperative CEA values <2.5 ng/m*l*: group 2 preoperative value >2.5 ng/m*l* postoperative value <2.5 ng/m*l*; group 3 preoperative and postoperative values >2.5 ng/m*l*). (From Oh and MacLean, *Can. J. Surg.,* 20, 64, 1977. With permission).

good measure of the adequacy of surgical treatment. However, radiation therapy and chemotherapy have less accurate monitors of disease control or progression. Often objective criteria by which to establish the effectiveness of therapy are completely lacking; serial CEA assays may, in many patients, provide the necessary objective criteria to monitor response, or failure to respond, to radiation and/or chemotherapy.

Vider et al.[85,86] reported a correlation of CEA levels and the clinical response to radiation therapy. Fifty seven of ninety-two cancer patients with a variety of primary tumors had CEA levels greater than 2.5 ng/m*l*. Curves defined by serial CEA assays were matched with a clinical evaluation of disease activity. Breast cancer showed an 89% correlation, lung carcinoma 80%, large bowel cancer 75%, and other organs less. Sugarbaker et al.[87] correlated serial CEA assays with the clinical course of 16 patients undergoing high dose (4500 to 7000 rads) radiation therapy for colorectal cancer. They concluded that high dose radiation therapy of localized colorectal cancer reliably reduced previously elevated circulating CEA titers. If CEA titers significantly decreased during therapy, the bulk of tumor was within the radiation treatment field; if CEA titers did not decrease a further search for disseminated disease revealed spread outside the treatment portal. This clinical observation was of value in patient management decisions. For example, a patient with rectal cancer in whom an elevated pretreatment CEA value falls to within the normal range after 4500 to 5000 rads is likely a good candidate for cure by abdomino-perineal resection. However, if CEA levels fail to significantly decrease, disease outside the pelvis must be suspected. Indeed if retroperitoneal or hepatic spread is documented by further clinical investigation, a lesser surgical procedure that will give local control (fulguration or intracavitary radiation) should be recommended rather than abdomino-perineal resection.

Sugarbaker and co-workers[87] also showed that in patients with elevated pretreatment CEA levels, persistently low CEA levels after therapy indicated disease control, but that a rapid rebound of elevated levels 6 to 8 weeks following completion of treatment occurred with disease progression. Because the rebound in circulating CEA likely respresents a regrowth of viable tumor, delay in surgical excision of tumor after completion of radiation therapy should not be delayed over 6 to 8 weeks.

Donaldson et al.[88] demonstrated similar CEA patterns in patients treated with radiation therapy for carcinoma of the cervix. In 32 patients followed during and after therapy with serial CEA determinations three patterns were seen: (1) decline to normal, associated with a disease free state, (2) decline but not to normal associated with heavy cigarette smoking or persistent disease, and (3) decline to normal, followed by a rise to abnormal, associated with tumor recurrence. Indeed, patterns of CEA seen during and after high dose radiation therapy closely resemble those seen following surgery.

Mulcare and LoGerfo[89] noted good correlations between the pattern of change of serial CEA assays and the patient's response to systemic chemotherapy. They defined three groups of patients. Some patients showed no significant change in their CEA levels, and clinically had a steady progression of disease. Pretreatment CEA in this group of patients was in the normal range or only slightly elevated. In these patients, circulating CEA is of nontumor origin and it is therefore not surprising that CEA assays are of no help in management.

A second group of patients showed a significant sustained increase in CEA levels. These patients also showed a steady progression of their disease. Occasionally as patients became terminal their CEA lvels were noted to fall for unknown reasons. A third group of patients showed significant decreases in their CEA levels and each also had marked clinical improvement during therapy. Vider et al.[86] reviewed the experience at Kentucky Medical Center with CEA monitoring of chemotherapy patients. They emphasize that the CEA test seems useful in those cancer patients with elevated CEA in the plasma.

Herrera et al.,[90] Young et al.,[91] and Mayer et al.[92] reviewed their institution's experience with CEA as a monitor of chemotherapeutic effects. Young et al.[91] defined a fourth pattern of response seen primarily in patients with colorectal cancer where 90 to 100% of patients eventually develop elevated CEA levels as disease progresses. They say patients not responding to chemotherapeutic agents change from normal to abnormal CEA with progressive disease.

Herrer and co-workers[90] offer an important *caveat* in interpreting serial CEA values in patients treated with nitrosourea compounds. In these patients they report a tendency to lower CEA levels regardless of the patient's tumor response to the drug. This could be due to the nitrosoureas producing a diffuse block of cellular activity including glycoprotein production both at the necleous and in the cytoplasm; while other compounds act as alkylating agents or by inhibition of enzymes involved in the metabolism of nucleic acids (i.e., 5-FU inhibiting thymidylate synthetase).

In summary serial CEA assays in patients whose tumors produce CEA elevations in the blood can be a valuable monitor of treatment. The adequacy of surgical resection, the likelihood of disease control by radiation therapy, and the response to systemic chemotherapy can be assessed in many patients. Of course, whenever possible a correlation of serial CEA levels with other clinical assessments should be made.

REFERENCES

1. Gold, P. and Freedman, S. O., Demonstration of tumor-specific antigens in human colonic carcinomata by immunologic tolerance and absorption techniques, *J. Exp. Med.,* 122, 467, 1965.
2. Banjo, C., Shuster, J., and Gold, P., Intermolecular heterogeneity of the carcinoembryonic antigen, *Cancer Res.,* 34, 2113, 1974.

3. Terry, W. D., Henkart, P. A., Coligan, J. E., and Todd, C. W., Structural studies of the major glycoprotein in preparations with carcinoembryonic antigen activity, *J. Exp. Med.,* 136, 200, 1972.
4. Coligan, J. E., Henkart, P. A., Todd, C. W., and Terry, W. D., Heterogeneity of the carcinoembryonic antigen, *Immunochemistry,* 10, 591, 1973.
5. Eveleigh, J. W., Heterogeneity of carcinoembryonic antigen, *Cancer Res.,* 34, 2122, 1974.
6. Vrba, R., Alpert, E., and Isselbacher, K. J., Carcinoembryonic antigen: Evidence for multiple antigenic determinants and isoantigens, *Proc. Natl. Acad. Sci. U.S.A.,* 72, 4602, 1975.
7. Arnon, R., Bustin, M., Calef, E., Chatchik, S., Hamovich, J., Novick, N., and Sela, M., Immunologic cross-reactivity of antibodies to a synthetic undecapeptide analogous to the amino-terminal segment of the carcinoembryonic antigen, with the intact protein and with human sera, *Proc. Natl. Acad. Sci. U.S.A.,* 73, 2123, 1976.
8. Burton, P., von Kleist, S., Sabine, M. C., and King, M., Immunohistological localization of carcinoembryonic antigen and nonspecific cross-reacting antigen in gastrointestinal normal and tumor tissues, *Cancer Res.,* 33, 3299, 1973.
9. Sherbet, G. V., Epigenetic processes and their relevance to the study of neoplasia, *Adv. Cancer Res.,* 97, 1970.
10. Freed, D. J. L. and Taylor, G., Carcinoembryonic antigen in feces, *Br. Med. J.,* 1, 85, 1972.
11. Elias, E. G., Holyoke, E. D., and Chu, T. M., Carcinoembryonic antigen in feces and plasma of normal subjects and patients with colorectal cancer, *Dis. Colon Rectum,* 1, 17, 38.
12. Martin, F. and Martin, M. S., Radioimmunoassay of carcinoembryonic antigen in extracts of human colon and stomach, *Int. J. Cancer,* 9, 641, 1972.
13. Khoo, S. K., Warner, N. L., Lie, J. T., and MacKay, I. R., Carcinoembryonic antigenic activity of tissue extracts: a quantitative study of malignant and benign neoplasms, cirrhotic liver, normal adult and fetal organs, *Int. J. Cancer,* 11, 681, 1973.
14. Molnar, I. G., Vandevoorde, J. P., and Gitnick, G. L., CEA levels in fluids bathing gastrointestinal tumors, *Gastroenterology,* 70, 513, 1976.
15. Dyce, B. J. and Haverback, B. J., Free and bound carcinoembryonic antigen (CEA) in feces and plasma of normal subjects and patients with colorectal carcinoma, *Dis. Colon Rectum,* 17, 8, 1974.
16. Schuster, J., Silverman, M., and Gold, P., Metabolism of human carcinoembryonic antigen in xenogeneic animals, *Cancer Res.,* 33, 65, 1973.
17. Primus, F. J., Goldenberg, D. M., and Hansen, H. J., Metabolism of carcinoembryonic antigen (CEA) in a human tumor-hamster model, *Fed. Proc. Fed. Am. Soc. Exp. Biol.,* 32 (Abstr.), 834, 1973.
18. Thomas, P. and Hems, P. A., The hepatic clearance of circulating carcinoembryonic antigen by the mouse, *Biochem. Soc. Trans.,* 5, 312, 1977.
19. Holyoke, E. D., Reynoso, G., and Chu, T., Carcinoembryonic antigen in patients with carcinoma of the digestive tract, in *Proc. 2nd Conf. Embryonic and Fetal Antigens in Cancer,* National Technical Information Service, U.S. Department of Commerce, Springfield, Va., 1972, 215.
20. Go, V. L. W., Ammon, H. V., Holtermuller, K. H., Krag, E., and Phillips, S. F., Quantitation of carcinoembryonic antigen-like activities in normal human gastrointestinal secretions, *Cancer,* 36, 2346, 1975.
21. Lurie, B. B., Lowenstein, M. S., and Zamcheck, N., Elevated circulating CEA levels in benign extrahepatic biliary tract obstruction and inflammation, *JAMA,* 233, 326, 1975.
22. Lowenstein, M. S., Rau, P., Rittgers, R. A., Adhi, B., Kupchik, H. Z., and Zamcheck, N., CEA in duodenal aspirates of patients with benign and malignant disease; preliminary observations, *J. Natl. Cancer Inst.,* in press.
23. Moore, T., Dhar, P., Zamcheck, N., Keeley, A., Gottlieb, L., and Kupchik, H. Z., Carcinoembryonic antigen(s) in liver disease. I. Clinical and morphologic studies, *Gastroenterology,* 63, 88, 1972.
24. Kupchik, H. Z. and Zamcheck, N., Carcinoembryonic antigen(s) in liver disease. II. Isolation from human cirrhotic liver and serum and from normal liver, *Gastroenterology,* 63, 95, 1972.
25. Delwiche, R., Zamcheck, N., and Marcon, N., Carcnoembryonic antigen in pancreatitis, *Cancer,* 31, 328, 1973.
26. Sharma, M. P., Gregg, J. A., Lowenstein, M. S., McCabe, R. P., and Zamcheck, N., Carcinoembryonic antigen (CEA) activity in pancreatic carcinoma and pancreatitis, *Cancer,* 38, 2457, 1976.
27. Gitnick, G. L. and Molnar, I. G., Carcinoembryonic antigen transmission by blood products, *Cancer,* 42, 1568, 1978.
28. LoGerfo, P., Krupey, J., and Hansen, H. J., Demonstration of an antigen common to several varieties of neoplasia. Assay using zirconyl phosphate gel, *N. Engl. J. Med.,* 285, 138, 1971.
29. Wight, D. G. D. and Gazet, J-C, Carcinoembryonic antigen levels in inflammatory disease of the large bowel, *Proc. R. Soc. Med.,* 65, 967, 1972.
30. Moore, T. L., Kantrowitz, P. A., and Zamcheck, N., Carcinoembryonic antigen (CEA) in inflammatory bowel disease, *Clin. Res.,* 20, 462, 1972.

31. Rule, A. H., Straus, E., Vandevoorde, J., and Janowitz, H. D., Tumor associated (CEA reacting) antigen in patients with inflammatory bowel disease, *N. Engl. J. Med.*, 287, 24, 1972.

32. Dilawari, J. B., Lennard-Jones, J. E., MacKay, A. M., Ritchie, J. K., and Sturzaker, H. G., Estimation of carcinoembryonic antigen in ulcerative colitis with special reference to malignant change, *Gut*, 16, 255, 1975.

33. Morson, B. C. and Pang, L. S. C., Rectal biopsy as an aid to cancer control in ulcerative colitis, *Gut*, 8, 423, 1967.

34. Yardley, J. H. and Keren, D. F., "Precancer" lesions in ulcerative colitis. A retrospective study of rectal biopsy and colectomy specimens, *Cancer*, 34, 835, 1974.

35. Cook, M. G., Path, M. R. C., and Golighan, J. C., Carcinoma and epithelial dysplasia complicating ulcerative colitis, *Gastroenterology*, 68, 1127, 1975.

36. Gardner, R. C., Feinerman, A. E., Kantrowitz, P. A., Gootblatt, S., Lowenstein, M. S., and Zamcheck, N., Serial carcinoembryonic antigen (CEA) levels in patients with ulcerative colitis, *Am. J. Dig. Dis.*, 23, 129, 1978.

37. Stevens, D. P. and MacKay, I. R., Increased carcinoembryonic antigen in heavy cigarette smokers, *Lancet*, 1, 1238, 1973.

38. Alexander, J. C., Silverman, N. A., and Chretien, P. B., Effect of age and cigarette smoking on carcinoembryonic antigen levels, *JAMA*, 235, 1975, 1976.

39. Pulimood, B. M., Knudsen, A., and Coghill, N. F., Gastric mucosa after partial gastrectomy, *Gut*, 17, 463, 1976.

40. Doos, W. G., Wolff, W. I., Shinya, H., DeChabon, A., Stenger, R. J., and Gottlieb, L. S., CEA levels in patients with coloretal polyps, *Cancer*, 36, 1996, 1975.

41. Alm, T. and Wahren, B., Carcinoembryonic antigen in herditary adenomatosis of the colon and rectum, *Scand. J. Gastroenterol.*, 10, 875, 1975.

42. Guirgis, H. A., Lynch, H. T., Harris, R. E., and Vandevoord, J. P., Carcinoembryonic antigen (CEA) in the cancer family syndrome, *Cancer*, 42, 1574, 1978.

43. Sugarbaker, P., Zamcheck, N., and Moore, F. D. K., Assessment of serial carcinoembryonic antigen (CEA) in post operative management of colon and rectal cancer, *Cancer*, 38, 2310, 1976.

44. McNeil, B. J. and Adelstein, S. J., Determining the value of diagnostic and screening tests, *J. Nucl. Med.*, 17, 439, 1976.

45. Joint National Cancer Institute of Canada/American Cancer Society Investigation, a collaborative study of a test for carcinoembryonic antigen (CEA) in the sera of patients with carcinoma of the colon and rectum, *Can. Med. Assoc. J.*, 107, 25, 1972.

46. Hansen, H. J., Snyder, B. S., Miller, E., Vandevoorde, J. P., Miller, O. N., Hines, L. R., and Burns, J. J., Carcinoembryonic antigen (CEA) assay, a laboratory adjunct in the diagnosis and management of cancer, *Hum. Pathol.*, 5, 139, 1974.

47. Chu, T. M. and Holyoke, E. D., Can CEA assay be used as a screening test for cancer? Proc. 11th Int. Cancer Congress, Florence, Italy, 1, 351, 1974.

48. Dykes, P. W. and King, J., Progress report: carcinoembryonic antigen, *Gut*, 13, 1000, 1972.

49. Laurence, J. J. R., Stevens, U., Bettelheim, R., Darcy, d. Leese, C., Turnerville, C., Alexander, P., Johns, E. W., and Neville, A. M., Evaluation of the role of plasma carcinoembryonic antigen (CEA) in the diagnosis of gastrointestinal, mammary, and bronchial carcinoma, *Br. Med. J.*, 3, 605, 1972.

50. Concannon, J. P., Dallow, M. H., and Frich, J. C., Carcinoembryonic antigen (CEA) plasma levels in untreated cancer patients and patients with metastatic disease, *Radiology*, 108, 191, 1973.

51. Ona, F., Zamcheck, N., Dhar, P., Moore, T., and Kupchik, H. Z., Carcinoembryonic antigen (CEA) in the diagnosis of pancreatic cancer, *Cancer*, 31, 324, 1973.

52. McCartney, W. H. and Hoffer, P. B., The value of carcinoembryonic antigen as an adjunct to the radiological colon examination in the diagnosis of malignancy, *Radiology*, 110, 325, 1974.

53. Sugarbaker, P. H., Beard, J. O., and Drum, D. E., Detection of hepatic metastases from cancer of the breast, *Am. J. Surg.*, 133, 531, 1977.

54. McCartney, W. H. and Hoffer, P. B., Carcinoembryonic antigen assay: an adjunct to liver scanning in hepatic metastases detection, *Cancer*, 42, 1457, 1978.

55. Goldenberg, D. M., Deland, F., Kim, E., Bennett, S., Primus, F. J., Van Nagel, J. P., Estes, N., DeSimone, P., and Rayburn, P., Use of radiolabeled antibodies to carcinoembryonic antigen for the detection and localization of diverse cancers by external photoscanning, *N. Engl. J. Med.*, 298, 1384, 1978.

56. Mach, J. P., Jaeger, P. H., Bertholet, M. M., Ruegsegger, C. H., Loosli, R. M., and Pettavel, J., Detection of recurrence of large bowel carcinoma by radioimmunoassay of circulating carcinoembryonic antigen (CEA), *Lancet*, 2, 535, 1974.

57. MacKay, A. M., Patel, S., Carter, S., Stevens, U., Laurence, D. J. R., Cooper, E. H., and Neville, A. M., Role of serial plasma CEA assays in detection of recurrent and metastatic colorectal carcinoma, *Br. Med. J.*, 4, 382, 1974.

58. **Herrera, M. A., Chu, T. M., and Holyoke, E. D.**, Carcinoembryonic antigen (CEA) as a prognostic and monitoring test in clinically complete resection of colorectal carcinoma, *Ann. Surg.*, 183, 5, 1976.

59. **Martin, E. W., James, K. K., Hurtubise, P. E., Catalano, P., and Minton, J. P.**, The use of CEA as an early indicator for gastrointestinal tumor recurrence and second-look procedures, *Cancer*, 39, 440, 1977.

60. **Ratcliffe, J. G., Wood, C. B., Burt, R. W., Malcolm, A. J., and Blumgart, L. H.**, Patterns of Change in Carcinoembryonic Antigen (CEA) Levels in Patients Developing Recurrent Colorectal Cancer, in 6th Meet. Int. Research Group for Carcinoembryonic Proteins, Marburg/Lahn, W. Germany, September 17—21, 1978.

61. **Wanebo, H. J., Rao, B., Pinsky, C. M., Hoffman, R. G., Stearns, M., Schwartz, M. R., and Oettgen, H. F.**, Preoperative carcinoembryonic antigen level as a prognostic indicator in colorectal cancer, *N. Engl. J. Med.*, 299, 448, 1978.

62. **Foster, J. H. and Berman, M. M.**, *Solid Liver Tumors*, W.B. Saunders, Philadelphia, 1977, 225.

63. **Martini, N., Huvos, A. G., and Mike, V.**, Multiple pulmonary resections in the treatment of osteogenic sarcoma, *Ann. Thorac. Surg.*, 12, 271, 1971.

64. **Rosenberg, S. A., Flye, M. W., Conkle, D., Seipp, C., Levine, A. S., and Simon, R.**, The treatment of osteogenic sarcoma. II. Aggressive resection of pulmonary metastases, *Cancer Treat. Rep.*, 63, 753, 1979.

65. **Rittgers, R. A., Steele, G., Zamcheck, N., Lowenstein, M. S., Sugarbaker, P. H., Mayer, R. J., Lokich, J. J., Maltz, J., and Wilson, R. E.**, Transient carcinoembryonic antigen (CEA) elevations following resection for colorectal cancer: a limitation in the use of serial CEA levels as an indicator for second look surgery, *J. Natl. Cancer Inst.*, 61, 315, 1978.

66. **Madden, J. L. and Kandalaft, S.**, Electrocoagulation in the treatment of cancer of the rectum, in *Surgery Annual*, Nyhus, L. M., Ed., Appleton Century Crofts, New York, 1974, 195.

67. **Booth, S. N., Jamison, G. G., King, J. P. G., Leonard, J., Oates, G. D., and Dykes, P. W.**, Carcinoembryonic antigen in the management of colorectal carcinoma, *Br. Med. J.*, 4, 183, 1974.

68. **Denk, H., Tappeiner, G., Eckerstorfer, R., and Holzner, J. H.**, Carcinoembryonic antigen (CEA) in gastrointestinal and extra-gastrointestinal tumors and its relationship to tumor cell differentiation, *Int. J. Cancer*, 10, 262, 1972.

69. **Shamberg, J. F.**, personal communication.

70. **Kalser, M. H., Barkin, J. S., Redlhammer, D., and Heal, A.**, Circulating carcinoembryonic antigen in pancreatic carcinoma, *Cancer*, 42, 1468, 1978.

71. **Wang, D. Y., Bulbrook, R. D., Hayward, J. C., Hendricks, J. C., and Frachimont, P.**, Relationship between plasma carcinoembryonic antigen and prognosis in women with breast cancer, *Eur. J. Cancer*, 11, 615, 1975.

72. **Haagensen, D. E., Kister, S. J., Vandervoord, J. P., Gates, J. B., Smart, E. K., Hansen, H. J., and Wells, S. A.**, Evaluation of carcinoembryonic antigen as a plasma monitor for human breast carcinoma, *Cancer*, 42, 1512, 1978.

73. **Meyers, R. E., Sutherland, D. J., Meakin, J. W., Kellen, J. A., Malkin, D. G., and Matkin, A.**, Carcinoembryonic antigen in breast cancer, *Cancer*, 42, 1520, 1978.

74. **Tormey, D. C. and Waalkes, T. P.**, Clinical correlation between CEA and breast cancer, *Cancer*, 42, 1507, 1978.

75. **Dent, P. B., McCulloch, P. B., Wesley-James, O., MacLaren, R., Muirhead, W., and Dunnett, C. W.**, Measurement of carcinoembryonic antigen in patients with bronchogenic carcinoma, *Cancer*, 42, 1484, 1978.

76. **Concannon, J. P., Dalbow, M. H., Hodgson, S. E., Headings, J. J., Markopoulos, E., Mitchell, J., Cushing, W. J., and Liebler, G. A.**, Prognostic value of preoperative carcinoembryonic antigen (CEA) plasma levels in patients with bronchogenic carcinoma, *Cancer*, 42, 1477, 1978.

77. **Apffel, C. A. and Peters, J. H.**, Regulation of antigenic expression, *J. Theoret. Biol.*, 26, 47, 1970.

78. **Lurie, B. B., Bull, D. M., Zamcheck, N., Steward, A. M., and Helms, R. A.**, Diagnosis and prognosis in colon cancer based on a profile of immune reactivity, *J. Natl. Cancer Inst.*, 54, 319, 1975.

79. **Araj, G. F., Rink, C. M., and Blakemore, W. S.**, Suppression of lymphocyte blastogenesis by carcinoembryonic antigen (CEA), *Fed. Proc. Fed. Am. Soc. Exp. Biol.*, 38, 1172, 1979.

80. **Dhar, P., Moore, T., Zamcheck, N., and Kupchik, H. Z.**, Carcinoembryonic antigen (CEA) in colonic cancer. Use in preoperative and postoperative diagnosis and prognosis, *JAMA*, 221, 31, 1972.

81. **LoGerfo, P., Herter, F., and Hansen, H. J.**, Tumor-associated antigen in patients with carcinoma of the colon, *Am. J. Surg.*, 123, 127, 1972.

82. **Livingstone, A. S., Hampson, L. G., Schuster, J., Gold, P., and Hinchey, E. J.**, Carcinoembryonic antigen in the diagnosis and management of colorectal carcinoma, *Arch. Surg.*, 109, 259, 1974.

83. **Sorokin, J. J., Sugarbaker, P. H., Zamcheck, N., Pisick, M., Kupchik, H. Z., and Moore, F. D.**, Serial carcinoembryonic antigen assays. Use in delection of cancer recurrence, *JAMA*, 228, 49, 1974.

84. **Oh, J. H. and MacLean, L. D.**, Prognostic use of preoperative and immediate postoperative carcinoembryonic antigen determinations in colonic cancer, *Can. J. Surg.*, 20, 64, 1977.

85. Vider, M., Kashmiri, R., Hunter, L., Moses, B., Meeker, W. R., Utley, J. F., and Maruyama, Y., Carcinoembryonic antigen (CEA) monitoring in the management of radiotherapeutic patients, *Oncology,* 30, 257, 1974.

86. Vider, M., Kashmiri, R., Meeker, W. R., Moses, B., and Maruyama, Y., Carcinoembryonic antigen (CEA) monitoring in the management of radiotherapeutic and chemotherapeutic patients, *Am. J. Roentgenol.,* 124, 630, 1975.

87. Sugarbaker, P. H., Bloomer, W. D., Corbett, E. D., and Chaffey, J. T., Carcinoembryonic antigen (CEA) monitoring of radiation therapy for colorectal cancer, *Am. J. Roentgenol.,* 127, 641, 1976.

88. Donaldson, E., Van Nagell, J. R., Wood, E. G., Peltsch, Q., and Goldenberg, D. M., Carcinoembryonic antigen in patients treated with radiation therapy for invasive aquamaous cell carcinoma of the cervix, *Ann. J. Roentgenol.,* 127, 829, 1976.

89. Mulcare, R. and LoGerfo, P., Tumor assiciated antigen in chemotherapy of solid tumors, *J. Surg. Oncol.,* 4, 407, 1972.

90. Herrera, M. A., Chu, T. M., Holyoke, E. D., and Mittelman, A., CEA monitoring of palliative treatment for colorectal carcinoma, *Ann. Surg.,* 185, 23, 1977.

91. Young, V. L., Kashmiri, R., Hazen, R., and Meeker, W. R., Usefulness of serial carcinoembryonic antigen (CEA) determinations in monitoring chemotherapy, *South. Med. J.,* 69, 1274, 1976.

92. Mayer, R. J., Garnick, M. B., Steele, G. D., and Zamcheck, N., Carcinoembryonic antigen (CEA) as a monitor of chemotherapy in disseminated colorectal cancer, *Cancer,* 42, 1428, 1978.

Chapter 11

HOST RESISTANCE AND RESPONSE OF TUMORS TO IONIZING RADIATION

Naresh Prasad and Luka Milas

TABLE OF CONTENTS

I. INTRODUCTION

Radiotherapy is, in general, a local treatment modality of nondiseminated cancer. Its success or failure to induce local control depends primarily on radiobiological factors. However, a significant amount of evidence indicates that host antitumor resistance factors may interact with the tumor and modify the radiation dose required for tumor control. Immunosuppression, specific immunization, and treatment of tumor-bearing hosts with biological response modifiers have all been shown to induce alterations in the radiosensitivity of tumors in experimental animals. Interestingly only few clinical studies, however, have been carried out that employed immunotherapeutic treatment as an adjunct to radiation therapy. This chapter will be a short overview of literature on this subject.

II. RESPONSE OF MAMMALIAN CELLS TO IONIZING RADIATION

The beneficial effect of radiation treatment on a malignant tumor depends not only on the lethal effect of irradiation on tumor, but also a host's normal tissues surrounding the tumors. Thus there are biological (host and tumor related) and physical (radiation) factors which can affect the outcome of radiation treatment on malignant tumors. We would like to summarize some of these factors.[1]

A. Cell Killing and Cell Survival Curve

The lethal effects of radiation on living cells are generally considered to be composed of two separate processes: one due to single-hit killing and the other to an accumulation of sublethal injuries to certain target sites in the cell. The mathematical model for this combined process rests on an assumption of randomness and independence in the action of radiation among target sites of the same cell, as well as among different cells.

The single-hit component is believed to be modeled according to a Poisson process wherein for a very small concentration (in space and time), the probability of two or more lethal hits on a single cell is negligible compared to the probability of a single hit. Furthermore, for nonoverlapping small intervals of the same size, the probabilities are identical and independent.[2-4] With these assumptions the probability distribution of lethal hits on a particular cell from a greater concentration of radiation exposure can be expressed as the Poisson distribution. Figure 1 illustrates observed values from random samples of size 100, along with expected frequencies according to Poisson distributions with different hit rates. Note that the probability of no hits decreases as λ increases, but is greater than zero for all λ.

The correspondence between observed and expected *frequencies* in Figure 1 is quite good even for a sample of 100 cells. When millions of cells are exposed, the agreement between observed and expected *proportions* would be virtually perfect, if all of the above assumptions apply.

Implied in the Poisson model is that the mean number of lethal hits per cell (λ) is proportional to the dose of radiation applied.[5] If this were the only mechanism for cell killing, the semilogarithmic plot of a cell survival curve would appear as a straight line throughout the range of radiation dose levels. However, a typical cell survival curve will tend to flatten out, or have a "shoulder", at low doses, and to become exponential in shape (i.e., linear on a semilogarithmic plot) for large doses (curve C of Figure 2). One hypothesized explanation for this type of curve is provided by a "target theory" model consisting of lethality due to single hits and to an accumulation of sublethal injuries to a fixed number of target sites.[6-8] The probability of sublethal damage is the same at each site, these probabilities are independent among sites and all sites must be hit during one radiation exposure for cell killing to occur.[4] This model

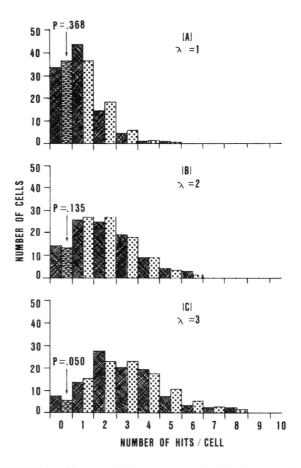

FIGURE 1. Observed ▨ and expected ▨ hits per cell for random samples of 100 cells with mean hit rates of $\lambda = 1$, $\lambda = 2$, and $\lambda = 3$; Respective probabilities of no hits are P = .368, P = .135, and P = .050; based on poisson distributions with the probability of K hits = $P(K) = \lambda^K e^{-\gamma}/K!$; k = 0,1,...,

is illustrated on Figure 2. Curve 2A is the exponential component due to single-hit killing; Curve 2B is the component due to accumulated sublethal injury; Curve 2C is the combined survival curve obtained as a product of the other two. Note the flatness of Curve 2B at low doses and the resultant shoulder on Curve 2C. The point (n) where the survival curve (2C) crosses the vertical axis called the "extrapolation number", and the dose D_q where the linear projection of this curve crosses the values PS = 1 is called the "quasithreshold dose".[9,10]

B. Repair of Sublethal Injury

Again assuming that the target theory model for accumulated sublethal cell injury applies, evidence suggests that most cells which have received injury to (n-1) or fewer sites, can experience essentially a full recovery within hours following a clinical dose of radiation.[11] The implication of this is that cell killing due to accumulated sublethal injury from two successive doses of moderate size (with a intervening recovery period) will be less than from a single dose of twice the size. Thus, if certain types of cells are more resistant to sublethal injury, or recover more readily from such injury than other cells they would be more amenable to survival from fractionated radiation exposure. In particular this would be an important fact to exploit if the cells that are intended

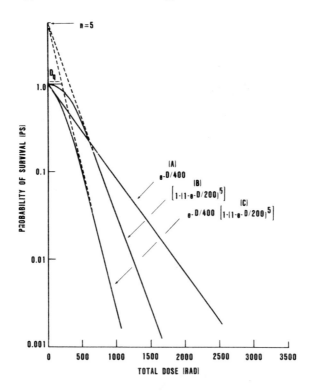

FIGURE 2.   Cell survival as a function of lethal single hits and accumulated sublethal injury. The mean lethal dose for single-hit killing (curve 2A) is shown as 400 rad, and the mean sublethal dose at each target site (curve 2B) is shown as 200 rad. The probability of cell survival (curve 2C) equals the product of the two component curves.

for killing (e.g., neoplastic) are less resistant to sublethal injury than those which are intended for survival (e.g., normal cells).[12]

If cells with sublethal injury recover completely in the interval between successive fractionated doses, if the assumption of independence and identical probabilities of cell lethality apply in successive doses, and if the target theory is assumed, then the probability of survival in K successive fractionated doses would be as illustrated on Figure 3 for a number of different fractionated dose levels. The survival curve for the total of several fractionated doses can be represented as exponential (the dashed line curves of Figure 3).[2] Note that the probability of survival increases at each total dose size as the size of the fractionated dose decreases, as illustrated for a total dose of 1200 rads. There are two limiting curves in this family: curve 3A represents the exponential curve for single-hit killing only, and is the limiting curve that is approached as the fractionated dose becomes infinitesimally small (according to the theoretical model); curve 3F represents the lower limit of cell survival and applies when the total dose is administered in a single application.

On all of the intermediate curves of Figure 3 the probability of survival should only be interpreted at the nodes which represent the increments of the fractionated doses. Dashed lines on Figure 3 represent the idealized exponential curves passing through the nodes.

The effect of varying the dose rate of continuous radiation is analogous to the effect of varying the fractionated dose size in successive radiation exposures: a high dose rate produces an effect similar to that produced by a single unfractionated dose, whereas

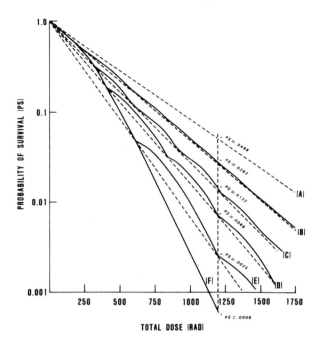

FIGURE 3. Cell survival curves for fractionated doses of various sizes: many small doses (curve 3A), 200 rad (curve 3B), 300 rad (curve 3C), 400 rad (curve 3D), 600 rad (curve 3E) and 1200 rad (curve 3F). Curves 3A and 3F are identical to curves 2A and 2C, respectively. Comparable survival at a total dose of 1200 rad is illustrated.

low dose rate produces effects like those caused by a series of relatively small fractionated doses. The explanation for this phenomenon is that at low dose rates the cells have the capability for repairing sublethal damage during radiation so cell mortality shifts towards single-hit killing. Conversely, at a high dose rate the cells do not have time to repair their damage during the period of exposure, so a large proportion of the cell mortality is accounted for by an accumulation of sublethal cell damage.

C. Tumor Response to Radiation

The term "tumor" simply means swelling, but historically it has been equated with neoplasm. Among the many definitions of neoplasm, a much more meaningful definition is that of Willis,[13] "A neoplasm is an abnormal mass of tissue, the growth which exceeds and is uncoordinated with that of the normal tissues and persists in the same excessive manner after cessation of the stimuli which evoke the change." A tumor may be benign or malignant. A benign tumor is rarely life-threatening, is slow in growth and progression, and does not metastize, whereas the malignant tumor is highly proliferative, infiltrative, and metastasizes throughout the body leading to death.

The degree of cell organization in tumors varies depending upon the tumor type. In most tumors, at any one point in time cells are present in various phase of the cell cycle. Those tumor cells which possess reproductive integrity and are capable of repopulating tumors, are called clonogenic cells or tumor stem cells. One of the major differences between normal stem cells and tumor stem cells is that the former are under homeostatic control, while the latter are not. The proportion of clonogenic cells varies depending upon the type of tumor. For a given type the number of clonogenic cells is correlated with tumor volume; also the radiation dose required for tumor control is directly related to tumor volume.[1]

Most solid tumors are highly cellular when small, but rapidly outgrow their blood supply; large tumors become shells of proliferating cells surrounding a necrotic center. The thickness of the proliferating zone of viable cells remains essentially constant but the central necrotic area increases in size. The vascularity is very poor in the necrotic area and consequently oxygen concentration is reduced and a hypoxic condition is created. Cells in the hypoxic area are viable and do not divide for long periods of time. These cells are radioresistant and ultimately may be responsible for recurrence of the tumor.[14-19]

For complete eradication of a tumor, there must be no surviving clonogenic cells. If we consider that cell killing by radiation is according to the target theory model described previously, then it is highly probable that at least small percentage of clonogenic cells will survive. Theoretically, this means that there is no absolute "tumoricidal dose" (i.e., one that will kill all cells with certainty) and that there is a finite probability (>0) that some clonogenic cells will always survive in a particular tumor.

It has been suggested that the number of clonogenic cell doublings is correlated with the number of tumor volume doublings, and also that the radiation dose required for tumor control is directly proportional to the number of doublings of clonogenic cells.[1]

D. Cell Cycle

Terasima and Tolmach[20] showed for the first time in vitro that cells are not uniformly radiosensitive throughout the cell cycle but have sensitive and resistant phases. Such phenomena have been investigated in many cell-lines by various investigators, and although results vary, the general features are that radiosensitivity increases as cells progress from one phase of the cell cycle to another. For example, the cells in G_2 are more radiosensitive than those in G_1 or S.[21]

E. Oxygenation

As we know, the presence of oxygen at the time of radiation enhances the radiation effect at cellular or tissue levels.[22,23] The state of oxygenation of tumor cells is mainly dependent on the vascularity of tumor cells. The poor vascularity at the center of a tumor in comparison to its periphery is responsible for a lower oxygen concentration at the center and consequently for the heterogeneities within tumor cell populations. Such hetergeneous populations of tumor cells reduce the prognosis of tumor control by radiotherapy. The mechanism of such radiosensitization by oxygen is not yet fully understood. For example, oxygen may "fix" the radiation damage which may otherwise be repairable.[1] The "oxygen effect" is highly utilized for treatment of hypoxic tumor cells by radiotherapy.[24] Some methods by which radioresistance of a hypoxic tumor can be reduced are

1. Increased Oxygenation of Tumor: Increased oxygenation of tumors can be attempted in the following ways:
   a. Inhalation of hyperbaric oxygen: The theory is that by increasing oxygen pressure in the blood, oxygen may diffuse into the hypoxic tissues of the tumor. Usually three atmospheres of O_2 pressure are utilized, but apparently oxygen never reaches the hypoxic cells.
   b. Carbogen: Du Sault[25] first suggested having patients breathe a mixture of 5% CO_2 and 95% O_2 during radiation treatment. CO_2 is a respiratory stimulant and causes vasodilation. At the same time increased O_2 tension in the tissues produces vasoconstriction, and O_2 is released more readily to the hypoxic cells. The oxygenation of tumors has been improved in this way,[26] but clinical trials have given inconclusive results with respect to tumor control.[27]
2. Decreased Oxygenation of Normal Tissues: Ellis[28] suggested that the patient should breath nitrogen for a short time and then air. Radiation treatment to the tumor would be applied while the patient is breathing air. Theoretically, normal tissues will be protected during radiation while malignant tissues will be affected. The use of controlled hypoxia is very risky even for a short period.
3. Hypoxic Sensitizers: There are many chemicals that sensitize the hypoxic cells of tumors but not the normal well-oxygenated tissues. These chemicals of the electron affinic have been described

by many authors.[29-31] Two such chemicals, Synkavit and metholtrexate, have been evaluated in radiotherapy trials. Krishnamurthi et al.[32] have shown significant improvement in disease-free survival rates at three years in patients with advanced cancer who were treated with Synkavit® in addition to radiotherapy. However, Mitchell[33] did not observe any benefit by treatment with Synkavit during radiotherapy.

4. Fractionation Schedules: A typical curative course of radio-therapy involves a high dose of radiation given daily in fractionated doses over 3- to 10-week period. Such a common dose is usually 4000 to 7000 rad given 200 rad per day, 5 days per week. The benefits of fractionation was mentioned earlier, are twofold. Each dose will result in the death analysis of tumor cells; therefore more space is available for proliferation of normal tissues and reoxygenation of tumor tissues. When the ratio of normal to tumor cells is increased by the accumulated dose, the effectiveness of further irradiation will be enhanced.

5. High Linear Energy Transfer Radiation: Linear Energy Transfer, abbreviated LET, is defined as the mean energy released by a charged particle per unit length that the particle traverses, and is affected by the velocity and charge of the ionizing particle. As the LET of radiation increases, the ability to produce biological damage also increases. This effect is called the relative biological effectiveness (RBE) and is defined as a ratio of dose of test radiation to dose of standard radiation which produce the same biological effect. Detailed discussion of LET and RBE, can be found in standard texts on radiation physics[23] or radiotherapy.[22] X and γ rays have low LET radiation while X-particles, neutrons and protons have high LET radiation. The high LET radiations are less dependent on oxygen and are more effective against hypoxic cells than low LET radiations. Three types of high LET radiations: (1) fast neutrons, (2) π-mesons, and (3) light atomic nuclei have been proposed for clinical application and are being investigated in many cancer treatment centers.

F. Therapeutic Ratio

Therapeutic ratio (TR) is the ratio between the largest radiation dose that will not have a serious effect on the structure or functionality of the normal surrounding tissues of the host (i.e., the normal tissues tolerance dose: NTTD) and the smallest dose that will be lethal to malignant tissues (i.e., the malignant tumor lethal dose: MTLD).

$$TR = \frac{\text{Normal Tissue Tolerance Dose (NTTD)}}{\text{Malignant Tumor Lethal Dose (MTLD)}}$$

If the TR ratio is greater than 1, the local tumor can be successfully controlled. The NTTD is subjectively determined; the radiotherapist must decide what degree of damage to normal tissues is acceptable in return for radiocurability of the tumor. Tolerance doses of various groups vary from a low of 1000 rad to 7500 rad or higher, and are affected by volume of tissues irradiated and fractionation schedules.

The Malignant Tumor Lethal Dose (MTLD) varies depending on the tumor type, size, extent, differentiation and pathological grades, and on its response to ionizing radiation. Some of these tumor-related factors have been discussed earlier in the chapter.

G. Immunological Status

It is believed that cancer patients with good general immunocompetence have favorable prognosis compared to cancer patients with poor general immunocompetence.[34] As we have seen in previous chapters of this book, it is clear that although radiotherapy reduces the tumor burden, it also exerts a negative influence on the host immune system. Such an impaired immune system causes a failure of the host to detect and/or destroy residual tumor cells.

III. IMMUNOLOGICAL BASIS FOR TUMOR IMMUNOTHERAPY

When under oncogenic stimuli, normal cells become transformed into malignant cells, they acquire new growth characteristics, and gain surface antigens recognized by the host immune system as foreign. Immune reaction develops to eliminate newly transformed cells thus protecting physiological integrity of the host. There is ample evidence indicating that development and growth of tumors in experimental animals is indeed often under immunological control.[35] Evidence, however, is still insufficient to allow the same statement to be made for malignant tumors in man, although several human tumors have been found to elicit antitumor immune resistance mechanisms.[35] Although both humoral and cell-mediated immune responses are elicited by tumor antigens, the latter is generally considered as being important in tumor rejection. T lymphocytes from mice immunized to the tumor exhibit in vitro specific cytoxicity for tumor cells and can transfer antitumor immunity to normal recipients.[36] In addition to T lymphocytes, other subpopulations of lymphocytes are also involved in destruction of tumor cells. K (killer) cells, which have receptors for the Fc portion of the IgG molecule, are cytotoxic for tumor cells in the presence of antibody molecules.[37] Natural killer (NK) cells, another lymphocyte subpopulation with antitumor activity, occur at high levels in lymphoid organs of several species including humans.[38] NK cells do not express surface markers for either B or mature T lymphocytes, and apparently they do not require specific information to become cytotoxic for tumor cells. These cells are assumed to be a first level of defense against tumor development. Beside different lymphocyte subpopulation, macrophages can also, as effector cells, participate in tumor rejection. Cytotoxicity of macrophages for tumor cells can be brought about either by activation in an immune specific manner or by a variety of nonspecific activating agents such as *Corynebacterium parvum (C. parvum),* Bacilus Calmette Guerin (BCG), and pyran-copolymer.[39,40]

Production of lymphoid cells and antibodies cytotoxic for tumor cells are not the only constituents of the immune response of the host to tumor antigens. If it were so, deviations from the immunological control would occur extremely seldom. However, escape from the immunological surveillance appears not to be such a rare event. It can be brought about by many factors, some of which will be mentioned briefly. Tumor host may respond by production of blocking antibodies that interfere in an inhibitory sense with cell-mediated mechanisms.[41] On the other hand, growing tumors release antigens into circulation, which by itself or as antigen antibody complexes, can block cell-mediated destruction of tumor cells.[42] Tumor cells also release factors which inhibit macrophage functions such as chemotoxis and phagocytosis.[43] The presence of a tumor may lead to the production of suppressor cells, which are mainly T lymphocytes and macrophages, that inhibit the production or expression of cytotoxic immune cells.[44] Other immune phenomena, such as immunological tolerance to tumor antigens, sneaking through, tumor growth immunostimulation, and antigen modulation, also participate in tumor escape from the immune surveillance.

Both tumor destructive and tumor protective immune mechanisms may be present within a single tumor host and further tumor progression depends on which of the two mechanisms prevail. This interaction between host and its tumor is complex and not yet fully understood to permit design rational approaches to immunotherapy. During the past decade or so, many different approaches and forms of immunotherapy have been developed in experimental tumor models and tested in clinical trials with variable success.

A. Nonspecific Immunostimulation

This form of therapy employs administration of agents capable of potentiating various responses of the immune system. Many factors, bacterial extracts, chemically defined compounds, and interferon, have been found to possess such properties and they are commonly called biological response modifiers (BRM) (Table 1). Treatment of

Table 1
MAJOR BIOLOGICAL RESPONSE MODIFIERS WITH ANTITUMOR ACTIVITY

Anaerobic corynebacteria *(C. parvum, C. granulosum)*
Bacillus-Calmette-Guerin (BCG)
Methanol-extraction residue of BCG (MER)
Bacterial cell walls
Anionic polymers (pyran-copolymer and MVE's)
Interferon and interferon inducers
Glucan
Levamisole

animals with BRM produces profound morphological and functional changes within lymphoreticuloendothelial tissues. There is an extensive proliferation of lymphophistocytic elements, and in particular, macrophages which become activated. Cellular and humoral immune responses to various antigens are modulated and mostly augmented. Treated animals have increased phagocytic activity and increased resistance to infections and malignant tumors. Our understanding of mechanisms by which BRM affect tumor growth has greatly increased during the past few years, although it still remains quite incomplete. Mechanisms are many but the following two seem to dominate: immunologically nonspecific response mediated by activated macrophages and potentiation of the specific antitumor resistance.[39,40] Interferon, an immunotherapeutic agent that recently arose great interest in clinical immunotherapy, has antiviral properties, inhibits proliferation of tumor cells, activates macrophages, and increases natural killer (NK) cell activity and antibody-dependent cell cytotoxicity.[45] Compared to other forms of immunotherapy, nonspecific immunostimulation, especially therapy with BCG and *C. parvum,* has been the most often used for treatment of cancer patients. They may be applied systemically, but inoculation of these compounds directly into neoplastic lesion is usually of a more therapeutic efficiency. This therapy approach is referred to as regional immunotherapy.

B. Active Specific Immunotherapy

This treatment employs vaccines containing tumor antigens with the aim to augment specific immune responses to a particular tumor. Tumor cells can be used alone or mixed with adjuvants (for example, with Freund's adjuvant). Cells are usually inactivated with high doses of ionizing radiation or less frequently by other means. Attempts have been made to increase antigenicity of tumor cells by treating them with neuraminidase, chemicals, etc. Instead of using whole cells, subcellular components of tumor cells can also be used for active immunotherapy. They include crude cell extracts, isolated cell membranes, and solubilized surface antigens. Specific immunotherapy of malignant tumors appeared quite nonefficient, and therapeutic efficacy of this treatment modality may be anticipated to be increased if combined with nonspecific immunostimulation.

Immunotherapy of malignant tumors can also be approached by transferring into tumor hosts syngeneic, allogeneic, xenogeneic sensitized or nonsensitized lymphocytes, or immune antitumor serum. Transfer of lymphocytes is referred to as adoptive and that if immune serum as passive immunotherapy. In general, both of these approaches are quite nonefficient and in the case of allogeneic and xenogeneic transfer, they are associated with damage of normal tissues. Recently, more attention has been paid to employment of extract from lymphoid cells such as transfer factor, thymosin, and immune RNA. These factors are capable of stimulating cellular immunity and have, even in clinical trials, exhibited certain antitumor efficacy.

Antitumor efficacy of tumor immunotherapy modalities depends on a variety of factors, which have been reviewed in detail elsewhere.[39,40] We shall point out here, however, that tumor mass at the time of commencement of immunotherapy is one of the most critical factors. Abundance of experimental animal studies show that only a limited number of tumor cells, usually less than 10^6, can be eliminated by antitumor immune reaction. Extremely seldom have tumors larger than 1 cm in diameter (containing approximately $10^{8.5}$ cells) been observed to undergo complete regression following immunotherapy.[39] At the time of tumor diagnosis, the mass of the majority of tumors is already larger than that which can be controlled by host antitumor immune reaction, and because of this, immunotherapy has to be combined with other cancer treatment modalities, including radiotherapy.

IV. COMBINATION OF IMMUNOTHERAPY WITH RADIOTHERAPY

Response of many malignant tumors of experimental animals to ionizing radiation is modified by changes in functional status of the immune system of tumor hosts. In general, immunosuppressive treatments reduce specific and nonspecific stimulation of the antitumor resistance mechanisms and enhance therapeutic efficacy of radiation. Manipulations of the immune resistance also affect the spread of tumors. Our intention is to give, in this section, a brief account on reported evidence dealing with the dependency of tumor radioresponse on the tumor host immune competence, and in particular, describe studies that investigated possibilities of combining immunotherapeutic and radiotherapeutic treatments. Illustrative figures are from our own studies.

A. Effect of Immunosuppression and Specific Immunization on Tumor Radioresponse

Different immunosuppressive procedures, including exposure of animals to sublethal whole body irradiation (WBI),[46-48] corticosteroids,[49] and depletion of T lymphocytes,[47] may decrease sensitivity to tumors to radiation. An example of this is shown in Figure 4. A murine fibrosarcoma growing in normal mice or in mice treated with 600 rad WBI one day prior to tumor cell transplantation was exposed to different doses of γ-radiation. Higher doses of radiation were required to control tumors in WBI than in normal mice. In former mice, TCD_{50} value (dose of irradiation yielding local tumor control in 50% of animals) was ∼5100 rad and in normal mice, ∼3050 rad. However, WBI delivered to mice after local tumor irradiation caused no change in tumor radiocurability,[46] implying that already existing antitumor immunity may not be sensitive to immunosuppressive procedures. This aspect of tumor radioimmunotherapy has so far been investigated only marginally.

Opposite to the effect of immunosuppressive treatments, specific immunization can increase the therapeutic response of tumors to radiation. This was observed by treatment of mice with radiation attenuated tumor cells,[46] or tumor tissue fragments,[49] and treatment of rats with autochthonous biopsied tumor pieces.[50] In certain instances, specific immunization can decrease tumor radiocurability,[51] a phenomenon that may be ascribed to formation of blocking factors (soluble tumor antigens, antibodies, antibody-antigen complexes). It should be mentioned that the effect of specific immunization greatly depends on tumor immunogenicity; less immunogenic tumors are expected to be less sensitive to the combined treatment modality.[52]

B. Combination of Tumor Radiation with Nonspecific Immunotherapy

Most reported studies dealth with *C. parvum* and BCG, agents that have dominated in the field of tumor immunotherapy during the past decade.

1. Corynebacterium parvum

Extensive studies were carried out by Suit and associated[53,54] and by our group.[55,56]

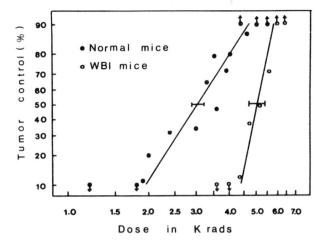

FIGURE 4.   Radiation dose response curves for local control of
8 mm fibrosarcoma in C₃Hf/Bu mice, normal or immunosuppressed by 600 rad whole body irradiation (WBI) 1 day before
tumor transplantation. Tumors were growing in the right hind
thighs of mice. Cross-bars indicate the TCD_{50} values and their
95% confidence limits. Symbols with arrows represent groups with
<10% or >90% of the tumors controlled.[48]

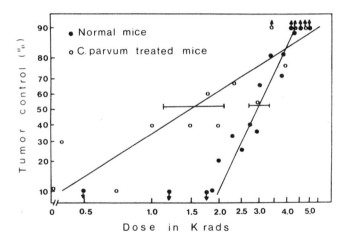

FIGURE 5.   Radiation dose response curves for local control of 8
mm fibrosarcomas in normal C. parvum-treated C₃Hf/Bu mice. C.
parvum was given to mice 2 to 3 days before tumor irradiation. Tumors were growing in the right hind thighs of mice. Cross-bars indicate the TCD_{50} values and their 95% confidence limits. Symbols with
arrows represent groups with <10% or >90% of the tumors controlled.[48]

Using a murine fibrosarcoma, these investigators observed that C. parvum significantly augmented response of that tumor to both single and fractionated doses of γ-
radiation. Figure 5 shows single dose response curves of 8 mm tumors growing in
normal and C. parvum treated mice. Treatment with C. parvum, which was given to
mice when tumors had grown to 6 mm in diameter, reduced TCD_{50} value from ∼3050
rad in normal mice to 1500 rad. The improvement in radiocurability was observed with
lower doses of radiation that did not exceed some 2500 rad. The nonefficiency of high

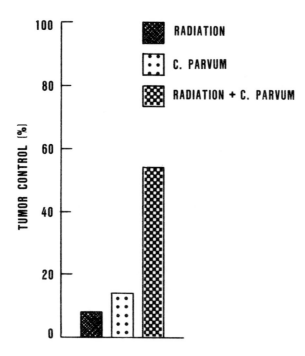

FIGURE 6.   Effect of *C. parvum* on radiocurability of 8 mm fibrosarcomas in C_3Hf/Bu mice. Tumors were growing in the right hind thighs of mice and were exposed to 500 rad daily for 6 days. *C. parvum* (0.25 mg) was given intravenously after the first dose of radiation.[56]

radiation doses was suggested to possibly have been due to radiation-induced injury of stromal tissues and alterations in the blood supply which in turn, may have reduced the access of immune effector cells into tumor.[55] In addition, higher radiation doses may have inactivated local lymphocytes and macrophages. In other tumor models, *C. parvum* was able to augment therapeutic efficiency of single doses of radiation higher than 5000 rad.[54]

Figure 6 shows that *C. parvum* greatly augments the response of a murine fibrosarcoma to fractionated radiation. The effect was synergistic. Tumors that did not undergo complete rejection following the combined treatment grew more slowly than tumors treated by either radiation or *C. parvum* alone. This resulted in the prolongation of survival of unsuccessfully treated mice. Also, *C. parvum* delayed the appearance of tumor metastases and reduced the overall incidence of metastases (Figure 7).

Many factors appear to determine the extent by which *C. parvum* increases response of tumors to ionizing radiation. They include dose and route of administration of bacteria, sequence of *C. parvum* treatment in relation to radiation exposure and immunogenicity, size and anatomic localization of tumors. Systemic application of 0.1 to 0.5 mg of bacteria was very effective, and in general, it is this treatment that causes the most profound effects upon the lymphoid tissues. Another efficient route of *C. parvum* is intratumoral.[53] In this case, lymphoproliferative changes occur predominantly in the local lymph nodes, which respond to tumor antigens by a more pronounced specific immune response.[39] Time relationships between treatments of *C. parvum* and radiation is a very important factor. In studies with a murine fibrosarcoma the greatest augmentation of tumor radiocurability was achieved when *C. parvum* was applied before irradiation.[55] A murine squamous cell carcinoma responded equally well to pre- and postirradiation treatments with *C. parvum*. Ullrich and Adams,[57] however,

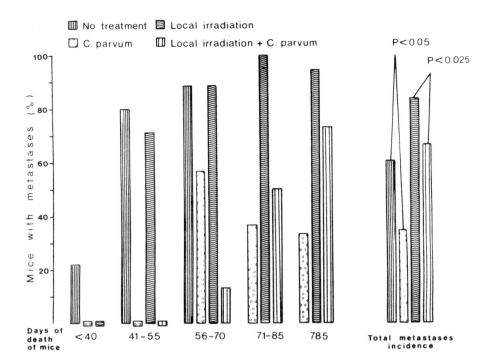

FIGURE 7. Effect of *C. parvum*, local tumor irradiation, or both on the incidence of fibrosarcoma metastases in the lungs of C_3Hf/Bu mice. Metastasis incidence was determined at the time of death of the mice. Varying schedules of fractionated radiation and *C. parvum* was employed (see Reference 56).

observed that *C. parvum* was more effective when given after irradiation. Tumor immunogenicity also influences the effect of *C. parvum* on tumor radiocurability. In general, more immunogenic tumors respond better than less immunogenic tumors.[53,56] In the case of weakly immunogenic tumors, the effect is usually evidenced by a moderate slowing in the growth of irradiated tumors and in prolongation of the survival of tumor hosts. As already mentioned, immune rejection responses to tumors are efficient against only a limited number of tumor cells. Therefore, even the combination of treatments small tumors are expected to be more easily controlled than large tumors. Combination of *C. parvum* and radiation resulted in higher percentage of cures of 4 to 6 mm fibrosarcomas than 8 mm fibrosarcomas.[53,55] Also, radiocurability of 5 and 8 mm, but not of 12 mm, squamous cell carcinomas was markedly increased by this bacterium.[54] In regard to tumor localization, it appears that tumors growing intradermally respond better to *C. parvum* than tumors growing intramuscularly.[55]

2. BCG

Haddow and Alexander[50] found no benefit of BCG treatment in augmenting sensitivity of a rat chemically induced sarcoma to radiation. In another rat sarcoma model, BCG improved the response of radiotherapy, but the effect was less profound than that caused by *C. parvum*.[58] Local tumor radiotherapy combined with BCG resulted in a significant reduction in the number of lung metastases of the Lewis lung carcinoma.[59] Also, methanol extraction residue fraction of BCG markedly increased the radioresponse of a murine fibrosarcoma and a mammary carcinoma.[60]

3. Other BRM

Pyromen (pseudomones polysaccharide),[58] glucan,[61] and vitamin A[62] were shown to

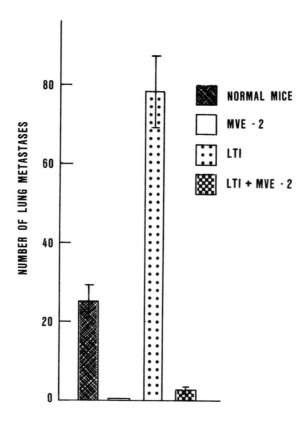

FIGURE 8.   Effect of MVE-2 fraction of pyran-copolymer (25 mg/kg, intravenously) on local thoracic irradiation (LTI)-induced enhancement of pulmonary metastases of a fibrosarcoma (designated NFSa) in C_3Hf/Bu mice. Mice were given iv injection of 2×10^5 NFSa cells one day after LTI with 1000 rad of γ-rays. MVE-2 was given 2 days before irradiation.

be capable to augmenting sensitivity of animal tumors to radiation, but the effect was less profound than that caused by *C. parvum.* Using the murine KHT fibrosarcoma, which induces no measurable host defense response, glucan did not improve tumor-free survival over radiation alone.[63] Similarly, MVE-2 fraction of pyran-copolymer failed to increase the mean survival time of mice with Lewis lung carcinoma over that achieved by the irradiation alone.[64] On the other hand, pyran-copolymer greatly increased the response of a murine fibrosarcoma to local X-irradiation.[65]

C. Protection Against Radiation-Induced Promotion of Tumor Metastasis Formation

Exposure of animals to WBI leads to profound destruction of lymphatic tissues and consequently to impaired immune response. Even localized irradiation can cause lymphopenia and impaired immune reaction, although the magnitude of the damage is far less than that of WBI. These aspects of radiation have been discussed in detail in previous chapters. The concern has been expressed that radiation-induced changes in the lymphoid tissues and immune reactivity may be conducive to tumor growth and spread.[66] So far, this contention received no firm clinical evidence. However, there is another aspect of radiation-induced enhancement of tumor metastases that has received a fair degree of attention. It has repeatedly been shown that exposures of the thorax of mice and rats to either single or fractionated radiation enhanced formation of metastases in the lung by tumor cells injected intravenously after radiation.[67-69]

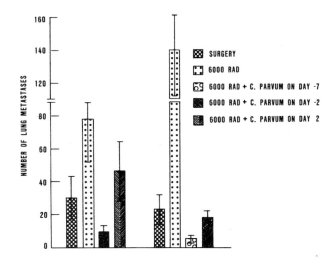

FIGURE 9. Protection by *C. parvum* against local tumor radiation-induced enhancement of spontaneous pulmonary metastases of a murine mammary carcinoma in C₃Hf/Bu mice. Primary tumors were amputated or irradiated with 6000 rad, when they reached 9 to 10 mm in diameter (designated as day 0), *C. parvum* was given intravenously in the dose of 0.25 mg. The number of metastasis was determined 28 days following amputation or irradiation of primary tumors.

Similar phenomenon can be produced by treatment of animals with chemotherapeutic agents, in particular with cyclophosphamide.[70] The phenomenon seems to be largely nonimmunological in its nature, (i.e., due to the damage of lung tissue and provides tumor cells with more favorable microenvironment for their proliferation than normal lung tissues.[68] However, when radiation or chemotherapeutic agents are initiated after tumor cells had already lodged in the lung, reduction in the number of metastases insues indicating that the metastases promoting effects of such treatments is outweighed by their tumor inhibiting activities.[69] Although clinical relevance of this phenomenon is uncertain at present, it may pose a threat in situations when relatively high doses of "prophylactic" irradiation are given without previous ablation of a primary tumor or its concomitant irradiation.[69] In the case of chemotherapy, enhancement of metastasis formation can be expected in situations of limited antitumor efficacy of applied compounds or when resistance of tumor cells to these drugs develop.

Taking the above into consideration, it appears important to search for possibilities of protecting against or reduce the metastasis promoting effects of radiation. A possibility may be to treat tumor hosts with BRM prior to radiation delivery. In this way, certain antitumor resistance responses, induced by BRM, such a macrophage activation, can resist to ionizing radiation and thus reduce tumor promoting aspect of radiation-induced damage. *C. parvum* can efficiently protect animals against enhancement of tumor metastases caused by WBI[71] and local thoracic irradiation (LTI).[72] Similar protective activity is exerted by MVE-2 fraction of pyran-copolymer, which is a potent macrophage activating agent (Figure 8).

Even local tumor irradiation can sometimes increase metastatic spread.[73] Treatment of animals with *C. parvum* can abolish this effect of radiation (Figure 9).

D. Clinical Studies on Combination of Tumor Radiotherapy and Immunotherapy

In comparison to the combination of immunotherapy with chemotherapy significantly fewer number of investigations have been performed to determine the therapeutic efficacy of the combination of BRM and radiotherapy. Sokal et al.[74] reported that yearly vaccination with BCG reduced the recurrence rate and prolonged the disease-free interval in patients with Stages IA and IIA lymphomas who were treated with local irradiation. Head and neck patients showed a slight increase in the survival rate if they received *C. parvum* in addition to radiotherapy with [60] Co.[75] Treatment with *C. parvum* commenced 6 weeks after completion of the radiation therapy; s.c. injections of bacteria were given weekly for the first 6 weeks, and then once every 2 weeks for the duration of the trial. Cheng et al.,[76] however, found no benefit in combining *C. parvum* with radiotherapy of head and neck carcinomas. Practically no studies on the therapeutic efficacy of other BRM have been reported when these were combined with radiotherapy.

REFERENCES

1. **Withers, H. R. and Peters, L. J.,** Biologic aspects of radiation therapy, in *Textbook of Radiotherapy,* Fletcher, G. H., Ed., Lea & Febiger, Philadelphia, 1980, 103.
2. **Elkind, M. M. and Whitmore, G. F.,** *The Radiobiology of Cultured Mammalian Cells,* Gordon and Breach Science Publishers, New York, 1967.
3. **Johns, H. E. and Cunningham, J. R.,** *The Physics of Radiology,* Charles C Thomas, Springfield, Ill., 1969.
4. **Lea, D. E.,** *Actions of Radiation on Living Cells,* 2nd ed., Gray, L. H., Ed., Cambridge University Press, Cambridge, 1956.
5. **Alper, T.,** Variability in the oxygen effect observed with microorganisms. III. Escherichia coli B, *Int. J. Radiat. Biol.,* 3, 369, 1961.
6. **Alper, T., Ed.,** *Cell Survival After Low Doses of Radiation: Theoretical and Clinical Implications,* John Wiley & Sons, Bristol, 1975.
7. **Elkind, M. M.,** Fractionated dose radiotherapy and its relationship to survival curve shape, *Cancer Treat. Rev.,* 3, 1, 1976.
8. **Neary, G. J.,** The dependence of the oxygen effect on the intensity of gamma irradiation in Vicia faba, in *Progress in Radiobiology,* Mitchell, J. S., Holmes, B. E., and Smith, C. L., Eds., Charles C Thomas, Springfield, Ill., 1955, 355.
9. **Alper, T., Gillies, N. E., and Elkind, M. M.,** The sigmoid survival curve in radiobiology, *Nature (London),* 186, 1062, 1960.
10. **Alper, T., Fowler, J. F., Morgan, R. L., Vonberg, D. D., Ellis, F., and Oliver, R.,** The characterizations of the "type C" survival curve, *Br. J. Radiol.,* 35, 722, 1962.
11. **Withers, H. R. and Mason, K. A.,** The kinetics of recovery in irradiated colonis mucosa of the mouse, *Cancer,* 34, 896, 1974.
12. **Withers, H. R.,** The 4 R's of radiotherapy, in *Advances in Radiation Biology,* Vol. 5 Lett, J. T. and Adler, H., Eds., Academic Press, New York, 1975, 241.
13. **Willis, R. A.,** *The Spread of Tumors in the Human Body,* Butterworth, London 1952.
14. **Powers, W. E. and Tomach, L. J.,** Demonstration of an anoxic component in a mouse tumor-cell population by in vivo assay of survival following irradiation, *Radiology,* 83, 328, 1964.
15. **Rubin, P. and Casarett, G. W.,** *Clinical Radiation Pathology,* Vol. 2, W. B. Saunders, Philadelphia, 1968, 903.
16. **Suit, H. and Maeda, M.,** Oxygen effect factor and tumor volume in C3H mouse mammary carcinoma; preliminary report, *Am. J. Roentgenol.,* 96, 177, 1966.
17. **Song, C. W. and Levitt, S. H.,** Vascular changes in Walker 256 carcinoma of rats following X irradiation, *Radiology,* 100, 397, 1971.
18. **Thomlinson, R. H.,** An experimental method for comparing treatment of intact malignant tumors in animals and its application to the use of oxygen in radiotherapy, *Br. J. Cancer,* 14, 555, 1960.
19. **Tanaka, Y.,** Regional tumor blood flow and radiosensitivity, in *Fraction Size in Radiobiology and Radiotherapy,* Sugahara, T., Revesz, L., and Scott, O. C. A., Eds., Igaku Shoin Ltd., Tokyo, 1974, 13.
20. **Terasima, T. and Tolmach, L. J.,** Variations in several responses of HeLa cells to X-irradiation during the division cycle, *Biophys. J.,* 3, 11, 1963.
21. **Sinclair, W. K.,** Dependence of radiosensitivities upon cell age, in *Time and Dose Relationships in Radiation Biology as Applied to Radiotherapy,* Brookhaven National Laboratory, BNL 50203 (C-57), Clearinghouse for Federal Scientific and Technical Information, Springfield, Va., 1970, 97.

22. **Andrews, J. R.**, *The Radiobiology of Human Cancer Radiotherapy,* University Park Press, Baltimore, 1978.
23. **Hall, E. J.**, *Radiobiology for the Radiologist,* Harper & Row, New York, 1978.
24. **Duncan, W.**, Exploitation of the oxygen enhancement ratio in clinical practice, *Br. Med. Bull.,* 29, 33, 1973.
25. **Du Sault, L. A.**, The effect of oxygen on the response of spontaneous tumours in mice to radiotherapy, *Br. J. Radiol.,* 36, 749, 1963.
26. **Johnson, R. J. R.**, A comparison of the effect of hyperbaric oxygen and oxygen plus 5% CO_2 on tissue circulation and oxygenation, *Radiology,* 98, 177, 1971.
27. **Rubin, P., Poulter, C. A., and Quick, R. S.**, Changing perspectives in oxygen breathing and radiation therapy, *Am. J. Roentgenol. Rad. Ther. Nucl. Med.,* 105, 665, 1969.
28. **Ellis, F.**, The use of hypoxia in radiotherapy, *Br. J. Radiol.,* 35, 506, 1962.
29. **Adams, G. E., Fowler, J. F., and Wardman, P.**, Hypoxic cell sensitizers in radiobiology and radiotherapy, *Br. J. Cancer,* 37, Suppl. 3, 1978.
30. **Adams, G. E.**, Hypoxic cell sensitizers for radiotherapy, *Int. J. Radiat. Oncol. Biol. Phys.,* 4, 135, 1978.
31. **Dische, S.**, Hypoxic cell sensitizers in radiotherapy, *Int. J. Radiat. Oncol. Biol. Phys.,* 4, 157, 1978.
32. **Krishnamurthi, S., Shanta, V., and Nair, M. K.**, Studies of chemical sensitization in the radiotherapy of oral and cervical carcinomas, *Cancer,* 20, 822, 1967.
33. **Mitchell, J. S.**, *Cancer: If Curable, Why Not Cured?* Heffer, Cambridge, 1971.
34. **Hersh, E. M., Gutterman, J. U., and Mavligit, G. M.**, Cancer and host defense mechanisms, in *Pathobiology Annual,* Joachim, H. L., Ed., Appleton-Century-Crofts, New York, 1975, 133.
35. **Klein, G.**, Immune and non-immune control of neoplastic development: contrasting effects of host and tumor evolution, *Cancer,* 45, 2486, 1980.
36. **Carottini, J. C. and Brunner, K. T.**, Cell mediated cytotoxicity, allograft rejection and tumor immunity, *Adv. Immunol.,* 18, 67, 1974.
37. **Perlman, P., Perlmann, H., Wahlin, B., and Hammarström, S.**, Quantitation, fractionation and surface marker Analysis of IgG- and IgM-dependent cytolytic lymphocytes (K cells) in human blood, in *7th Int. Symp. Immunopathology,* Miescher, P. A., Ed., Schwabe and Co., Basel, 1977, 321.
38. **Heberman, R. B. and Holden, H. T.**, Natural cell-mediated immunity, *Adv. Cancer Res.,* 27, 305, 1978.
39. **Milas, L. and Scott, M. T.**, Antitumor Activity of *Corynebacterium parvum, Adv. Cancer Res.,* 26, 257, 1978.
40. **Baldwin, R. W. and Pinn, M. V.**, BCG in tumor immunotherapy, *Adv. Cancer Res.,* 28, 91, 1978.
41. **Baldwin, R. W. and Robins, R. A.**, Induction of tumor-immune responses and their interaction within the developing tumor, *Contemp. Topics Mol. Immunol.,* 6, 177, 1977.
42. **Currie, G. A. and Basham, C.**, Serum-mediated inhibition of the immunological reactions of the patient to his own tumor: a possible role for circulating anitgen, *Br. J. Cancer,* 26, 427, 1972.
43. **James, K.**, The influence of tumor cell-products on macrophage funtion *in vitro* and *in vivo:* a review, in *The Macrophage and Cancer,* James, K., McBride, W., and Stuart, A., Eds., Econoprint, Edinburgh, 1977, 225.
44. **Broder, S., Munel, L., and Waldman, T. A.**, Suppressor cells in neoplastic disease, *J. Natl. Cancer Inst.,* 61, 5, 1978.
45. **Colby, B.**, Interferon systems — an overview, in *Interferons and Their Actions,* Stewart, W., Ed., CRC Press, Boca Raton, Fla., 1977, 1.
46. **Suit, H. D. and Kastelan, A.**, Immunologic status of host and response of methylcholanthrene-induced sarcoma to local X-irradiation, *Cancer,* 26, 232, 1970.
47. **Stone, H. B., Peters, L. J., and Milas, L.**, Effect of host immune capability on radiocurability and subsequent transplantability of a murine fibrosarcoma, *J. Natl. Cancer Inst.,* 63, 1229, 1979.
48. **Stone, H. B. and Milas, L.**, Modification of radiation response of murine tumors by misonidazole (Ro-07-0589), host immune capability, and *Corynebacterium parvum, J. Natl. Cancer Inst.,* 60, 887, 1978.
49. **Cohen, A. and Cohen, L.**, Estimation of the cellular lethal dose and the critical cell number for the C_3H mammary carcinoma from radiosensitivity studies *in vivo, Nature (London),* 185, 262, 1960.
50. **Haddow, A. and Alexander, P.**, An immunological method of increasing the sensitivity of primary sarcomas to local irradiation with X-rays, *Lancet,* 1, 452, 1964.
51. **Jurin, M. and Suit, H. D.**, *In vivo* and *in vitro* studies of the influence of the immune status of C_3Hf/Bu mice on the effectiveness of local irradiation of a methylcholanthrene induced fibrosarcoma, *Cancer Res.,* 32, 2201, 1972.
52. **Suit, H. and Kastelan, A.**, Tumor control by irradiation: a C_3H/He mouse mammary carcinoma in mammary-tumor-agent-positive and mammary-tumor-agent-free mice, *J. Natl. Cancer Inst.,* 40, 945, 1968.

53. Suit, H. D., Sedlacek, R., Wagner, M., Orsi, L., Silobrcic, V. and Rothman, K. J., Effect of *Corynebacterium parvum* on the response to irradiation of A C₃H fibrosarcoma, *Cancer Res.*, 36, 1305, 1976.
54. Suit, H. D., Sedlacek, R. S., Silobrcic, V., and Linggood, R. M., Radiation therapy and *Corynebacterium parvum* in the treatment of murine tumors, *Cancer*, 37, 2573, 1976.
55. Milas, L., Hunter, N., and Withers, H. R., Combination of local irradiation with systemic application of anaerobic corynebacterium in therapy of a murine fibrosarcoma, *Cancer Res.*, 35, 1274, 1975.
56. Milas, L., Hunter, N., Stone, H. B., and Withers, H. R., *Corynebacterium parvum*. Effect of radiocurability of murine tumors, *Cancer Immunol. Immunother.*, 5, 109, 1978.
57. Ullrich, R. L. and Adams, G. D., The combined use of local and *Corynebacterium parvum* in the treatment of line 1 carcinoma, *Radiat. Res.*, 73, 267, 1978.
58. Moroson, H. and Schechter, M., Treatment of rat fibrosarcoma by radiotherapy plus immune adjuvants, *Biomedicine*, 25, 97, 1976.
59. Dubois, J. B. and Serrou, B., Treatment of the mouse lewis lung tumor by the association of radiotherapy and immunotherapy with *Bacillus-Calmette-Guerin*, *Cancer Res.*, 36, 1731, 1976.
60. Yron, I., Weiss, D. W., Robinson, E., Cohen, D., Adelberg, M. G., Mekory, T., and Haber, M., Immunotherapeutic studies in mice with the methanol-extraction residues (MER) fraction, *Natl. Cancer Inst. Monogr.*, 39, 33, 1973.
61. Suit, H. D., Elman, A., Sedlacek, R., and Silobrcic, V., Comparative evaluation of tumor-inhibitory activity of glucan and *C. parvum* in a mouse fibrosarcoma model, *Prog. Cancer Res. Ther.*, 7, 235, 1978.
62. Tannock, I. F., Suit, H. D., and Marshall, N., Vitamin A and radiation response of experimental tumors: an immune-mediated effect, *J. Natl. Cancer Inst.*, 48, 731, 1972.
63. Stewart, C. C., Valeriote, F. A., and Perez, C. A., Preliminary observations on the effect of glucan in combination with radiation and chemotherapy in four murine tumors, *Cancer Treat. Rep.*, 62, 1867, 1978.
64. Morahan, P. S., Barnes, D. W., and Munson, A. E., Relationship of molecular weight to antiviral and antitumor activities and toxic effects of maleic anhydride-divinil ether (MVE) polyanions, *Cancer Treat. Rep.*, 62, 1797, 1978.
65. Collins-Tsui, A. L. and Song, C. W., Effects of combined radiotherapy and immunotherapy with the use of pyran copolymer on murine fibrosarcoma, *J. Natl. Cancer Inst.*, 60, 1477, 1978.
66. Stjernsward, J., Radiotherapy, host immunity and cancer spread, in *Secondary Spread in Breast Cancer*, Stoll, B. A., Ed., William Heinemann, London, 1977, 139.
67. van den Brenk, H. A. S., Burch, W. M., Orton, C., and Sharpington, C., Stimulation of clonogenic growth of tumor cells and mestastases in the lungs by local X-irraduation, *Br. J. Cancer*, 27, 291, 1973.
68. Withers, H. R. and Milas, L., Influence of preirradiation of lung on development of artificial pulmonary metastases of fibrosarcoma in mice, *Cancer Res.*, 33, 1931, 1973.
69. Peters, L. J., Mason, K. A., and Withers, H. R., Effect of lung irradiation on metastases: radiobiological studies and clinical correlations, in *Radiation Biology in Cancer Research*, Meyn, R. E. and Withers, H. R., Eds., Raven Press, New York, 1979, 515.
70. van Putten, L. M., Kram, L. K. J., Van Dierendenck, H. H. C., Smink, T., and Fwzy, M., Enhancement by drugs of metastatic lung nodule formation after intravenous tumor cell injection, *Int. J. Cancer*, 15, 588, 1975.
71. Milas, L., Hunter, N., Vasic, I., and Withers, H. R., Protection by *Corynebacterium granulosum* against radiation-induced enhancement of artificial pulmonary metastases of a murine fibrosarcoma, *J. Natl. Cancer Inst.*, 52, 1875, 1974.
72. Peters, L. J., Mason, K., McBride, W. H., and Patt, Y. Z., Enhancement of lung colony forming efficiency by local thoracic irradiation: interpretation of labelled cells studies, *Radiology*, 126, 499, 1978.
73. Milas, L., Mason, K., and Withers, H. R., Therapy of spontaneous pulmonary metastases of a murine mammary carcinoma with anaerobic corynebacteria, *Cancer Immunol. Immunother.*, 1, 233, 1976.
74. Sokal, J. E., Aungst, C. W., and Synderman, M., Delay in progression of malignant lymphoma after BCG vaccination, *N. Engl. J. Med.*, 291, 1226, 1974.
75. Mahe, E., Bourdin, J. S., Gest, H., Saracino, R., Brunet, M., Halpern, G., Debaud, B., and Roth, F., Therapeutic trial with reticulostimulin in patients with ear, nose, or throat cancers, in *Corynebacterium Parvum: Applications in Experimental and Clinical Oncology*, Halpern, B., Ed., Plenum Press, New York, 1975, 376.
76. Cheng, V., Suit, H. D., Wang, C. C., Raker, J., Keuman, S., and Rothman, K., Clinical trial of *C. parvum* and radiation therapy in the treatment of head and neck carcinomas, in *Second Int. Conf. on Immunotherapy of Cancer: Present Status of Trials in Man*, Book of Abstracts, Washington, D. C., 1980, 15.

INDEX